BLACKWELL'S BASICS OF MEDICINE

Heart Failure

BLACKWELL'S BASICS OF MEDICINE

Books in the series:

Acid-Base

Potassium

Salt & Water

Heart Failure

Renal Failure

Heart Failure

Horacio J. Adrogué, MD, FACP
Professor of Medicine
Baylor College of Medicine
Department of Veterans Affairs Medical Center
Houston, Texas

Donald E. Wesson, MD, FACP
Professor of Medicine and Physiology
Texas Tech University Health Sciences Center
Lubbock, Texas

Blackwell
Science

Blackwell Science

EDITORIAL OFFICES:
238 Main Street, Cambridge, Massachusetts
02142, USA
Osney Mead, Oxford OX2 0EL, England
25 John Street, London WC1N 2BL, England
23 Ainslie Place, Edinburgh EH3 6AJ,
Scotland
54 University Street, Carlton, Victoria 3053,
Australia
Arnette Blackwell SA, 1 rue de Lille, 75007
Paris, France
Blackwell Wissenschafts-Verlag GmbH,
Kurfürstendamm 57, 10707 Berlin,
Germany
Blackwell MZV, Feldgasse 13, A-1238
Vienna, Austria

DISTRIBUTORS:
North America
Blackwell Science, Inc
238 Main Street
Cambridge, Massachusetts 02142
(Telephone orders: 800-215-1000 or
617-876-7000)

Australia
Blackwell Science Pty Ltd
54 University Street
Carlton, Victoria 3053
(Telephone orders: 03-347-5552)

Outside North America and Australia
Blackwell Science Ltd
c/o Marston Book Services, Ltd
P.O. Box 87
Oxford OX2 0DT
England
(Telephone orders: 44-865-791155)

Acquisitions: Victoria Reeders
Development: Coleen Traynor
Production: Kathleen Grimes

Typeset by M & N Toscano,
Somerville, MA
Printed and bound by Braun-Brumfield, Inc,
Ann Arbor, MI

Notice: The indications and dosages of all
drugs in this book have been recommended in
the medical literature and conform to the
practices of the general medical community.
The medications described do not necessarily
have specific approval by the Food and Drug
Administration for use in the diseases and
dosages for which they are recommended. The
package insert for each drug should be
consulted for use and dosage as approved by
the FDA. Because standards of usage change,
it is advisable to keep abreast of revised
recommendations, particularly those
concerning new drugs.

*Library of Congress Cataloging-in-
Publication Data*
Adrogué, Horacio J.
    Heart Failure/ Horacio J. Adrogué,
    Donald E. Wesson.
        p.   cm.
    Blackwell's Basics of Medicine
    Includes bibliographical references and
    index.
    ISBN 0-86542-429-2
    1. Heart Failure.
    2. Heart Failure—Pathophysiology.
    I. Wesson, Donald E.
    II. Title.   III. Series.
    [DNLM: 1. Heart Failure, Congestive.
    2. Cardiac Output, Low.   WG 370
    A243h 1995]
    RC685.C53A34   1995
    616.1'29—dc20
    DNLM/DLC
    for Library of Congress   94-21186
                                       CIP

To our families

Sarita
Sofía, Horacio, Soledad,
Matías and Marcos Adrogué

Wanda
David and Donald Wesson

Contents

The practice of medicine is rapidly moving from health care delivered by multiple specialists, each responsible for a single problem, toward comprehensive patient management provided by a single practitioner. A proper response to this trend mandates that health care providers successfully integrate knowledge from multiple disciplines and skillfully apply it to patient care. Yet, past and current education compels students to swallow sizable amounts of information on each of the various basic science disciplines (i.e., anatomy, biochemistry, etc.), and within a short time thereafter, they are force-fed the various components of clinical sciences. Thus, acquisition of clinical knowledge is accomplished with simultaneous loss of fundamental concepts of basic sciences. This undesirable effect is due to our outdated educational curriculum that does not allow proper digestion, incorporation, and integration of knowledge, as well as fails to develop and nurture the skills required to deliver comprehensive health care.

This issue, entitled *Heart Failure*, represents the fourth of the Blackwell's Basics of Medicine Series, a book collection that examines relevant topics in Medicine using concepts that pertain to the basic sciences, as a starting point. The doctrine on which this series has been formulated dictates that two critical elements should be present in order to acquire the skills necessary for optimal patient management. These two elements are: a thoughtful approach based on solid pathophysiological knowledge and the ability to apply common sense generously while acquiring basic medical principles. If properly combined, the presence of these two elements allows the unraveling of difficult and/or obscure clinical situations. This series uses simple questions followed by short answers as well as case presentations to illustrate the various topics presented. The sequential order of the questions chosen provides the reader with layers of knowledge that will steadily increase his/her understanding of each topic. The application of the various concepts mentioned above in the analysis of each case helps to consolidate theoretical principles with practical facts.

Heart Failure, like the previous issues of this series, examines a carefully selected topic that is germane to the daily practice of medicine. In it, readers will find the tools for an intelligent interpretation of clinical data based on sound pathophysiological concepts enabling them to provide quality care.

The teaching approach used in this series is at variance with that of the traditional system of medical education that advocates the acquisition of an encyclopedic knowledge as the critical weapon to deal with medical problems. Our belief is, instead, that the time and energy spent by science students in knowledge acquisition should be limited and the emphasis should be placed in expanding the student's ability to integrate theory and practice.

H.J.A.
D.E.W.

Acknowledgments

The authors want to extend their gratitude and indebtedness to the Debbie S. Verrett for her patience, secretarial expertise, and dedication in deciphering and typing the manuscript.

ESSENTIALS OF HEMODYNAMICS

1   What is the role of the circulatory system with respect to whole body homeostasis?

☐ The role of the circulatory system is to maintain an appropriate composition of all body fluids for optimal survival and function of the cells. This function involves the transport of oxygen and other nutrients, removal of metabolic waste products, humoral communication throughout the body, and regulation of body temperature. Coordination and integration of all body tissues require participation of the circulatory as well as the endocrine and nervous systems. The latter is primarily concerned with communications, whereas the endocrine system regulates body functions.

2   Describe the major body fluid compartments.

☐ The intracellular fluid (ICF) contains approximately two thirds of total body water and the remaining one third is held in the extracellular fluid (ECF). The latter is further subdivided into the interstitial and intravascular compartments, which have two thirds and one third, respectively, of the ECF volume.

3   What is the major determinant of the size of each compartment for a given total body fluid content?

☐ The quantity of solutes in each compartment determines its size, so that a deficit or excess of solutes in a particular fluid space will shrink or swell, respectively, that space in comparison with other compartments. The partition of water is determined by the osmotic activity of the solutes confined to each compartment. One major solute predominantly accounts for the size of each fluid compartment. These solutes are potassium and sodium for the intracellular and extracellular spaces, respectively. Because the hydraulic permeability of most cell membranes is very high, water freely and rapidly moves among all body compartments.

4   Explain the determinants of the size of the intravascular compartment.

☐ Because the intravascular compartment is a subdivision of the ECF (the other major subdivision of ECF is the interstitial compartment), the overall size of ECF is a critical determinant of the intravascular volume. Thus, ECF expansion causes hypervolemia (increased intravascular volume), whereas ECF contraction causes hypovolemia (decreased intravascular volume). The second major determinant of the size of intravascular volume is the net force that controls the partition of fluids between interstitial and intravascular spaces. This net force is determined by the combined effects of the following elements acting across the vessel wall: permeability, net hydrostatic pressure, and net oncotic pressure. How these factors yield the net force is established by the Starling law of fluid exchange. This law determines the size of the intravascular volume for a given ECF volume.

5   What are the main reservoirs of blood volume in the circulatory system?

☐ The veins contain most of the blood in the systemic circulation and approximately two thirds of the total body blood volume. In contrast, the blood volume is equally divided among the arterial, capillary, and venous conduits in the pulmonary circulation, which contains only about one tenth of the total body blood volume. Consequently, blood normally held in the large capacitance system (venous compartment of the systemic circulation) can be mobilized to the arterial and capillary compartments whenever homeostatic needs demand it.

6   What are the functional elements or parts of the circulation?

☐ The circulation includes the heart and a series of interconnected tubes or vessels. The heart consists of two pumps in series: the right ventricle to propel blood through the lungs for exchange of oxygen and carbon dioxide (pulmonary circulation) and the left ventricle to propel blood to all tissues of the body (systemic circulation). The vessels connected to each pump are the arteries (high-pressure distributing tubes), arterioles (stopcocks and control valves of the vascular tree), capillaries (where exchange of diffusible substances between blood and tissues occurs), and veins (low-pressure collecting tubes and blood reservoir).

7 What determines the direction, velocity, and the pulsatile/steady character of blood flow in the circulatory system?

☐ Appropriate flap valves within the heart secure unidirectional blood flow. The velocity of blood (linear velocity in cm/sec, not to be confused with volume flow in cm^3/sec) is inversely related to the cross-sectional area so that the very large capillary bed (many capillaries branch out from each arteriole and coalesce to form venules) produces a very slow blood flow in the capillaries. Whereas the cross-sectional area of the aorta is $2.5 \, cm^2$, that of the capillaries is about $2500 \, cm^2$. The intermittent nature of cardiac contraction and arterial blood flow is associated with steady, slow flow at the capillary level because of frictional resistance in the arterioles, distention of the aorta and its branches during ventricular contraction (systole), and forward propulsion of blood during ventricular relaxation (diastole) due to elastic recoil of the walls of large arteries.

8 What are the determinants and the levels of blood pressure in the various compartments of the systemic and pulmonary circuits?

☐ Because the left and right ventricles pump blood directly into the aorta and pulmonary artery, respectively, these vessels have the highest pressure within each circuit. The systolic and diastolic pressure in the aorta and systemic arteries are about 120 and 75 mmHg, respectively, and mean value about 90 mmHg. Normal blood pressure for adults is less than 130 mmHg systolic and less than 85 mmHg diastolic and high-normal is 130 to 139 mmHg systolic and 85 to 89 mmHg diastolic. The blood pressure associated with the lowest cardiovascular risk in adults is less than 120 mmHg systolic and less than 80 mmHg diastolic. The systolic and diastolic pressure in the pulmonary artery are about 25 and about 10 mmHg, with a mean pressure of about 15 mmHg. The mean arterial pressure in each circuit can be estimated as the sum of systolic pressure, plus diastolic pressure multiplied by two, and the value obtained is divided by three. The large resistance to blood flow through the arterioles is responsible for the major decrease in pressure that occurs when blood flows from arteries to capillaries (about 17 and about 7 mmHg in the systemic and pulmonary capillaries, respectively). The lowest blood pressure in the circulation occurs at the termination of the venae cavae in the right atrium (about 0 mmHg) and at the entrance of pulmonary veins in the left atrium (about 2 mmHg).

---

9   What is cardiac output?

☐ Cardiac output is the volume of blood pumped per unit of time (usually expressed as L/min) by the heart into the systemic or pulmonary circulation and is the product of stroke volume and heart rate. The two pumps in series, right and left ventricles, propel equal amounts of blood per minute and are responsible for the blood flow in the entire system. Consequently, the same volume of blood flows through each segment of the circulation each minute (cardiac output), and the velocity of blood in arteries, capillaries, and veins is inversely proportional to their respective cross-sectional area. Cardiac output can be measured in patients by the Fick method (based on the Fick principle that states that blood flow through an organ or the whole body is equal to the amount of a substance taken up per unit of time such as oxygen, divided by the arterial minus the venous level of the substance, known as the A-V difference), and the indicator dilution method. In the latter technique, a known amount of an indicator (e.g., dye such as indocyanine green or radioactive isotope) is injected into an arm vein, and the concentration of the indicator in serial samples of arterial blood is measured (i.e., cardiac output is equal to the amount of indicator injected divided by its average concentration in arterial blood after a single circulation through the heart). The indicator dilution technique most commonly used is based on thermodilution and the indicator injected is cold saline solution (i.e., injected into the right atrium via a double-lumen catheter and the temperature change of blood is measured by a thermistor probe located in the pulmonary artery). Cardiac output is best expressed per unit of body surface area (usually m^2), known as cardiac index (normal value is 2.3 to 3.9 $L/min/m^2$). A cardiac index of less than 2.0 $L/min/m^2$ produces severe tissue hypoperfusion.

---

10   What is stroke volume?

☐ Stroke volume is the amount of blood pumped out of the left or right ventricle with each cardiac contraction (systole). Its normal value in resting adults expressed per unit body surface area, known as stroke index, is 30 to 65 $mL/m^2/beat$, and this volume is pumped in about 0.25 sec. The determinants of stroke volume are: preload, afterload, inotropic state of the myocardium (cardiac contractility), frequency of contraction (heart rate), and uniformity (or lack of it) of electrical and mechanical function of the ventricle.

---

11   What is the normal heart rate?

☐ Heart rate ranges between 50 and 150 beats/min in most normal adults during daily activities. Cardiac output might decrease when heart rate reaches 180 to 200 beats/min because of an impairment in cardiac filling during the shorter diastole, as well as with lower heart rates because of an insufficient compensatory increase in stroke volume that accompanies bradycardia. Because adults under resting conditions have a normal sinus rhythm with rates of 60 to 100 beats/min, sinus bradycardia and sinus tachycardia are present if the rate is less than 60 and more than 100 beats/min, respectively.

---

12   What is the sinoatrial (SA) node of the heart?

☐ The SA node of the heart is a band of specialized myocardial tissue, located in the wall of the right atrium near its junction with the superior vena cava, that serves as the normal cardiac pacemaker. Depolarization in this area initiates a propagated wave of activation that spreads into the remaining regions of the heart.

---

13   What is the importance of the automaticity of the heart?

☐ Automaticity of the heart is a basic property in which the cardiac tissue initiates its own stimulus for myocardial contraction (and therefore pumping action) to deliver blood to all tissues. Because pumping blood through tissues provides nutrients and removes waste products, even a brief interruption of cardiac function might result in distress or death of critical tissues (e.g., brain). Thus, the heart has mechanisms that ensure its continuous function independently of influences from other tissues (e.g., brain). Multiple backup systems help to secure the continuous function of the heart that include several pacemakers in reserve, ready to be activated as needed (i.e., atrioventricular [AV] node or ventricle-initiated rhythms). Because the rate of firing by the SA node normally is the highest compared with other automatic cells of the heart, the SA node overrides the action of all the reserve pacemakers under normal circumstances. Consequently, the SA node is normally the commander of the heart rhythm. Failure of the SA node to fire (i.e., to initiate a propagated stimulus throughout the heart) or a major depression of its own automaticity allows other automatic cells to take over the heart rhythm. In this setting, those automatic cells with the highest firing rate will command the cardiac rhythm. In the event of failure of automaticity of the substitute pacemaker, another set of automatic cells kicks in as the pacemaker of the heart. Consequently, redundant mechanisms secure continuous depolarizing stimuli, leading to myocardial contraction and relaxation (systole and diastole, respectively), and securing pumping of blood.

---

14   Is the blood flow produced by the left ventricle identical to that of the right ventricle?

☐ The left ventricular output is theoretically slightly higher than that of right ventricle due to the small blood flow of bronchial arteries that drain into the pulmonary veins and the coronary blood flow that drains into the left atrium and ventricle through thebesian veins. In addition, changes in body position, changes in respiration cycle (inspiration and expiration), and physiologic adjustments might cause transient and very short-lasting periods (seconds) in which a substantial differential in left and right ventricular outputs develops. However, the mean cardiac output of left and right ventricle is, for practical purposes, identical.

15   Are the functions of the right and left ventricle of equal importance in maintaining the circulation under normal conditions?

☐ No. In experimental settings, the right ventricle is not required for maintenance of pulmonary blood flow and arterial pressure at rest. When this chamber is excluded from the circulation (i.e., experimentally bypassed), the left ventricle maintains the entire circulation although fluid retention and a mild increase in venous pressure develops. By contrast, right ventricular function is important to maintain adequate circulation during exercise, in states of increased pulmonary vascular resistance, and during hypovolemia.

16   What are the general determinants of arterial blood pressure?

☐ The determinants of arterial blood pressure are conveniently grouped as physical and physiologic. The physical determinants of arterial pressure are: (1) the blood volume within the arterial system (arterial blood volume) and (2) the elastic characteristics (pressure-volume relationship or compliance) of the arterial compartment. The physiologic determinants modify the physical ones, that is, the arterial blood volume and/or compliance, through changes in total circulating blood volume, arterial "inflow" or cardiac output, arterial "outflow" or peripheral run-off, and properties of the vascular wall (structural and functional changes). Thus, physiologic factors operate on the physical determinants of arterial blood pressure.

17   What are the specific determinants of arterial blood pressure?

☐ Mean arterial pressure is determined by cardiac output and peripheral or vascular resistance (impediment to blood flow through the vessels) according to Ohm's law (electric circuit theory) and Poiseuille's law (flow of fluids theory). Ohm's law applied to the circulation establishes that:

$$\dot{Q}(\text{fluid flow}) = \frac{\Delta P(\text{pressure difference})}{R(\text{resistance})}$$

in which $\dot{Q}$ is blood flow or cardiac output, ΔP is the pressure difference between the beginning and end of the circulation (since the systemic circulation ends in the right atrium, which has a pressure of about 0 mmHg, ΔP is identical to mean arterial pressure), and R is peripheral or vascular resistance. Poiseuille's law specifically applies to straight and rigid tubes filled with homogeneous fluid and having steady laminar flow. Although these conditions do not strictly apply to blood vessels in vivo, the law is often used to describe blood flow in vivo. Poiseuille's law establishes that:

$$\text{Fluid flow} = \frac{\pi \times (\text{pressure difference}) \times (\text{radius})^4}{8 \times (\text{vessel length}) \times (\text{fluid viscosity})}$$

where π and 8 are constants of proportionality. The hydraulic resistance according to this law is:

$$R = \frac{\text{pressure difference}}{\text{fluid flow}}$$
$$= \frac{8 \times (\text{vessel length}) \times (\text{fluid viscosity})}{\pi \times (\text{radius})^4}$$

Consequently, Poiseuille's law allows for further dissection of the various components responsible for vascular resistance in the circulation.

---

18   What principles governing the circulation derive from Ohm's and Poiseuille's laws?

☐ These laws and corresponding equations establish that: (1) blood flow is directly proportional to the pressure difference but inversely proportional to the vascular resistance; (2) vascular resistance is dramatically and inversely influenced by vessel radius because the latter is raised to the fourth power; (3) blood vessels connected in parallel (an advantageous arrangement found in most capillary beds) have less resistance to flow than if they are connected in series; in addition, parallel arrangement of blood vessels provides a greater total cross-sectional area with the same resistance as a single wide tube (i.e., the total resistance of 16 small tubes with four times the total cross-sectional area is the same as that of a single wide tube); and (4) blood viscosity, which might be altered by changes in hematocrit, serum proteins, and temperature, might have a significant effect on flow and circulatory pressure when acting on small vessels.

---

19   How is the resistance to blood flow, known as vascular resistance, measured and expressed?

□ The impediment to blood flow through vessels (simply called vascular resistance) cannot be measured directly but must be calculated from measurements of blood flow and pressure differences along the circulation. Vascular resistance is calculated by dividing mean pressure difference between two points in the vascular system by the blood flow between them (i.e., mean amount of blood passing from one point to the other per unit time). Vascular resistance might be expressed in various units including: (1) peripheral resistance units (PRU) in which the pressure gradient is expressed in mmHg and blood flow in mL/sec; since in normal adults at rest the pressure difference between the systemic arteries and veins is about 100 mmHg, and the simultaneously measured cardiac output is about 100 mL/sec (i.e., 6 L/min amounts to 6000 mL flowing through the circulatory system in 60 sec), the total peripheral resistance is about 1 PRU $(100/100 = 1)$; (2) CGS (cm-gram-sec) units, obtained by multiplying PRU units by a conversion factor of 1332 and allow for expression of vascular resistance in $dyn \cdot sec \cdot cm^{-5}$, which is the conventional unit used in both fluid mechanics and hemodynamic monitoring; and (3) R units in which the pressure gradient is expressed in mmHg and blood flow in L/min; this unit may be converted to CGS units by multiplying its value times 80. Calculation of vascular resistance in R units and subsequent multiplication by 80 is the standard method used in clinical settings including intensive care units and hemodynamics laboratories. Normal systemic vascular resistance is 770 to 1500 $dyn \cdot sec \cdot cm^{-5}$.

20   What are the major factors that control the caliber or lumen diameter of blood vessels?

☐ The caliber of blood vessels is controlled by the vascular smooth muscle, which contracts and relaxes in response to various stimuli, a process known as vasomotion. The major factors that influence vasomotion include: (1) the autonomic nervous system whose fibers innervate the blood vessels and locally release norepinephrine or acetylcholine; (2) metabolic, chemical, and hormonal substances locally produced and/or carried in the blood stream; and (3) the vascular endothelium that produces vasodilatory (e.g., nitric oxide, also known as endothelium-derived relaxing factor or EDRF) and vasoconstrictor (e.g., endothelin-1) substances that are involved in the local modulation of vascular smooth muscle contraction. The relative importance of these mechanisms varies markedly from one vascular bed to another. In most organs the autonomic nervous system works synergistically with nonneural influences (e.g., PO_2, PCO_2, K^+, prostaglandins, nitric oxide) to regulate regional blood flow.

21   What nerve terminals of the autonomic nervous system control the lumen diameter or caliber of blood vessels?

☐ Constriction and relaxation of vascular smooth muscle is regulated by nerve fibers of three main types that reach arteries and veins throughout the body, as follows: (1) sympathetic vasoconstrictor type that release norepinephrine at the nerve endings which acts on α_1 receptors in vascular smooth muscle; (2) sympathetic vasodilator type that release acetylcholine from nerve endings and play a role in the myocardium, skeletal muscle, sweat glands of the skin, and some cutaneous areas; and (3) parasympathetic vasodilator type that release acetylcholine at the nerve endings (i.e., in erectile vessels of the genital organs) or kallikrein (i.e., in the salivary glands where this substance acts on a plasma protein to produce the potent vasodilator bradykinin).

22 What are the effects of K^+ on vascular resistance of arterioles?

☐ Potassium depletion causes arteriolar constriction in several vascular beds, whereas K^+ administration has vasodilatory effects. Hypokalemia due to K^+ deficit can induce constriction of coronary and cerebral vessels, possibly leading to ischemic damage of these tissues.

23 Describe the link between systemic blood pressure and the level of K^+ stores.

☐ Increased systemic vascular resistance, producing hypertension, has been postulated to occur in states of K^+ depletion. Potassium repletion can decrease peripheral vascular resistance and diminish systemic blood pressure.

24 Compare the normal levels of systemic and pulmonary vascular resistance.

☐ The mean normal systemic vascular resistance (SVR) expressed in CGS units in an adult is about 1200 units (i.e., [90 mm Hg ÷ 6 L/min] × 80 = 1200 units) and the range, as previously indicated, is 770 to 1500 $dyn \cdot sec \cdot cm^{-5}$. SVR can be transiently as high as four times the mean normal value (about 5000 units) in the presence of generalized vasoconstriction. Conversely, SVR can be transiently as low as one fourth of the mean normal value (about 300 units) in the presence of generalized vasodilation. SVR is calculated from hemodynamic monitoring data as follows:

$$SVR = \frac{MAP\,(mmHg) - CVP\,(mmHg)}{cardiac\ output\,(L/min)} \times 80$$

where MAP (mean arterial pressure) might be calculated as follows:

$$MAP = (systolic\ BP - diastolic\ BP)1/3 + diastolic\ BP$$

and CVP (central venous pressure) is either measured or estimated. The mean normal pulmonary vascular resistance (PVR) expressed in CGS units in an adult is about 70 units (i.e., [5 mmHg ÷ 6L/min]×80 = 67 units). The conventional normal range of PVR is 20 to 120 dyn·sec·cm^{-5}. PVR is calculated from hemodynamic monitoring data as follows:

$$PVR = \frac{MPAP\ (mmHg) - PAOP\ (mmHg)}{cardiac\ output\ (L/min)} \times 80$$

where MPAP is mean pulmonary artery pressure (e.g., 13 mmHg), and PAOP is pulmonary artery occlusion pressure that measures mean pulmonary wedge pressure, which is approximately equal to the left atrium pressure (e.g., 8 mmHg, range is 2 to 12 mmHg).

---

25 Should increased and decreased vascular resistance be equated with arteriolar constriction and dilation, respectively?

☐ No. The interpretation of increases and decreases in vascular resistance (VR) as indicative of vasoconstriction and vasodilation, respectively, is a gross oversimplification. Other factors including vascular occlusion (that increases VR), active bleeding (that decreases VR), and changes in blood viscosity, modify calculated levels of VR.

---

26 What physiologic factors control pulse pressure?

☐ The pulse pressure generated with each heartbeat has a systolic zenith and diastolic nadir that depend on factors other than those controlling mean arterial pressure including: (1) the stroke volume ejected by the ventricle; and (2) the capacitance of the arterial tree. The terms capacitance and compliance applied to the blood vessels describe important properties with clinical implications. Capacitance refers to the blood volume within the vasculature at a given transmural pressure. Thus, capacitance is modified by the geometry of the vessels (volume at zero transmural pressure or unstressed volume) and their viscoelastic properties (i.e., compliance). The term compliance refers to the change in blood volume within the vasculature due to a change in pressure (C = ΔV / ΔP). Thus, compliance represents the slope of the pressure-volume relationship. Pulse pressure increases directly with stroke volume. An increase in the amount of blood entering the arterial tree during systole and leaving in diastole produces, as expected, a bigger rise and fall in arterial pressure during systole and diastole, respectively. Pulse pressure decreases when stroke volume is reduced. The effects of arterial capacitance (sum of unstressed volume and compliance) are opposite to those resulting from changes in stroke volume. The lower the capacitance of the arterial system, the larger will be the rise in pressure for a given stroke volume pumped by the ventricle, producing a wider pulse pressure. The rigid aorta (low compliance) of old age increases pulse pressure. A third factor that controls pulse pressure is how brisk is ventricular ejection, although this factor is of smaller importance compared to the previous factors discussed.

27 Explain further the relationship among volume, compliance, and capacitance of arteries and veins.

□ The blood volume held by a vein at zero transmural pressure is about three times that of a corresponding artery because of the different size or geometry of these vessels. In addition, veins have weaker walls than arteries, such that for a comparable size, veins can hold approximately eight times more blood at a given rise in transmural pressure (vascular compliance of veins is about eight times larger than arteries). The composite effect of the two previously mentioned characteristics, geometry and compliance, determines the capacitance of the vascular system. Thus, the capacitance of veins is about 24 times that of corresponding arteries since veins have a larger volume (about three times) and are more distensible (about eight times). The capacitance of arteries and veins increases if the lumen diameter increases because of structural changes (e.g., aortic aneurysm, vein varicosities), or by relaxation of vascular smooth muscle (e.g., sympathetic blockade produces venodilation, augmenting venous capacitance).

28   What physiologic factors modify the volume-pressure relationships of the arterial and venous systems?

☐ Sympathetic stimulation increases the pressure per unit blood volume contained in the arteries and veins, whereas the opposite occurs with sympathetic blockade. Consequently, the increased vascular tone that follows sympathetic activation shifts blood from large veins to the heart, allowing the circulation to operate almost normally when up to 25% of blood volume has been lost (e.g., hemorrhage). The capacitance of the circulatory system, especially the veins, is under sympathetic control and this regulatory system alters the volume-pressure relationship by its effect on vascular smooth muscle tone. Physiologic adjustments in the capacitance of the circulatory system help to maintain adequate tissue perfusion under conditions of circulatory stress (e.g., physical exercise, pregnancy, and intravascular volume depletion).

29   What are the two mechanisms by which cardiac output (quantity of blood pumped by each ventricle per unit time) might change?

☐ Cardiac output might change because of alterations in the frequency of contractions (heart rate) or the volume of blood ejected per contraction (stroke volume). In most settings where an increased cardiac output is needed, both mechanisms are recruited. Yet, the relative contribution of each of these two mechanisms varies depending on the circumstances or specific disease states of the circulatory system.

30   Describe the role of heart rate as a determinant of cardiac output.

☐ Heart rate and three other variables that control stroke volume (i.e., preload, afterload, and myocardial contractility) are the critical determinants of cardiac output. Nevertheless, a faster heart rate is the major mechanism by which cardiac output increases in response to a moderate increment in tissue demands. The higher cardiac output observed with tachycardia requires a commensurate increase in venous return or preload. A faster heart rate decreases the duration of each systole, yet the total time per minute spent in systole is longer because there are more systoles per minute. When heart rate reaches 180 to 200 beats/min, however, the obligatory shortening of the duration of diastole leads to decreased ventricular filling and a fall in cardiac output.

---

31   What is the Starling law of the heart, also known as the Frank-Starling law or phenomenon?

☐ Starling's law of the heart establishes that the intact ventricle has the capacity to vary its force of contraction on a beat-to-beat basis as a function of its preload reflected in the end-diastolic size (i.e., resting myocardial fiber length). This length-force relationship established by Starling's law secures equal cardiac output of the two pumps in series despite the effect of changes in intrathoracic pressure on preload of the ventricles. If the right ventricle temporarily pumps more blood than the left ventricle because of decreased intrathoracic pressure (e.g., inspiration), the proper balance between the two pumps is soon achieved because the consequent augmented venous return to the left atrium and ventricle enhances left ventricular end-diastolic fiber length, increasing left ventricular stroke volume. Achievement of balance between the two pumps is only one of the multiple hemodynamic effects that this law exerts on the circulation.

---

32   Why does the length-force relationship established by the Frank-Starling law apply to both cardiac and skeletal muscle in the isolated preparation as well as in the intact organism?

☐ The force of contraction varies with initial muscle length in both cardiac and skeletal muscle in all conditions because it depends on the relative position of the two sets of myofilaments (thick and thin) within the sarcomere or contractile unit. The structural and functional characteristics of the sarcomere are similar (not identical) in cardiac and skeletal muscle. The thick filaments are 1.5 μm in length (about 110 Å in diameter) while the thin filaments measure 1.0 μm in length (about 50 Å in diameter). Maximal force develops at resting sarcomere lengths of about 2.2 μm (cardiac muscle), wherein the number of crossbridge attachments between overlapping thick and thin filaments is maximal. At normal filling pressure of the ventricles (left 3 to 12 mmHg, right 2 to 7 mmHg), the sarcomere length varies from 2.1 μm at end of diastole to 1.8 μm at normal end-systole or 1.6 μm after maximal systolic emptying. When ventricular filling pressure reaches the upper limit of normal (left 12 mmHg, right 7 mmHg), the sarcomere length is about 2.2 μm and maximal ventricular contraction develops at that preload.

---

33   What parameters or measurements are used to graphically express the Frank-Starling "function curves" of isolated papillary muscle and intact heart?

☐ Myocardial resting fiber (and sarcomere) length is plotted on the horizontal axis (x-axis or abscissa) because this property is the independent variable, whereas force of contraction (the dependent variable) is plotted on the $y-$ or vertical axis known as the ordinate. The corresponding parameter for the intact heart plotted on the x-axis can be left atrial mean pressure, left ventricular end-diastolic pressure, or left ventricular end-diastolic volume (which is more difficult to measure) because each of them can substitute for resting fiber or sarcomere length. Left ventricular stroke volume or systolic pressure is plotted on the y-axis as a substitute for force of contraction. Consequently, a pressure-volume diagram plot is commonly used to examine "function curves" in the intact heart. They reflect the effects of end-diastolic volume (resting myocardial fiber length) on contractility of the heart.

---

34   What are the two basic function curves that describe the passive and active states of the contractile unit in the isolated papillary muscle and in the intact heart?

☐ The two basic function curves in papillary muscle and intact heart are: (1) the passive, resting, or diastolic curve; and (2) the active or systolic curve. The two functional states are usually depicted in a single diagram in which the lower curve represents the resting or diastolic function while the upper curve illustrates the active or systolic function. The tension or force (measured in grams) before contraction stretches the papillary muscle and therefore increases sarcomere length. This length-tension relationship yields a basic function curve of passive or resting tension. Electric stimulation causes contraction, and the tension or force (measured in grams) increases with moderate stretching (extreme stretching might decrease maximal tension during contraction). Thus, contraction produces a new basic function curve of active tension. Evaluation of the intact heart allows drawing of the diastolic and systolic function curves that correspond precisely to resting and active tension curves of the isolated papillary muscle preparation.

---

35 What are the main characteristics of the resting or diastolic function curve of the heart (e.g., left ventricle)?

□ The diastolic function curve of the heart is remarkably flat at low and intermediate levels of resting sarcomere length or diastolic volume. In these conditions, which resemble those found in the normal state, diastolic volume can substantially increase with only a small rise in diastolic pressure (i.e., pregnancy, physical exercise). By contrast, a steep rise of the diastolic curve develops at large intraventricular volumes (i.e., congestive heart failure with cardiac enlargement) because the ventricle becomes much less compliant with further distention (i.e., a small volume increase produces a large rise in pressure). The steep upward diastolic curve may eventually join the systolic curve in an exhausted ventricle that is unable to contract because extreme stretching might decrease maximal contractile tension while steadily increasing resting tension.

---

36 Compare diastolic distensibility and compliance of the ventricles.

□ The pressure-volume relationship (plotted on the *y*- and *x*-axis, respectively) of the ventricle during diastole allows for examination of both distensibility and compliance of this cavity in the basal state compared to the changes induced by disease. An upward displacement of the diastolic pressure-volume curve represents a reduction of ventricular distensibility because a higher pressure develops at any given volume. Conversely, a downward displacement of this curve indicates increased ventricular distensibility because a lower pressure is found at any given volume. Thus, changes in ventricular distensibility modify the pressure-volume relationship such that the new curve is displaced along the *y*-axis but remains parallel to that found in the normal state. Ventricular compliance, on the other hand, is the ratio of change in ventricular diastolic volume in response to change in ventricular pressure so that the slope of the curve (rather than the previously mentioned upward or downward displacement of the curve) is modified when this parameter is altered. A larger than normal rise in diastolic pressure for any given increment in volume indicates increased ventricular stiffness or decreased ventricular compliance. Most commonly, disease states simultaneously reduce diastolic distensibility and compliance (e.g., pericardial restraint, fibrosis of endocardium and myocardium).

---

37   What are the determinants of ventricular relaxation in diastole?

☐ Relaxation of the heart in diastole depends on factors that are intrinsic as well as extrinsic to the ventricular chamber. The intrinsic factors include: (1) passive elasticity of the wall, (2) active elasticity due to residual sarcomere tension from previous contraction, (3) diastolic suction, and (4) stress relaxation (also known as "delayed compliance" that allows the ventricle to receive a larger diastolic volume without a significant rise in diastolic pressure). The extrinsic factors include the pericardium, fullness of coronary vessels, loading of the contralateral ventricle, and extrinsic compression (e.g., pleural pressure). The term lusitrophy is used to describe the diastolic properties of the myocardium and cardiac chambers.

---

38   Compare the compliance (i.e., the slope of the diastolic pressure-volume relationship or $\Delta V / \Delta P$) and volume during diastole and systole of the two ventricles.

☐ The normal right ventricle is more compliant than the left due to its thinner wall. Yet, the end-diastolic volume (75 ± 15 mL/m^2), end-systolic volume (25 ± 8 mL/m^2), stroke index (50 ± 15 mL/m^2), and ejection fraction (ratio of stroke volume to end-diastolic volume, SV / EDV, mean value 0.67 and range 0.55 to 0.78) of the two ventricles are approximately equal. The greater compliance of the right ventricle is responsible for its lower end-diastolic pressure in comparison with the left. The upper limit of normal for right ventricular end-diastolic pressure is 7 mmHg; that of the left ventricle is 12 mmHg.

39 What are the main characteristics of the active or systolic function curve of the heart (e.g., left ventricle)?

☐ The active or systolic function curve of the heart represents the Frank-Starling relationship of force (or pressure) development by the ventricle as a function of initial fiber length (or diastolic volume). The systolic curve is remarkably steep at low and intermediate levels of resting sarcomere length (or diastolic volume) so that considerable active tension (also ventricular stroke volume or systolic pressure) develops in response to very small changes in diastolic volume or pressure. Thus, the steep shape of the early and intermediate phases of the systolic curve contrast with the flat shape of the corresponding periods of the diastolic curve, as previously described. The normal heart operates on the ascending portion (upper half) of the systolic function curve and on the flat portion of the diastolic function curve. Consequently, the normal heart takes full advantage of the Starling law, allowing for substantial increases in cardiac output in response to increased venous return that occurs with a minimal rise in diastolic filling pressure. This arrangement helps to avoid passive congestion in the pulmonary and systemic circulations during circumstances that demand an increased cardiac output. At larger than normal left ventricular diastolic volume or pressure (e.g., greater than 12 mmHg for left ventricular end-diastolic pressure), passive tension rises markedly without an increment in active tension. Further increments in left ventricular diastolic pressure might lead to depression of myocardial contractility so that systolic function is accurately represented by a descending curve (e.g., end-diastolic pressures exceeding 30 mmHg in the presence of increased aortic pressure).

40   What are cardiac preload and afterload, two major determinants
        of stroke volume and of performance of the intact ventricle?

□ Preload is the cardiac filling at the end of diastole (i.e.,
end-diastolic filling pressure) which, according to Starling law
of the heart, helps determine the force of ventricular contraction during systole. Afterload is the resistance to ejection of
blood at the initiation of ventricular contraction during systole
(e.g., aortic blood pressure for left ventricle, pulmonary artery
pressure for right ventricle). The concepts of preload and afterload arise from in vitro studies of papillary muscle or atrial
myocardium in which one end of the muscle is attached to a
tension transducer and the other end is attached to a lever that
is free to move. A small weight, termed "preload" is placed
on the lever to stretch the muscle and a "stop" is applied so
that any added weight to the lever will neither stretch the
muscle nor will be sensed by this tissue until it starts contracting in response to electric stimulation. Loads added once the
"stop" has been applied represent the "afterload." Total load
imposed on the preparation equals the sum of preload and afterload.

41   What are the differences, if any, between left and right ventricu-
        lar function curves (i.e., indexes of ventricular performance or
        pump performance derived from Frank-Starling curves) in re-
        sponse to changes in preload and afterload?

□ The "function curves" of the intact heart usually evaluate
the left ventricle, which is the dominant pump of the circulatory system. Nevertheless, a comparable function curve can
be obtained to assess the right ventricle. The overall shape of
right and left ventricular function curves in response to
changes in preload (i.e., for the right ventricle may be estimated from central venous pressure, whereas for the left
ventricle is obtained from left ventricular end-diastolic pressure and estimated clinically from pulmonary capillary wedge
pressure or pulmonary artery diastolic pressure) are similar
although the right ventricle has a steeper systolic function if
stroke volume (or cardiac output) is plotted on the y-axis of
the length-tension relationship. Nevertheless, the responses of
the two ventricles to changes in afterload (i.e., pulmonary ar-

tery pressure for right ventricle, aortic blood pressure for left ventricle) are substantially different. The right ventricle is incapable of immediately adjusting to an increasing afterload. In addition, diastolic volume and ejection fraction of the right ventricle are very sensitive to increasing afterload, which causes tricuspid regurgitation (reversal of blood flow to the right atrium).

---

42   What are the functions of cardiac atria?

☐ Cardiac atria have mechanical and endocrine functions. Mechanical functions include the role of each atrium as a reservoir that facilitates rapid ventricular filling and as a pump (the atrial kick) that increases end-diastolic volume and pressure. Like the ventricles, the atria increase the force of contraction in response to an increase in fiber length. Loss of effective atrial pumping function (e.g., atrial fibrillation) in an otherwise normal heart does not decrease cardiac output at rest but limits the increase of cardiac output to vigorous exercise. If ventricular disease is present and the compliance of this chamber is diminished, cardiac output might be decreased at rest. Endocrine functions include the production of atrial natriuretic peptides (ANP) that increase diuresis (urine volume), natriuresis (urine sodium excretion), and relax intestinal smooth muscle.

---

43   How important is the atrial contribution to ventricular preload?

☐ Atrial contraction at the end of ventricular diastole augments ventricular filling (preload) and increases end-diastolic volume and pressure. Like the ventricle, the atrium responds to increasing stretch with a more forceful contraction that secures adequate emptying of this chamber leading to a low mean atrial pressure throughout most of diastole. The low mean atrial pressure during most of the cardiac cycle (except for the period of atrial systole) facilitates venous return to the heart from the systemic and pulmonary circulations. The absence of effective atrial contraction due to atrial fibrillation or an ill-timed atrial systole from failed coordination between atrial and ventricular contraction (i.e., in AV dissociation or nodal rhythm) increases mean atrial pressure, leading to reduced venous return and ultimately impairing ventricular performance. The atrial contribution to ventricular preload is of major importance in the presence of stenotic AV valves, ventricular hypertrophy, and other states of reduced ventricular compliance, especially at rapid ventricular rates (i.e., shortened ventricular filling period).

---

44 Elaborate further on the relative importance of atrial systole to ventricular filling during slow compared to fast heart rates.

☐ Atrial systole (or contraction) contributes more to ventricular filling during fast heart rates as compared to slow ones. Contraction of the atria occurs while ventricles are in diastole, the AV valves are open, and after a significant fraction of total end-diastolic filling of the ventricle has occurred. Most ventricular filling during diastole occurs immediately after opening of the AV valves, a time period called the rapid filling phase. This initial phase of diastole is followed by a period of slow ventricular filling, also called diastasis, during which blood returning from the systemic veins flows into the right ventricle and blood from the pulmonary veins flows into the left ventricle through open AV valves. At slow heart rates, ventricular filling is nearly complete at the end of diastasis and subsequent atrial contraction adds little additional blood to the ventricle before this chamber contracts during systole. At rapid heart rates, the period of ventricular diastole is shortened such that filling of this chamber is incomplete (i.e., disappearance of diastasis as well as shortening of rapid ventricular filling), and the atrial contribution to ventricular filling is substantially increased. The atrial contribution to ventricular filling is large when atrial contraction occurs immediately after the rapid filling phase because the pressure gradient between the atria and ventricles is maximal (the ventricle is not filled to capacity).

---

45 How is ventricular preload estimated and what are its determinants?

☐ Preload of the left ventricle may be assessed from the left ventricular end-diastolic pressure or estimated from the pulmonary capillary wedge pressure or pulmonary artery diastolic pressure. Preload of the right ventricle may be evaluated from central venous pressure. Determinants of preload are total circulating blood volume, distribution of blood between the intra- and extrathoracic compartments, venous tone, diastolic filling time, atrial contribution to ventricular filling, ventricular compliance, and changes in venous return caused by alterations in peripheral vascular resistance.

---

46 How do changes in total blood volume and fraction of blood volume held in the thorax modify cardiac preload?

□ A decreased and increased total blood volume will decrease and increase preload, respectively, in the absence of compensatory mechanisms. However, activation of the adrenergic nervous system allows maintenance of a constant preload if reductions of blood volume are small (less than 15% of total volume) or gradual. At any given total blood volume, preload increases when a greater fraction of blood is held in the thorax (e.g., recumbent posture, deep inspiration, head-out water immersion, inflation of a lower body positive-pressure suit, absence of gravitational force during space flight). Conversely, preload decreases when a greater fraction of blood is held outside the thorax (e.g., upright posture, suction applied to the lower extremities and trunk, increased intrathoracic pressure due to pneumothorax or application of positive-pressure ventilation). Increased pericardial pressure due to effusion within this cavity and constrictive pericarditis also reduce preload. The effect of changes of other determinants of ventricular preload on the level of this parameter are examined in the answer to subsequent questions.

---

47 What are the effects of decreased systemic venous tone, diastolic filling time, and atrial contribution to ventricular filling on cardiac preload?

□ Dilation of the venous capacitance system, substantial shortening of cardiac diastole that reduces rapid ventricular filling, and absence of appropriately timed atrial contraction decrease cardiac preload, and consequently, reduce stroke volume and cardiac output. Compensatory mechanisms might preserve a normal preload if only one of these alterations is observed, but they fail to counterbalance the effect on preload if two or more defects are present simultaneously.

---

48   What is the effect of diminished ventricular compliance on cardiac preload?

☐ Ventricular compliance is the ratio of change in ventricular volume to change in ventricular diastolic pressure ($\Delta V / \Delta P$); ventricular stiffness is the reciprocal of this ratio (the change in pressure for a given change in volume or $\Delta P / \Delta V$). Diminished ventricular compliance reduces preload because higher diastolic pressure is produced with a given initial fiber length (the relatively small fiber length for the associated high diastolic pressure decreases force of contraction according to Starling's law) and venous congestion of the systemic and pulmonary circulation are apt to develop. Ventricular stiffness increases with aging, ischemia, cardiac hypertrophy due to chronic hypertension as well as other causes, fibrosis, infiltrative diseases, pericardial disease, and other conditions. The diminished ventricular compliance observed in the previously mentioned disease states is responsible for the development of the so-called diastolic dysfunction.

---

49   Do changes in peripheral vascular resistance significantly alter cardiac preload and, as a consequence, cardiac output?

☐ Yes. Physiologic and pathologic states characterized by a low peripheral vascular resistance increase venous return and thereby augment cardiac output due to a higher preload. Physiologic conditions with these features are physical exercise and pregnancy. Pathologic states that have low peripheral vascular resistance and augmented venous return include fever, hypoxemia, anemia, Paget's disease of bone, beriberi, patent ductus arteriosus, opening of an arteriovenous fistula, and other conditions. A diminished impediment to blood flow through the vessels (i.e., decreased vascular resistance) also increases cardiac output by facilitating stroke volume during ventricular systole.

50   What is preload reserve?

☐ Preload reserve, also known as stroke volume reserve, is the blood volume that might be ejected per systole in addition to the normal stroke volume. Contributors to preload reserve include an increased end-diastolic volume due to higher preload as well as a reduced ventricular end-systolic volume due to augmented cardiac contraction (according to Starling's law) because these mechanisms produce a larger than normal stroke volume. A preload reserve of approximately 30% can be made available at low levels of exercise because of an increase in end-diastolic volume. By contrast, ventricular end-diastolic volume decreases at the very high heart rates (the shorter diastole reduces ventricular filling time) associated with vigorous exercise. In this circumstance, a reduction of ventricular end-systolic volume due to stimulation of myocardial contractility allows for the maintenance of constant stroke volume.

51   Explain further ventricular afterload and enumerate its determinants for the left ventricle.

☐ Ventricular afterload is the sum of loads that oppose shortening of myocardial fibers of this chamber during systole. The single most important determinant of left ventricular afterload is arterial blood pressure. This factor is a key modulator of the quantity of blood ejected by the ventricle. The specific determinants of left ventricular afterload are: (1) peripheral vascular resistance (mostly arteriolar constrictor tone); (2) viscoelastic properties of the wall of aorta and larger arteries; (3) arterial blood volume at the onset of ventricular ejection; (4) myocardial wall stress, a determinant that increases as a function of ventricular pressure and internal radius of this chamber; and (5) blood viscosity. Abrupt alterations in arterial pressure or in any individual component of ventricular afterload cause reciprocal changes in wall shortening and stroke volume of the left ventricle, if preload is kept constant.

52   Does an increase in arterial pressure reduce stroke volume of the normal left ventricle?

☐ No. An elevated afterload increases ventricular end-diastolic volume (i.e., a rise in ventricular preload reserve), which enhances ventricular contraction. The higher diastolic volume, however, increases afterload further because of enhanced wall stress (due to higher internal radius of the ventricle), which in turn reduces myocardial fiber shortening. This new status of a larger ventricle in diastole, due to geometrical factors, allows for the maintenance of constant stroke volume in this setting of decreased myocardial fiber shortening. Thus, increased aortic pressure will not reduce stroke volume in the normal heart as long as preload and force of cardiac contraction can increase. In this condition, adaptation of the heart will lead to augmented left ventricular end-diastolic volume and pressure, constant stroke volume, and increased stroke work. Patients with impaired heart function due to either decreased myocardial contractility or hypovolemia (reduced preload) in association with normal contractility will reduce stroke volume in response to increased arterial pressure. The ability to maintain a constant stroke volume when arterial pressure increases occurs with moderate hypertension, but a severe rise in blood pressure will cause an immediate decrease in stroke volume in the normal as well as abnormal heart.

53   How do peripheral resistance, impedance of the aorta and large arteries, and arterial blood volume at onset of ventricular ejection contribute to ventricular afterload?

☐ Because peripheral resistance is one of the two critical determinants of arterial pressure (cardiac output is the other), changes in resistance due to constriction or dilation of arterioles increase and decrease, respectively, ventricular afterload. The impedance (stiffness) of the aorta and large arteries opposes cardiac ejection and dampens pulsatile blood flow because the viscoelastic properties of the vessel walls contribute to ventricular afterload. The mass of the blood column within the arterial system has an inertia that must be overcome by the myocardial contraction, and therefore it also contributes to ventricular afterload.

---

54 Explain the concept of myocardial wall stress or tension and how it contributes to ventricular afterload.

☐ Passive stretching of isolated papillary muscle increases sarcomere length producing a higher resting tension (measured in grams). In a comparable manner, passive stretching of the intact ventricle increases wall tension or stress. The increased wall tension is associated with higher diastolic pressure in the classic function curves of the heart (pressure-volume relationship). The higher wall tension in the resting state due to a larger diastolic volume is the starting point for the development of active tension at the onset of myocardial contraction (total tension equals its active value plus the resting one). The elevated basal tension caused by a larger end-diastolic ventricular volume increases myocardial oxygen consumption. Wall tension or stress is directly related to the product of intraventricular pressure and internal radius and is inversely related to wall thickness (Laplace's law). Laplace's law allows for the calculation of average circumferential wall tension (force per unit of cross-sectional area of wall) using different geometrical shapes (e.g., spherical or ellipsoidal ventricle). It must also be recognized that wall tension or stress falls during ventricular ejection (despite the concomitant small rise in the aortic pressure) because of the declining internal ventricular radius as well as the systolic thickening of the wall of this chamber.

---

55 How does blood viscosity contribute to ventricular afterload?

☐ Ventricular afterload increases in states of high blood viscosity because of frictional drag of this fluid against the ventricular walls. The percentage of red cells in the blood, known as hematocrit, is the major determinant of its viscosity, which is normally about three times that of water (i.e., hematocrit about 40%). However, blood viscosity can become as much as 10 times that of water when the hematocrit rises to

60% to 70%. The concentration and types of proteins in plasma also modify blood viscosity, but these effects are less important than that of the hematocrit.

---

56 How can left ventricular response to increased afterload be assessed?

☐ The infusion of a pressor agent (which induces systemic arteriolar constriction) such as angiotensin II transiently increases left ventricular afterload allowing for examination of the response of stroke volume, stroke work, and ventricular end-diastolic pressure to this challenge. The normal left ventricle responds to this stress with an increase in stroke work, a small rise in end-diastolic volume and pressure, and minor changes in stroke volume.

---

57 What is myocardial contractility (also called inotropic state or contractile state), and how might it be evaluated?

☐ The contractility or inotropic state of the heart describes the speed and shortening capacity of myocardial fibers during systole at a given force or total load (preload plus afterload). When total load is increased, both velocity and extent of shortening are reduced at constant contractility. The speed of contraction depends on the rapidity of cross-bridge cycling (formation and dissipation), and the degree of shortening during contraction is determined by the amount of cross-bridge formation. The inotropic state is evaluated by the so-called indexes of myocardial contractility that examine the mechanical performance of the heart [speed and degree of fiber shortening, that might be assessed by parameters such as the change in pressure per unit time factored for diastolic pressure, that is, $(dP/dt)/DP$] independently of both preload and afterload. On the other hand, the so-called indexes of ventricular performance (i.e., Frank-Starling relation) examine the volume of blood ejected by the heart in association with changes in preload or afterload. Consequently, indexes of ventricular performance do not reliably evaluate myocardial contractility.

58 Does measurement of cardiac output reliably evaluate myocardial contractility in patients with known or suspected heart disease?

□ No. Measurement of cardiac output alone, a time-honored method of assessing cardiac function, provides useful information of the pumping ability of the heart but fails as a measure of myocardial contractility. Its inadequacy stems from the critical dependency of cardiac output on preload and afterload, in addition to myocardial contractility. Furthermore, cardiac output in the normal human heart is less dependent on myocardial contractility than on ventricular preload and afterload as demonstrated by the unchanged (or even decreased) cardiac output observed in response to powerful stimulation of contractility (i.e., digitalis glycosides, paired electrical stimulation). By contrast, these stimuli might increase cardiac output in patients with documented heart failure secondary to diminished contractility (e.g., myocardiopathy). Consequently, demonstration of a reduced cardiac output alone does not allow one to conclude that contractility is depressed. Measurement of cardiac output and total body oxygen consumption during exercise is a more sensitive method to detect impaired ventricular performance. Evaluation of myocardial contractility requires measurements that are independent of preload and afterload, such as the maximum rate of pressure change in systole (dP/dt).

59 Describe the two phases (or components) of active myocardial tension during systole, known as isometric and isotonic contractions.

□ Isometric contraction refers to the phase of active tension during a ventricular systole in which no external shortening of myocardial fibers occurs. During this phase, force is maximal and velocity is zero. Although external shortening is absent in this phase, the development of force is accompanied by an internal shortening of the contractile element of sarcomere and stretching of the elastic element in series (that represents the elastic connections of the muscle to its points of fixation) to a comparable degree so that total length remains unchanged. Isotonic contraction describes the phase of active tension during ventricular systole in which external shortening occurs.

The velocity of shortening is inversely related to the load so that maximal velocity (V_{max}) develops at zero load. These phases of contraction are most commonly described for the isolated papillary muscle studied in vitro. In the intact ventricle, isometric and isotonic phases of contraction correspond to the systolic phases of isovolumetric contraction and ejection, respectively.

60   Compare the effects of increased initial fiber length, faster heart rate, and positive inotropic agents (i.e., digitalis glycosides, norepinephrine) on parameters that evaluate myocardial contractility.

☐ The maximal force that myocardial fibers can develop (i.e., isometric contraction in which velocity of shortening is zero), known as P_0, increases with positive inotropic agents and with increased initial fiber length but is unaltered with a faster heart rate. The maximal velocity of shortening (i.e., isotonic contraction in which the load, force, or tension, is zero), known as V_{max} increases with positive inotropic agents and a higher heart rate but is unaltered with an increased initial fiber length. Thus, P_0 and V_{max} increase simultaneously with positive inotropic agents (e.g., Ca^{++}, cardiac glycosides, isoproterenol, dopamine, dobutamine, other sympathomimetic agents, caffeine, theophylline, and their derivatives) but not with any of the other interventions. A faster heart rate increases the speed of contraction (dP/dt), also called force-frequency relation or Bowditch phenomenon, and the speed of relaxation (negative dP/dt).

61   How might myocardial contractility be evaluated during isometric contraction? What factors modify the inotropic state?

☐ Myocardial contractility during ventricular isometric (or isovolumetric) contraction might be evaluated with indexes that examine the force-velocity relation including: (1) maximum left ventricular dP/dt (normal 1650 ± 300 mm Hg/sec); (2) maximum left ventricular dP/dt factored for pressure level [(dP/dt)/P normal 44 ± 8 sec^{-1}]; and (3) (dP/dt)/DP at diastolic pressure (DP) of 40 mmHg (normal 38 ± 12 sec^{-1}). The previously mentioned indexes of myocardial contractility still have some limitations related to non-uniformities in the ventricular wall as well as being partially affected by changes in preload or afterload. Inotropic agents (e.g., digitalis preparations, etc.) increase the indexes of myocardial contractility, whereas physiologic depressants (e.g., severe myocardial hypoxia, ischemia, hypercapnia, acidosis) and pharmacologic depressants (e.g., high dosages of certain calcium antagonists, quinidine, procainamide, disopyramide, alcohol, barbiturates, local and general anesthetics) have the opposite effect. Loss of ventricular mass due to necrosis and intrinsic myocardial depression diminish all indexes of myocardial contractility. High-fidelity catheter-tip micromanometers are used during cardiac catheterization to measure the above-mentioned indexes of myocardial contractility during the isovolumetric phase of cardiac systole.

62   How might myocardial contractility be evaluated during isotonic contraction or ejection phase? What factors modify the inotropic state?

☐   Myocardial contractility during ventricular ejection (isotonic phase) might be evaluated with angiography, using indexes that examine the velocity-length relation including: (1) mean normalized systolic ejection rate (normal 3.3 ± 0.8 end-diastolic volumes per second); and (2) mean velocity of circumferential fiber shortening (normal 1.7 ± 0.4 circumferences per second). In a comparable manner to that previously described for isometric contraction, the indexes of myocardial contractility that evaluate the ejection phase have some limitations related to non-uniformities in the ventricular wall as well as being partially affected by changes in preload or afterload. Inotropic agents increase the above-mentioned indexes of myocardial contractility, whereas a depression of these indexes is observed with physiologic depressants, pharmacologic depressants, loss of ventricular mass, and intrinsic myocardial depression.

63   How reliable is measurement of ejection fraction (ratio of stroke volume and end-diastolic volume) in the evaluation of myocardial contractility?

☐ Ejection fraction is a commonly used and reliable index of cardiac performance that can be estimated by different techniques including radionuclide or radiocontrast angiography, two-dimensional echocardiography, and cinemagnetic resonance imaging. However, ejection fraction is significantly altered by changes in ventricular loading conditions, both preload and afterload, thereby precluding its use as a reliable index of myocardial contractility. Thus, a decreased ejection fraction and cardiac output may be observed with reduced preload (e.g., hypovolemia) or increased afterload (e.g., systemic hypertension with acute exacerbation) despite normal myocardial contractility. The ejection fraction (normal range 0.55 to 0.78, mean value 0.67, significant depression less than 0.50) remains a useful clinical index of ventricular contractility despite the limitations. The prognosis of heart failure, as well as that of coronary and valvular diseases, has been correlated with the ejection fraction.

64   What other measures of ventricular and myocardial function might be used?

☐ Because ventricular and myocardial function are commonly altered in disease states by a combination of abnormal loading and depression or loss of myocardium, evaluation of cardiac performance might require use of measures for each specific component. Consequently, estimation of preload, afterload, and ejection fraction help to define ventricular and myocardial function. In addition, myocardial performance might be evaluated by plotting a measure of ventricular mechanical activity (i.e., ventricular pressure, stroke volume, or their product known as stroke work) inserted in the y-axis (ordinate) against ventricular end-diastolic pressure or volume inserted in the x-axis (abscissa). This pressure-volume relationship represents a Frank-Starling curve in which stroke work varies with changes in preload. The position of the curve with respect to the x– and y-axes describes a specific level of ventricular contractility. Differences among points along this curve indicate the effects of changing preload on ventricular mechanical activity (e.g., an increase or decrease in ventricular stroke volume while contractility remains unchanged). By contrast, upward or downward displacement of the curve corresponds to a positive or negative inotropic effect, respectively, indicative of augmentation or depression of contractility, respectively. In addition, a steeper curve (increased slope) denotes enhanced contractility and a flatter one (decreased slope) indicates depressed contractility. A positive inotropic effect produces an upward displacement and a steeper slope (e.g., β-adrenergic agonists) of the curve, whereas a negative inotropic effect produces a downward displacement and a flatter slope (e.g., heart failure). Consequently, a family of ventricular function curves that reflects a spectrum of contractile states might be generated using these parameters. The evaluation of left ventricular function in patients can be performed during cardiac catheterization as well as with radionuclide techniques, radiocontrast angiography, and other methods.

---

65   Describe a commonly used approach to evaluate ventricular performance in the intensive care unit.

□ Examination of the response of cardiac output, arterial pressure, and pulmonary capillary wedge pressure to rapid expansion of blood volume in patients with low cardiac output or hypotension provides information about myocardial performance. If the abnormal hemodynamic status is due to hypovolemia, an elevated preload will increase cardiac output, cardiac work (i.e., product of cardiac output and the difference between arterial and atrial pressures), and the slope of the relationship between cardiac work and filling pressure. None of these changes will be observed if the patient's abnormal hemodynamic condition is due to decreased myocardial contractility.

---

66   What is cardiac reserve and which are its mechanisms?

□ Cardiac reserve is the capacity of the heart to pump more blood per unit of time in response to body needs. The normal heart can increase its output five- to sixfold to meet body demands (e.g., exercise). The mechanisms of cardiac reserve are: (1) increased heart rate (up to 170 to 180 or 120 to 140 beats/min in normal young and old individuals, respectively, but might reach 200 to 220 in trained athletes) due to decreased vagal tone on the sinus node and during vigorous stress by concomitant sympathetic stimulation; (2) increased stroke volume produced by recruiting preload reserve, increased end-diastolic fiber length of the atria and ventricles, increased myocardial contractility, or decreased afterload; (3) increased oxygen extraction from hemoglobin; this mechanism is important in skeletal muscle but of less value in the myocardium because the latter normally extracts about 75% of arterial blood oxygen content; (4) redistribution of blood flow to the heart, brain, and tissues that acutely require increased supply of nutrients (e.g., skeletal muscle in physical exercise) while that directed to other organs (e.g., splanchnic and renal circulation) is sacrificed; and (5) dilatation and hypertrophy of the heart, which help to sustain a given cardiac output under some physiologic (e.g., athletes) and pathologic (e.g., arterial hypertension) conditions but might represent long-term counterproductive mechanisms.

CONTROL OF HEART FUNCTION

67 What are myocytes, myofibrils, and sarcomeres?

☐ Myocytes are the myocardial cells or fibers. They contain many cross-banded bundles called myofibrils that are composed of longitudinally arranged repeating units termed sarcomeres. The normal size of ventricular myocytes is 100 to 120 μm in length and 15 to 25 μm in diameter. Myocytes from the conduction system or Purkinje cells are larger, whereas those from the atria are smaller. Adjacent myocardial cells are connected end to end by a thickened portion of the sarcolemma or cell membrane termed the intercalated discs. A segment of the disc known as the gap junction is a low-resistance pathway that transmits electrical activity among cells (functional syncytium). The myofibrils occupy about 50% of cell volume and the units or sarcomeres that they contain are separated by dark lines known as Z lines. The sarcomere is the contractile unit which has, in the resting state, a length of about 2.2 μm that might decrease to about 1.6 μm during contraction.

68 Name the various bands and lines of the myofibrils observed under light microscopy.

☐ Under light microscopy, cardiac myofibrils consist of alternating dark and light bands known as A bands (anisotropic) and I bands (isotropic), respectively. The A band contains a lighter zone centrally located, termed the H band, that is bisected by a darker M line. The I band is similarly bisected by a dark Z line. The sarcomere is the portion of the myofibril found between two adjacent Z lines. The properties and specific role of each of these structures are examined in the answers to pertinent questions.

69 Provide further details on the structure of the sarcomere or contractile unit.

☐ The sarcomere has two main bands termed A and I bands with lengths of 1.5 μm (constant length) and about 0.5 μm (variable length depending whether contraction or relaxation is present), respectively. The A band (dark or anisotropic band) rotates polarized light and occupies the center of the sarcomere. It contains both thick and thin filaments, composed of contractile proteins, and is flanked by two lighter bands termed I or isotropic ones. Only thin filaments are present in the I bands and extend from a Z line (at one end of the sarcomere) through the I band and into the A band. Thus, thin filaments of a sarcomere extend from the outer limit of the contractile unit toward its center. The inner endings of the thin filaments finish before (within the A band) reaching the corresponding inner ending of the thin filaments coming from the opposite Z line (or side) of the sarcomere. The zone located in the central area of the A band that is demarcated by the endings of the thin filaments (so that thin filaments are absent) is known as the H zone. The thick (about 1.5 μm in length) filaments are composed of myosin and the thin ones (about 1.0 μm in length) contain actin and other proteins (e.g., tropomyosin, troponin).

70   Summarize the characteristics and composition of the bands and lines of the sarcomere.

☐ The dark bands (A) are located in the center of the sarcomere, their length is constant, and they contain both contractile proteins myosin and actin. The light or I bands are on the sides of the sarcomere, their length is variable, and they contain only actin. The H zone, located at the center of the sarcomere, contains myosin exclusively. The Z lines are at each end of the sarcomere, they represent the point of insertion of the thin filaments (actin) and are located in the light or I bands that belong to adjacent sarcomeres. The M line of the sarcomere, which bisects the H band, is the region where the myosin rods come together and are linked by a variety of proteins (e.g., M protein, C and H proteins, creatine phosphokinase). The M line is surrounded by another protein termed myomesin.

71   What is the spatial arrangement of the thin (actin) and thick (myosin) filaments that allows for contraction and relaxation to occur?

☐ Each thick filament of the sarcomere is surrounded by six thin filaments and the area of juxtaposition of the two types of filaments is maximal during contraction (band I having only thin filaments is at its smallest length) and minimal at resting or relaxation state (band I is at its longest state). Interactions between the thick and thin myofilaments in the A band generate force and shortening of the sarcomere with the two types of filaments sliding on each other, maintaining a constant length for each filament. The interdigitating sliding of thick and thin filaments during contraction and relaxation is explained by formation and disruption of cross-bridges between myosin and actin due to complex reactions that consume energy.

---

72   Provide additional information about the thick and thin filaments.

☐ The thick filament consists essentially of myosin (about 400 molecules), a fibrous protein capable of adenosine triphosphate (ATP) hydrolysis on activation by actin in the presence of magnesium (Mg^{++}). Myosin can also bind directly with actin. Each myosin molecule has a rodlike single tail and two globular heads. The latter interact with the grooves of actin filaments during contraction, causing shortening of the sarcomere. The thin filament consists of two chains of globular actin arranged in a double helix and having the troponin-tropomyosin complex (regulatory proteins that constitute about 10% of the myofilaments) inserted in the grooves of the actin helix. In the resting, noncontractile state, muscle shortening is prevented by tropomyosin covering the actin site required for activation/interaction with myosin. In response to a rise in intracellular Ca^{++} (10^{-7} to 10^{-5} M) that develops with a cardiac action potential, Ca^{++} binds with troponin, which releases tropomyosin. Exit of these proteins from the grooves of actin enables actin to contact the myosin heads. Consequently, in the presence of ATP and Mg^{++}, the myosin heads "swivel" such that the thin filaments are pulled toward the center of the sarcomere.

---

73   Describe the actin-myosin interaction in cardiac contraction and relaxation.

☐ A "rowing motion" develops with the juxtaposition and subsequent "flexing" of the myosin heads on the actin grooves.

Simultaneously, the myosin head ejects the products of ATP hydrolysis (adenosine diphosphate, or ADP, and inorganic phosphate) and binds another molecule of ATP repeating a similar cycle. As long as intracellular $[Ca^{++}]$ remains high enough, the myosin head is free to interact with another groove of the actin molecule, resulting in further shortening of the sarcomere. At the end of systole intracellular $[Ca^{++}]$ decreases, the troponin-tropomyosin complex returns to its initial position in the grooves of the actin helix, preventing further actin-myosin interaction thereby leading to relaxation. Thus a "repressor" mechanism released by increased intracellular $[Ca^{++}]$ controls the contractile apparatus of the heart.

---

74   What are the major proteins of the myofibrils and what fraction of total protein content is accounted for by each of them?

□ Myofibrils contain contractile (i.e., myosin, actin), regulatory (i.e., tropomyosin and troponins C, I, and T), and structural (i.e., C protein, M line protein, α actinin, β actinin) proteins that account for 80%, 10%, and 10%, respectively, of total protein content in myofibrils. Myosin is located in the thick filaments, has a molecular weight (MW) of 500,000 daltons, and represents about 60% of total protein content. Actin is found in the thin filaments; its MW is 43,000 and accounts for about 20% of total proteins. Tropomyosin and troponin have MWs of approximately 70,000 and 86,000, respectively, and are located in the thin filaments. The various structural proteins have a wide range of MWs (40,000 to 750,000) and are located in the thick filaments (e.g., C protein), thin filaments (e.g., β actinin), M lines (e.g., M line proteins), and other areas of the myofibrils.

---

75   What is the role of the various organelles of the cardiac myocytes?

□ The myofibrils (about 50% of cell volume) are directly responsible for contraction and relaxation because they contain the sarcomeres or contractile units. The source of energy for the contraction cycle is made available by the mitochondria (about 20% of cell volume) in the form of ATP molecules. ATP stores are in equilibrium with the high-energy phosphate contained in cytosolic creatine phosphate. The T system is a network of tubules located in the cytoplasm (about 1% of cell volume), continuous with the extracellular space, and comprised of invaginations of the sarcolemma. This system transmits the electric signal of the membrane action potential to the cell interior. The sarcoplasma or cytosol contains ions and small solutes, surrounds the sarcomere and other organelles, and is characterized by rapid changes in $[Ca^{++}]$. The sarcoplasmic reticulum is a complex labyrinth of anastomosing intracellular tubules that surround each myofibril, releasing Ca^{++}, and taking up this ion during the contraction/relaxation cycle. In contrast with the T system, the sarcoplasmic reticulum is not continuous with the cell membrane or sarcolemma. The terminal cisternae (also called vesicles or lateral sacs) of the sarcoplasmic reticulum are involved in the release of Ca^{++} that triggers the myocardial contraction. The cell nucleus (about 5% of cell volume) is involved in protein synthesis, whereas lysosomes perform intracellular digestion and proteolysis. The outer envelope of the cardiac myocytes that contains all organelles is the sarcolemma or cell membrane. Its role includes control of ionic gradients by channels and pumps, harboring of receptors for hormones and drugs, and maintenance of cell integrity.

---

76 Explain the ionic determinants of the resting membrane potential of the myocardial cell.

☐ The resting potential of the myocardial cell is largely due to the electrical and chemical (electrochemical) gradient for potassium (K^+) across the cell membrane. Intracellular K^+ concentration ($[K^+]_i$) is much higher than its extracellular concentration ($[K^+]_e$) due to the influence of impermeable intracellular anions (Donnan equilibrium) and the action of the Na^+, K^+-ATPase located in the plasma membrane. The plasma membrane is highly permeable to K^+ allowing this cation to flow "downhill" out of the cell, increasing intracellular electronegativity. In general, processes that increase the rate of K^+ flow from the cell to the ECF (positive charge exiting the cell) produce a more negative cell interior that, by convention, is referred to as an increase in membrane potential. Such change in membrane potential is also referred to as hyperpolarization, in which the electrical potential is more negative with respect to ground (or ECF) that is taken as zero potential. By contrast, a decreased rate of K^+ flow from the cells to the ECF has the opposite effect. The contribution of other ions to the resting membrane potential is comparatively small. Although resting membrane potential is mostly a "K^+ diffusion potential," cell membrane pumps and exchangers that translocate ions in an "electrogenic" fashion (e.g., the Na^+,K^+-ATPase, and Na^+/Ca^{++} exchanger, respectively), play an additional role, albeit a comparatively minor one, as determinants of resting potential. The transport of the pump and exchanger is called "electrogenic" because both translocate different amounts of positive charges between the cell and ECF in each cycle of activity, changing the membrane potential. The Na^+, K^+-ATPase extrudes 3 Na^+ ions while pumping 2 K^+ ions into the cell, increasing cell electronegativity. By contrast, the Na^+/Ca^{++} exchanger allows the entry of 3 Na^+ ions for every Ca^{++} ion extruded (normal orientation of transport), decreasing cell electronegativity.

---

77   What is the role of Na^+ in the membrane potential of myocardial cells?

☐ The role of Na^+ as well as that of any ion as determinant of membrane potential depends on its electrochemical gradient across the cell membrane and its permeability. Although in the resting state the electrochemical gradient for Na^+ is substantial (since the cell interior is electronegative and the chemical gradient between the ECF and ICF is large, and these two mechanisms favor the cellular entry of Na^+), the very low cell membrane permeability accounts for the minor contribution of Na^+ to the resting membrane potential. Nevertheless, the "Na^+ diffusion potential" is responsible for the brisk depolarization (phase zero of action potential) that occurs during cell activation and is due to opening of cell membrane Na^+ channels. In addition, the spontaneous depolarization observed in some pacemaker cells (e.g., His-Purkinje system) is partially due to a relatively high cell membrane permeability to Na^+ allowing movement of this cation from the ECF to the ICF.

78 What is the role of Ca^{++} in comparison to that of Na^+ and K^+ in the action potential of cardiac muscle?

☐ Sodium and calcium, two cations having much higher concentration in the ECF as compared to their cellular levels, are responsible for inward currents during the action potential of cardiac muscle. Activation (opening) of Na^+ channels produces a large inward Na^+ current due to cellular Na^+ entry, which causes the rapid upstroke of depolarization (phase 0). A brief period of rapid and limited repolarization (phase 1) follows, which is partly due to inactivation of Na^+ channels. Thereafter, a new phase of stable depolarization (i.e., the plateau or phase 2) develops, which is due to competing influences of opposing currents (e.g., inward Ca^{++} and outward K^+ currents). Finally, a period of repolarization (phase 3) occurs and is due to an outward K^+ current that returns the membrane potential to its resting level (phase 4). Thus, activation of both Na^+ and Ca^{++} channels participates in the cardiac action potential, producing measurable inward currents.

79 Are the forces that favor cellular entry of Na^+ larger than those for Ca^{++} entry, considering their respective extracellular concentrations of about 140 mM and 1 mM?

☐ No. The forces that favor inward currents of Na^+ and Ca^{++} during the action potential depend on the electrochemical gradient of each ion, which is partially based on their respective concentrations outside and inside cells as determined by the Nernst equation. Let us examine their value for Na^+ assuming extracellular and intracellular concentrations of 140 mM and 15 mM, respectively. Thus,

$$E_{Na^+} = 58 \log \frac{\left[Na^+ \right]_e}{\left[Na^+ \right]_i} = 58 \times \log \frac{140}{15} - +56mV$$

where E_{Na^+} is the equilibrium potential for the distribution of Na^+. The cation with the higher E_{ion} will have the greater inward current during the cardiac action potential. Fifty-eight is a constant, and +56 mV is the predicted membrane potential that on channel activation causes an inward (depolarizing) current. Let us now examine the equilibrium potential for Ca^{++} ($E_{Ca^{++}}$) assuming extracellular and intracellular levels of 1 mM and 0.0001 mM, respectively. Thus,

$$E_{Ca^{++}} = \frac{58}{2} \log \frac{\left[Ca^{++} \right]_e}{\left[Ca^{++} \right]_i} = \frac{58}{2} \log \frac{1}{0.0001} = +116 \text{ mV}$$

where 2 is a factor determined by the valence of the cation, and +116 mV is the predicted membrane potential. Consequently, the driving force for Ca^{++} movement into the cell is larger than that for Na^+ despite the lower extracellular Ca^{++} concentration.

---

80 Compare the inward currents that result from activation of Na^+ and Ca^{++} channels.

☐ Inward currents due to Na^+ are characteristically fast, whereas those due to Ca^{++} entry are distinctly slow. The Na^+ and Ca^{++} channels involved in cardiac action potential are voltage dependent (i.e., open or closed state, known as gating, is modified by membrane potential), yet their threshold potential (i.e., membrane potential at which channel is activated) in mV differs substantially (−60 mV for Na^+ channels and −35 mV for Ca^{++} channels). Thus, an action potential develops when membrane potential (−80 mV at rest) reaches −60 mV, a level that opens Na^+ channels. When the additional depolarization caused by Na^+ entry reaches threshold potential for the Ca^{++} channels, the latter open and generate a new depolarizing current. The Ca^{++} current more slowly activates (5 to 20 msec and about 1 msec for Ca^{++} and Na^+ channels, respectively) and thereafter inactivates (30 to 300 msec and 2 to 10 msec for Ca^{++} and Na^+ channels, respectively) the myocytes and provides the inward current ("slow inward current") that maintains the cell membrane in a depolarized state during the plateau (phase 2) of the action potential.

81   Are the concentration gradients for Na^+, Ca^{++}, and K^+ dissipated during the action potential?

☐ No. Only a minor decrease in the concentration gradient of each of these ions develops with their translocation across the cell membrane in the process of myocardial depolarization/repolarization. The maintenance of ionic gradients is largely due to: (1) the relatively small fraction of the total available pool of these electrolytes that is actually translocated across the cell membrane and (2) counterbalancing processes that correct the redistribution of these ions simultaneously during tissue activation.

82   Summarize the major ionic currents that contribute to each phase of the cardiac action potential.

☐ Phase 0 (zero) is the rapid upstroke of the cardiac action potential (depolarization phase), due to activation (opening) of plasma membrane Na^+ channels, and is completed within a few milliseconds. This activation allows the rapid cellular entry of Na^+, which decreases (depolarizes) the membrane potential. The large depolarization of membrane potential inactivates (closes) these channels, thereby inhibiting Na^+ entry and contributing to the conclusion of this phase. Phase 1 (early repolarization phase) is the brief phase of rapid repolarization that follows the peak of the cardiac action potential and is due to the combined effect of a diminished positive inward current (Na^+ entry), a newly developed negative inward current (Cl^- entry), and a positive outward current (K^+ exit). Phase 2 (plateau phase) is characterized by a stable membrane potential (its stability accounts for the name of this phase as plateau phase) that is substantially lower than the resting membrane potential (sustained depolarization) and is due to a balance among currents caused by the slow cellular entry of Na^+, Cl^-, and Ca^{++}, and cellular exit of K^+. Phase 3 (late repolarization phase) is the period of repolarization that brings membrane potential to the more negative value observed at the resting state. This phase is due to discontinuation of inward currents of the previous phase and augmentation of outward K^+ current (exit of cellular K^+). Phase 4 (resting potential phase), the last of the cycle of electrical events, is characterized by a membrane potential at the resting level. Maintenance of membrane potential is due predominantly to an outward K^+ current (cellular exit of K^+), as described previously.

---

83   How large are the changes in cellular electrolyte composition caused by ion movements across the cell membrane that mediate the cardiac action potential?

☐ Although the previously described ion movements largely modify the cell membrane potential, these ion exchanges do not cause substantial alterations in the cellular concentrations of K^+ and Na^+. Each cellular depolarization associated with the cardiac action potential involves the movement of a relatively small number of ions. Consequently, the concentration gradients for these ions are only minimally decreased by the action potential. For example, when repetitive firing of the action potential is induced in sheep Purkinje fibers, cytosolic $[Na^+]$ increases by only about 10%.

---

84   What is the threshold potential?

☐ The threshold potential is a membrane potential that, when reached, produces cell activation characterized by the initiation of the action potential. The threshold potential is lower (more depolarized) than the membrane potential and is reached by partial depolarization of membrane potential. By contrast, the action potential involves complete depolarization of the membrane potential. When the threshold potential is reached, the action potential fires in an "all or none" fashion. This means that an action potential either fails to develop ("none") or this electrical event is fully expressed ("all"); intermediate stages do not occur. The threshold potential reflects the voltage sensitivity of membrane Na^+ channels that carry the inward Na^+ current responsible for phase 0 (zero) of the cardiac action potential. At the threshold potential, Na^+ channels are activated, initiating the action potential. The new level of cell membrane depolarization activates additional Na^+ channels, promoting expression of the phase 0 upstroke. By contrast, membrane repolarization closes (or deactivates) Na^+ channels, which reach the inactive or closed state observed when the membrane potential is at its resting state.

85   What factors are responsible for a cessation of the inward Na^+ current, manifested by the peak of the phase 0 upstroke?

☐ Attainment of the Na^+ equilibrium potential (due to cellular Na^+ entry) as predicted by the Nernst equation as well as time-dependent voltage inactivation of Na^+ channels are the main factors responsible for cessation of the inward Na^+ current. The major ions of the ICF and ECF are unequally distributed across the cell membrane. Large intracellular concentrations of impermeant anions (mostly phosphate and proteins) and ion pumps in the plasma membrane contribute to the maintenance of vastly different concentrations of Na^+, K^+, Cl^-, and Ca^{++} in the ICF compared to ECF compartments. The Nernst equation allows for quantification of the electric force that would be necessary to maintain the existing chemical gradients. This quantity is known as the equilibrium potential for a given ion. The equilibrium potential for Na^+ (E_{Na^+}) has been calculated in the answer to a previous question and amounted to +56 mV. Thus, an intracellular voltage of +56 mV would be required to maintain the observed chemical distribution for Na^+ in the resting state. Because the intracellular compartment in the resting state is electronegative (e.g., –80 mV), opening of Na^+ channels promotes cellular Na^+ entry driven by electrochemical forces, moving the membrane potential toward the electrochemical equilibrium for this ion. A time-dependent inactivation of Na^+ channels also participates in the termination of phase 0 of the cardiac action potential.

86   What is the importance of the prolonged myocardial depolarization with respect to cardiac function?

☐ The prolonged depolarization period (phase 2 of the cardiac action potential) produces a long refractory period during which activation, and therefore contraction of the myocardial muscle, does not occur. This period of ventricular relaxation (lack of contraction) allows for filling of the ventricle during diastole and facilitates an orderly cycle of activation followed by a short-lasting contraction of myocardium, therefore avoiding a condition known as tetany (abnormal state of persistent contraction). The function of the heart as a pump requires cycles of ventricular relaxation (ventricular filling during diastole) followed by contraction (ventricular emptying during systole). Thus, sustained contraction prevents meaningful pumping action by the heart. By contrast, sustained contraction might be required to perform specific tasks imposed on skeletal muscle.

---

87   What is the refractory period of the cardiac action potential?

☐ The refractory period is that time during which depolarizing stimuli are unable to initiate a propagated action potential. The refractory period occurs during passage of the cardiac action potential and immediately thereafter. Because the degree of unresponsiveness of the heart during the refractory period decreases with time, two distinct periods are recognized: the absolute or effective refractory period (ERP) and the relative refractory period (RRP). The ERP begins with cardiac depolarization and is characterized by the complete absence of a propagated action potential in response to a depolarizing stimulus of any magnitude. During the RRP that begins at the end of ERP, only stimuli of an intensity that exceeds the normal threshold can initiate a propagated action potential. Electrical stimuli of normal intensity occurring during the refractory periods (ERP and RRP) might elicit an action potential only at the point of stimulation (local response) that fails to propagate throughout the heart. Such local responses, however, can contribute to the development of cardiac arrhythmias.

---

88   How does the action potential of the sinoatrial node differ from that previously described for the main conduction system of the heart (Purkinje fibers)?

☐ The action potential of the SA node has an upstroke (phase 0) characterized by a smaller amplitude and longer duration than that of the Purkinje cells. The upstroke of the SA node action potential is due to an inward Ca^{++} current, whereas the upstroke of the Purkinje fiber action potential is due to an inward Na^+ current. The high levels of intracellular cyclic adenosine monophosphate (AMP) characteristic of SA myocardial cells lead to increased phosphorylation of Ca^{++} channels and thereby augment the flow of Ca^{++} current into these cells, enhancing automaticity. Interventions that decrease intracellular cyclic AMP levels of SA myocytes (such as stimulation of the muscarinic receptor by acetylcholine) has the opposite effect, decreasing Ca^{++} entry and the rate of firing of the SA node (diminished automaticity).

---

89   What cardiac cells exhibit automaticity and what are the main determinants of this property?

☐ Cardiac cells from the SA node, AV node, and those of the His-Purkinje system exhibit automaticity, that is, spontaneous depolarization during phase 4 of the cardiac membrane potential cycle. The spontaneous depolarization of phase 4 in automatic tissues is due to either an inward Ca^{++} current during this phase or a higher Na^+ conductance (i.e., a greater number of Na^+ channels in their open state) of automatic tissues compared with non automatic tissues. The inward Ca^{++} current (that occurs in the SA and AV nodes) and the inward Na^+ current (that occurs in the His-Purkinje cells) overcomes the outward K^+ current of these automatic cells, producing the characteristic spontaneous depolarization of phase 4. The progressive decrease in membrane potential of phase 4 triggers an action potential that propagates throughout the heart once its level reaches threshold potential.

---

90   How does the action potential of the AV node differ from that of other automatic cardiac cells (SA node and His-Purkinje system)?

☐ The action potential of the AV node as well as that of the SA node are characterized by a smaller amplitude and longer duration than that of the Purkinje cells. The AV node functions to delay impulse conduction between the atria and ventricles so that the ventricles remain in diastole (relaxation state of the myocardium), whereas the atria complete their contractile function, emptying their load into the corresponding ventricles. The same electrical impulse that led to atrial contraction promotes the sequential activation of the ventricles, securing coordination of these pumps in series. The sequential activation of atria and ventricles by the same impulse is due to the delay of impulse conduction through the AV node whose action potential has a slowly rising upstroke and therefore a slow linear velocity for conduction of the stimulus.

---

91   Characterize the action potentials of myocardial cells in the atria and ventricles that do not belong to the excitation system of the normal heart (i.e., SA node, AV node, His-Purkinje fibers).

☐ Most cells of the atria and ventricles do not belong to the excitation system of the normal heart; they lack pacemaker activity and are called nonspecific cardiocytes. Nevertheless, these cells can occasionally develop automaticity, generating "ectopic" systoles ("extra" systoles). The action potential of nonspecific cardiocytes differs in the atria as compared to the ventricles. The atrial action potential has a very brief plateau phase (phase 2) that merges into the repolarization phase (phase 3), making the distinction between these two phases difficult and contributing to the short duration of the action potential of atrial cells. This short phase of depolarization in atrial cells is due to a rapidly rising K^+ permeability mediated by channels that are controlled, in part, by the autonomic nervous system. This effect is demonstrated by vagal stimulation that opens K^+ channels leading to cellular K^+ exit, which shortens both duration of the action potential and the refractory period in the atria. In contrast with the atrial action potential, the ventricular action potential has a long duration of the plateau phase.

---

92   Compare the consequences of hyperkalemia and hypokalemia on the electrophysiologic properties of the heart.

☐ Whereas hyperkalemia characteristically depresses most electric properties of the heart, hypokalemia increases these properties. Thus, automaticity, duration of action potential refractory period, and resting membrane potential are all decreased in hyperkalemia and increased in hypokalemia. The altered electrophysiologic properties of the heart with these two electrolyte abnormalities are responsible for the development of arrhythmias.

---

93 What are the effects of hyperkalemia on cardiac excitability?

☐ Hyperkalemia alters cardiac excitability by depolarizing the resting membrane potential. Hyperkalemia also increases the cell membrane permeability to K^+, shortening the duration on the action potential, because cellular exit of K^+ is responsible for returning the depolarized cell membrane to its resting state. Furthermore, pacemaker activity is depressed because the spontaneous depolarization characteristic of pacemaker cells is inhibited because larger outward K^+ current opposes the normal inward Ca^{++} current (SA and AV nodes) and Na^+ current (His-Purkinje cells).

---

94 Review the ionic basis of pacemaker activity and the effects of plasma K^+ levels.

☐ The process of spontaneous depolarization characteristic of pacemakers is due to a persistent imbalance between cellular Ca^{++} or Na^+ entry and cellular K^+ exit. A greater rate of entry of cations (Ca^{++} or Na^+) than the exit rate of other ones (K^+) is responsible for the spontaneous depolarization found in pacemaker cells in the normal state. Hyperkalemia inhibits the spontaneous depolarization because it causes a persistently high permeability of K^+ leading to increased cellular exit of this ion, thereby counterbalancing the depolarization induced by Ca^{++} or Na^+ movement into the cell. Consequently, hyperkalemia inhibits automaticity of the cardiac pacemaker. As expected, hypokalemia produces the opposite effect because it reduces cell membrane permeability to K^+, thereby increasing automaticity of the heart.

---

95 Describe the impact of hyperkalemia on the T wave of the electrocardiogram (ECG).

☐ The T wave of the ECG is the expression of ventricular repolarization. Hyperkalemia narrows the base and increases the amplitude of the T wave ("peaked" T wave). This effect, observed when $[K^+]_p$ is above 6 mEq/L, is due to a shorter duration of ventricular repolarization.

---

96   Elaborate further on the cardiovascular influences of hyperkalemia.

☐ The cardiac effects of hyperkalemia are usually the dominant manifestations and most frequently precede other signs and symptoms. ECG monitoring allows recognition of the characteristic changes including peaked T waves, prolonged PR interval, depressed ST segment, shortened QT interval, widening of the QRS complex, absence of P waves, development of "sine waves," and possible asystole or ventricular fibrillation. Hyperkalemia also causes dilation of the blood vessels.

---

97   What are the effects of hypokalemia on cardiac excitability?

☐ The effects of hypokalemia on cardiac excitability are generally opposite to those described for hyperkalemia. Consequently, hypokalemia alters cardiac excitability by hyperpolarizing the resting membrane potential. Hypokalemia also decreases the cell membrane permeability to K^+ ions, prolonging the duration of the action potential, because cellular exit of K^+ is responsible for returning the depolarized cell membrane to its resting state. Furthermore, pacemaker activity is increased because the spontaneous depolarization characteristic of pacemaker cells is stimulated because a smaller outward K^+ current opposes the normal inward Ca^{++} current (SA and AV nodes) and Na^+ current (His-Purkinje cells).

---

98   Describe further the cardiovascular impact of hypokalemia.

☐ The cardiac effects include an increased risk of digitalis toxicity, supraventricular tachyarrhythmias (atrial, junctional), ventricular arrhythmias (isolated beats, bigeminal rhythm, tachycardia, or fibrillation), other characteristic ECG changes (flat or inverted T waves, depressed ST segments, prominent U waves, and a prolonged "QU" interval that resembles the prolonged "QT" interval characteristic of hypocalcemia), and structural myocardial damage (myocardial necrosis). The vascular effect of hypokalemia is constriction of arterioles (resistance vessels). Increased systemic vascular resistance, producing hypertension, has been postulated to occur in states of K^+ depletion. Potassium repletion can decrease peripheral vascular resistance and diminish systemic blood pressure.

99 **What are the major structural and functional differences between skeletal and cardiac muscle?**

☐ The lateral position of the cell nucleus in skeletal muscle contrasts with the myocardium in which the nucleus is centrally placed within its cells. Because contraction is an inherent property of cardiac tissue that does not require intervention of the nervous system, only free nerve endings are found in the myocardium. By contrast, activation of skeletal muscle contraction requires motor nerves that have special nerve endings known as motor plates at the myoneural junctions. Myocardial cells are smaller than skeletal muscle cells and the intercellular collagen is more abundant in heart muscle. These characteristics might explain the greater resting stiffness of cardiac muscle. Furthermore, the sarcomeres of cardiac muscle resist stretching beyond 2.2 μm, whereas in skeletal muscles the sarcomere allows stretching up to 3.6 μm (active tension falls in a linear fashion between 2.2 and 3.6 μm of sarcomere length and at the latter length, the overlap of thick and thin filaments completely disappears). The elastic component in series with the sarcomere is compliant in cardiac muscle (but not in skeletal muscle) so that during isometric contraction, substantial shortening of the sarcomeres occurs on the steep portion of the length-active tension curve. In summary, the sarcomeres of cardiac muscle function at a less variable length that secures a higher active tension in most physiologic conditions.

100 **Contrast the cardiac action potential with that of skeletal muscle.**

☐ The skeletal muscle action potential is a two-phase event consisting of a rapid depolarization (the cell interior becomes less electronegative with respect to ground or cell exterior) followed immediately by repolarization (cell interior regains its original electronegativity). This rapid upstroke (depolarization) is followed by a fast downstroke (repolarization) and these two events last 2 to 3 msec. Subsequently, a period called the "afterpotential" occurs lasting about 10 msec during which the membrane potential remains more positive than the resting potential as it slowly returns to baseline. By contrast, the cardiac action potential in the conduction system that propagates the excitation stimuli to the ventricles (i.e., Purkinje fibers) lasts 300 to 400 msec and has been divided into five phases. The rapid upstroke of the cardiac action potential is called phase zero. A short early repolarization phase (phase 1) is followed by a sustained depolarization phase (phase 2) that is mostly responsible for the long duration of the cardiac compared with skeletal muscle action potential. This depolarization plateau is followed by repolarization (phase 3) and return to the baseline membrane potential. Phases 1 and 2 of the cardiac action potential have no clear counterpart in the skeletal muscle. Phase 4 describes the resting membrane potential.

---

101   Contrast the specialized function of the two major forms of striated muscle known as "white" and "red" types and provide examples of each one.

□ White muscles are a "fast" type, designed for intense contraction over a short time period after which they must rest before contracting with the same intensity. They are typified by some skeletal muscles that allow an animal or human to sprint for short distances to escape danger. Red muscles are a "slow" type designed for sustained periods of activity without rest periods. Cardiac muscle typifies this type of muscle. Grossly, red muscles are darker than white muscles due to their higher myoglobin content, which facilitates the transfer and utilization of oxygen. The high myoglobin content is indicative of the importance of oxidative metabolism in red muscles to provide the large and continuous supply of energy necessary for the sustained activity of this type of striated muscle. In addition, red muscles contain large numbers of mitochondria, which are also important for oxidative metabolism. These structures occupy space that might otherwise be filled by contractile proteins, contributing to the relative weakness of red as compared with white muscles. Pale fibers characterize the gross appearance of white muscles, which have lower myoglobin content and fewer mitochondria but a greater number of contractile proteins. The lower oxidative metabolism of white muscles makes them dependent on local energy stores and anaerobic metabolism; these fuel sources can be rapidly exhausted, forcing the muscle to rest while it replenishes energy stores.

---

102 Contrast the regulation of Ca^{++} released by sarcoplasmic reticulum (SR) in skeletal muscle cell with that of cardiac muscle cell.

☐ The contraction of the mammalian skeletal muscle cell is an "all or none" mechanical process wherein the large amount of Ca^{++} released by the SR saturates the receptors of troponin C. Thus, regulation of contraction in the skeletal muscle occurs primarily by recruitment of varying numbers of active motor units by the central nervous system because each skeletal muscle cell, once activated, contracts with its maximal intensity. By contrast, variations in the force of contraction occur in cardiac muscle cells (it is not an "all or none" mechanical process), which are caused by changes in the amount of Ca^{++} made available for binding troponin C. It follows that there is an intricate system for regulating the amount of Ca^{++} released from SR in response to a stimulus in myocardial cells.

---

103 What are the major determinants of the large concentration gradient for Ca^{++} between the extracellular and the intracellular (10^{-3} M and 10^{-7} M, respectively) compartments?

☐ The large transmembrane ionic gradient for Ca^{++} is accounted for by: (1) a low resting permeability to Ca^{++} of cell membrane; (2) a Na^+ / Ca^{++} exchange mechanism that normally extrudes intracellular Ca^{++} in exchange for the "downhill" entry of extracellular Na^+ due to the large electrochemical gradient of Na^+ directed toward the cell interior; the Na^+, K^+ pump participates in this process by helping to maintain the normal electrochemical gradient for Na^+; and

(3) an ATP-dependent pump that extrudes cytosolic Ca^{++} (Ca^{++}-ATPase). The interplay of these mechanisms, as well as that of voltage-sensitive Ca^{++} channels that couple excitation and contraction, determine the concentration gradient for Ca^{++} across the sarcolemma.

---

104   What are the mechanisms that control the cytoplasmic $[Ca^{++}]$ in the myocardium?

☐ The cellular entry and exit of Ca^{++} occur by different pathways that are under physiologic control. The inward movement of Ca^{++} across the sarcolemma (cellular membrane) along its concentration gradient occurs through voltage-dependent channels (i.e., the movement of Ca^{++} through these pores is controlled by electrical potentials) and receptor-operated channels (i.e., the movement of Ca^{++} through these pores is controlled by cell membrane receptors sensitive to physiologic messengers or drugs). The outward movement of Ca^{++} across the sarcolemma depends on the Na^+ / Ca^{++} exchange mechanisms and active pumping by a Ca^{++}-ATPase. The Na^+ / Ca^{++} exchanger can operate in either direction (allowing either exit or entry of Ca^{++} and the opposite movement of Na^+) depending on the relative concentrations of extracellular and intracellular Na^+ and Ca^{++}. Nevertheless, the downhill movement of Na^+ into the cell along its electrochemical gradient present under physiologic conditions provides the energy (and mandates the direction of ion movement) for the translocation of Ca^{++} out of the cell against its concentration gradient. Calcium kinetics within the cell is modulated by several mechanisms that include: (1) uptake and release by intracellular structures such as the mitochondria, the internal surface of the sarcolemma, and the sarcoplasmic reticulum; (2) Ca^{++} buffering by intracellular proteins such as calmodulin, troponin C, and myosin-P light chains; and (3) a Ca^{++}-stimulated Mg^{++}-ATPase located within the membranes of the SR that removes Ca^{++} from the cytosol and sequesters it within these structures through an energy-requiring process.

105 How does the cell membrane Na^+/Ca^{++} exchanger alter the cellular pool of Ca^{++}?

☐ The Na^+/Ca^{++} exchanger located at the cell membrane mediates the facilitated bidirectional exchange of Na^+ for Ca^{++}. The net movement of electric charges due to the operation of this exchanger is asymmetric because three Na^+ ions are exchanged for every Ca^{++} ion. Thus, the exchange is not electroneutral but electrogenic (two positive charges of Ca^{++} moving out of the cell are exchanged for three positive charges of Na^+ moving into the cell) and, as a consequence, is sensitive to changes in the membrane potential. Depolarization of the cell membrane (e.g., cytosol becoming less electronegative with respect to the ECF because of cellular entry of Na^+ during action potential or other means of cell activation) promotes the exit of Na^+ and the entry of Ca^{++} through the Na^+/Ca^{++} exchanger. Repolarization of the membrane (e.g., cytosol becoming more electronegative with respect to the ECF during cell recovery from activation) has the opposite effect, promoting the exit of Ca^{++} and the entry of Na^+. Cardiac glycosides depolarize the cell membrane and thereby facilitate cellular Ca^{++} entry via the Na^+/Ca^{++} exchanger. During normal diastole (cardiac relaxation), repolarization of the cell membrane promotes Ca^{++} extrusion from the cell in exchange for Na^+ entry through the Na^+/Ca^{++} exchanger. On the contrary, during normal systole (cardiac contraction), depolarization of the cell membrane promotes Ca^{++} entry in exchange for Na^+ exit.

106 Compare the Na^+/Ca^{++} exchanger and the Ca^{++}-ATPase located in the cell membrane.

☐ The Na^+/Ca^{++} exchanger is a high-capacity and low-affinity transporting system that is energized by the ionic gradients between compartments separated by the plasma membrane (intra- and extracellular concentrations of Na^+ and Ca^{++}). On the contrary, the Ca^{++}-ATPase is a low-capacity and high-affinity system that derives the energy required for Ca^{++} extrusion from cardiac cells by ATP hydrolysis. The

Ca^{++}-ATPase pumps Ca^{++} out of the cells against a large electrochemical gradient and participates in the maintenance of a low $[Ca^{++}]$ in the cytosol during diastole.

---

107   What is excitation-contraction coupling?

☐ Excitation-contraction coupling is the series of interlocking steps that transmit a signal from the plasma membrane to the contractile proteins of the cardiac cell to initiate contraction. It begins with depolarization of the plasma membrane by the action potential and ends with binding of Ca^{++} to its troponin receptor. The latter reaction inhibits the binding of troponin to actin, enabling actin to interact with the myosin heads, starting the "rowing" motion of thin filaments over the thick ones. The multiple interlocking steps allow for modulation of cardiac performance in response to a variety of physiologic and pharmacologic stimuli. The steps include: (1) activation of Ca^{++} entry to the cytosol from the extracellular space through "voltage-dependent" Ca^{++} channels. This ion movement produces the "slow" inward current and is initiated by membrane depolarization caused by the "fast" inward current carried by Na^+ ions during the so-called "phase zero" of the action potential; and (2) release of Ca^{++} from intracellular stores. The movement of Ca^{++} entering the cytosol from the extracellular space into the cytosol does not activate contraction directly but instead induces release of a much larger amount of Ca^{++} stored in the SR. This mechanism is the so-called Ca^{++}-induced Ca^{++} release; and (3) Ca^{++} binding to its receptor on troponin, deactivating it and thereby allowing for the contractile process to begin.

---

108   What is the major source of the cytosolic Ca^{++} that inactivates troponin C to begin the contractile process?

☐ Calcium released from intracellular stores, primarily the SR, is the major source of the increment in cytosolic Ca^{++} that initiates the contractile process. The Ca^{++} that enters the cytosol from the extracellular space acts primarily to stimulate Ca^{++} release from the SR. Intracellular Ca^{++} release causes a rapid increase in the concentration of this cation throughout the muscle cell, allowing for rapid and simultaneous initiation of the contractile process throughout the cell. Exclusive reliance on extracellular Ca^{++} entry to cause the necessary increase in $[Ca^{++}]$ to produce cardiac contraction would depend on diffusion to distribute this cation throughout the cytosol, a process that is too slow and therefore would fail to induce a rapid and simultaneous contractile response of the myocardium.

---

109 Briefly describe the main membrane proteins involved in the increase and subsequent decrease of cytosolic $[Ca^{++}]$ that occur during contraction and relaxation, respectively, of cardiac muscle cells.

□ Cytosolic $[Ca^{++}]$ is substantially lower than that in both the extracellular space and the SR. Thus, movement of Ca^{++} into the cytosol is a "downhill" process (following its concentration gradient), whereas removal of Ca^{++} from the cytosol into either of these two compartments is against a concentration gradient ("uphill") and therefore requires expenditure of energy. Calcium entry from the extracellular space triggered by membrane depolarization (cardiac action potential) occurs primarily as the so-called "slow current" through the voltage-sensitive Ca^{++} channels. These channels are also referred to as dihydropyridine receptors because of their high affinity for this class of Ca^{++}-channel drugs (e.g., nifedipine). Cellular extrusion of Ca^{++} across the plasma membrane is done primarily by two Ca^{++}-transporting proteins. The first is a Ca^{++}-ATPase, which as its name implies, consumes energy in the form of ATP to extrude Ca^{++}. The second is a Na^+ / Ca^{++} exchanger, which uses the energy of the large extracellular-to-intracellular Na^+ gradient to extrude Ca^{++} in exchange for cellular Na^+ entry. The Ca^{++}-ATPase has a low capacity for Ca^{++} transport but a high affinity for this cation. By contrast, the Na^+ / Ca^{++} exchanger has a lower affinity for Ca^{++} but a much greater capacity than the Ca^{++}-ATPase for Ca^{++} extrusion from the cell. Calcium release from the SR occurs through a calcium channel or "foot" protein within the SR. This channel is often referred to as the ryanodine receptor because of its high affinity for binding this plant alkaloid. Calcium reuptake into the SR is done by a Ca^{++}-ATPase that is structurally different from the one in the plasma membrane.

Quantitatively, most of the Ca^{++} responsible for the increment of cytosolic $[Ca^{++}]$ and its subsequent decrease comes from and returns to the SR.

---

110   Summarize the most important characteristics of each of the major systems that modulate Ca^{++} homeostasis in myocardial cell membranes.

□ The "slow Ca^{++} channel" is a voltage-sensitive protein that transports Ca^{++} producing the slow inward Ca^{++} current during phase 2 of the cardiac action potential. It provides the pulse of intracellular Ca^{++} that triggers the release of a much larger amount of Ca^{++} from intracellular stores contained in the SR. The "Ca^{++}-release channel" of the SR is responsible for most of the Ca^{++} that activates the myofilaments for contraction in systole. The "fast Na^+ channel," a voltage-sensitive channel like the "slow Ca^{++} channel," is responsible for the upstroke of the cardiac action potential. The depolarization caused by activation of the "fast Na^+ channel" in turn triggers activation of the "slow Ca^{++} channel." A "nonspecific cation channel" that is activated by intracellular Ca^{++} produces depolarizing inward currents that account for the arrhythmias observed with toxic doses of cardiac glycosides (digitalis preparations). The "Na^+/Ca^{++} exchanger" located in the cell membrane mediates the facilitated (secondary active transport) bidirectional exchange of Na^+ for Ca^{++} across the sarcolemma. This exchange process is sensitive to the membrane potential because the charge movement across the sarcolemma is asymmetric (i.e., three Na^+ exchanged for one Ca^{++}). The "Na^+ pump" or Na^+,K^+-ATPase of the cell membrane mediates the active transport of Na^+ (out of the cell) and K^+ (into the cell) against their respective concentration gradients. The outward-facing surface of the α subunit of this enzyme is the binding site for cardiac glycosides. The "Na^+/H^+ exchanger" is an amiloride-sensitive protein that mediates the electroneutral exchange of Na^+ for H^+ and facilitates accumulation of intracellular Na^+ (and consequently accumulation of intracellular Ca^{++}). The "sarcolemmal Ca^{++} pump" is a low-capacity but high-affinity ATP-dependent protein that extrudes cellular Ca^{++} against a large electrochemical gradient and helps to maintain the low intracellular

intracellular [Ca^{++}] observed in diastole. The "ATP-dependent Ca^{++} pump" of the SR is responsible for myocardial relaxation in diastole by rapid sequestration of Ca^{++} at the end of systole.

---

111 Recapitulate the linkage among excitation, contraction, and relaxation of the myocardium.

☐ The cardiac cell membrane (also known as sarcolemma) is an effective barrier between the ECF and ICF, the latter bathing the contractile proteins. On excitation, the sarcolemma depolarizes (i.e., the cytosol becomes less electronegative) and extracellular Ca^{++} moves into the cytosol through specific Ca^{++} channels known as "slow" or "L-type" channels. This initial Ca^{++} current triggers the release of a larger quantity of Ca^{++} from the SR a tubular network that surrounds the myofilaments and comprises an important intracellular Ca^{++} store. The increase in cytosolic [Ca^{++}] causes a conformation change in inhibitory proteins (troponin C) located on the thin filaments (actin). Myocardial contraction occurs on detachment of troponin C, allowing cross-bridge cycling. At the end of systole, cytosolic [Ca^{++}] decreases, allowing for myocardial relaxation to occur. Calcium removal from the cytosol during relaxation is mainly due to reuptake into the SR (by Ca^{++}-ATPase pumps located in their membranes) and, additionally, to extrusion into the ECF across the sarcolemma by Ca^{++}-ATPase pumps and by Na^+ / Ca^{++} exchange. Transport proteins in the membrane of the SR and those in the sarcolemma help to maintain a concentration gradient of 10,000:1 between the ECF and the cytosolic [Ca^{++}] (10^{-3} M and 10^{-7} M, respectively).

---

112 What cellular messengers regulate function of contractile proteins?

☐ The force generated with each cardiac contraction is directly dependent on the quantity of Ca^{++} that is bound to troponin (its complete name is troponin C). Changes in cyclic AMP (e.g., due to activation or suppression of β-adrenergic receptors) as well as other substances/drugs can also modify the activity of protein kinases. These protein kinases phosphorylate (causing activation) one or more of the various contractile proteins, regulating their function. In addition, structural changes within the contractile proteins can modify their action in physiologic and pathologic states.

---

113   Is myocardial relaxation an active process that consumes cellular energy?

☐ Yes. The level of free or ionized cytosolic Ca^{++} that surrounds the myofilaments is the key determinant of both myocardial contraction and relaxation. A rapid rise in intracellular $[Ca^{++}]$ from 10^{-7} to 10^{-5} mol/L causes a conformation change in the regulatory proteins (i.e., troponin C) of the myofilaments. In the presence of ATP, this conformation change allows the cross-bridges between actin (thin filaments) and myosin (thick filaments) to dissipate and re-form, causing the filaments to slide over one another, leading to contraction. Myocardial relaxation, by contrast, is controlled by mechanisms that decrease intracellular $[Ca^{++}]$ to its normal value (10^{-7} mol / L). The retrieval of Ca^{++} into storage sites that promotes myocardial relaxation is largely due to active pumping of this ion into the SR by a Ca^{++}-transporting ATPase. Consequently, both myocardial contraction and relaxation are active processes that require energy (i.e., availability of ATP) and are critically dependent on precisely timed modulations of the intracellular $[Ca^{++}]$.

---

114   What determines the total tension and the rate of tension development by the contractile proteins?

☐ The quantity of Ca^{++} available for binding to troponin modulates the total tension developed by the contractile units while the rate of Ca^{++} delivery to troponin controls the rate of tension development. In addition, an increase in muscle length augments the sensitivity of the myofilaments to Ca^{++} and might also enhance the release of Ca^{++} by the SR. However, an increase in muscle length does not change or might actually decrease the cellular entry of Ca^{++}. The rate of tension decline during relaxation is modulated by the rate at which Ca^{++} is removed from troponin. The critical importance of Ca^{++} kinetics in the control of the inotropic state of the heart is also evident in disease states in which an alteration in the Ca^{++} fluxes or cytosolic $[Ca^{++}]$ leads to an augmented or depressed contractile state of the heart (e.g., severe hypocalcemia depresses myocardial contractility that is repaired with Ca^{++} infusions).

115　What changes in myocardial cells explain the more forceful than normal cardiac contraction that might follow a premature beat?

□　Changes in Ca^{++} kinetics are responsible for the augmented myocardial contractility observed with a shortened time interval between two cardiac contractions (the so-called postextrasystolic potentiation) as well as with some pharmacologic agents and disease states. The shortened time interval between contractions might be either limited to a "premature" or early contraction or generalized as in the case of tachycardia. Postextrasystolic potentiation describes the more forceful than normal contraction that immediately follows a premature depolarization of cardiac muscle. Although a premature depolarization produces a contraction of less than normal force, the ensuing depolarization produces a more forceful contraction. The different force of contraction of the two consecutive beats is due to differences in the quantity of Ca^{++} released from internal stores in response to each depolarization. The much larger amount of Ca^{++} released during the postextrasystolic beat produces a more forceful contraction. The greater contractility of the postextrasystolic beat is also associated with a longer diastolic filling period (i.e., increased preload), which further augments stroke volume in accordance with Starling's law.

116　What is the common pathway for the cardiac inotropic effects (positive or negative) of digitalis, β-adrenergic agents, and acidemia?

□　Changes in myocyte cytosolic $[Ca^{++}]$ influence the total tension developed by the contracting cell, the rate at which the tension is developed, and the rate of tension decline during myocardial relaxation. Furthermore, these functions are determined by the quantity of Ca^{++} available for binding to troponin, the rate at which Ca^{++} is delivered to this regulatory protein, and the rate at which Ca^{++} is removed from troponin (the removal of Ca^{++} from troponin allows this protein to inhibit the contractile process). Consequently, pharmacologic interventions and some clinical conditions alter cardiac contractility as a result of changes in $[Ca^{++}]$, including therapy with cardiac glycosides, β-adrenergic receptor stimulation or blockade, and acidemia. Cardiac glycosides increase cytosolic $[Na^+]$ by inhibiting Na^+, K^+-ATPase. The increased cytosolic $[Na^+]$ decreases the gradient for cellular Na^+ entry leading to inhibition of Ca^{++} extrusion by the Na^+ / Ca^{++} exchanger. The resulting increase in cellular $[Ca^{++}]$ increases myocardial contractility. β-adrenergic receptor stimulation increases cellular cyclic AMP, which augments cytosolic Ca^{++} entry through voltage-dependent channels; inhibition of these receptors has the opposite effect. Acidemia (decreased blood pH) of even moderate severity diminishes the amount of Ca^{++} released from SR, thereby reducing myocardial contractility. The mild stimulation of myocardial contractility that might be observed in acidemic states is due to the associated sympathetic activation.

---

117   How do acid-base disturbances and dysfunction of the thyroid gland modify cardiac contractility?

☐ Acidemia decreases and alkalemia increases myocardial contractility and these effects are partly accounted for by changes in Ca^{++} kinetics. Acidemia (decreased blood pH) decreases the quantity of Ca^{++} released from the SR and decreases Ca^{++} binding by troponin, whereas alkalemia (increased blood pH) has the opposite effects. Although acidemia has also been reported to increase myocardial contractility, this effect is likely due to the associated sympathetic overactivity (activation of $\alpha-$ and β_1-adrenoreceptors in the heart). Hypothyroidism decreases cardiac contractility and this effect is due to a slower release and uptake of Ca^{++} as well as the synthesis of slower myosin isoenzymes. Conversely, hyperthyroidism increases cardiac contractility and the underlying mechanisms involve changes comparable to those described for hypothyroidism but having the opposite direction.

118 Briefly describe how an extracellular signal causes an intracellular response that might alter the function of tissues and organs including the heart.

□ Many substances including hormones, neurotransmitters, and pharmacologic agents can influence the function of cells in tissues and organs including the heart without entering the cell interior. The hormones and neurotransmitters (known as first messengers), as well as drugs, can bind with molecules on the cell surface called receptors. The cell membrane receptors will bind some but not all messenger substances demonstrating specificity for a given first messenger, drug, or a class of pharmacologic agents. Binding of the first messenger or pharmacologic agent to the cell membrane receptor generates a "second messenger" (such as cyclic AMP, among others) by the interaction of the receptor with a coupling protein. These coupling proteins are often bound to the cell membrane. It is the second messenger that transmits the signal to appropriate cell organelles/enzymes to promote a change in cell function. The cascade of events initiated by an extracellular message that promotes a change in cell function is known as signal transduction.

119 What are G proteins and how do they relate to cellular signal transduction?

□ G proteins, also known as GTP-binding proteins, are coupling proteins distributed among a wide variety of body tissues including the myocardium. Their name derives from their unique properties to bind guanine nucleotides (i.e., GTP or guanine triphosphate), substances that play a critical role in modulation of cell function. The G proteins can have either stimulatory or inhibitory effects on the cellular level of the second messenger, and these properties account for their name as G_s (stimulatory) and G_i (inhibitory) proteins, respectively. G_s stimulates and G_i inhibits the catalytic unit of cellular adenylate cyclase, the enzyme that promotes the formation of cyclic AMP from $ATP\text{-}Mg^{++}$. The G proteins are a most important family of coupling proteins associated with a wide variety of cellular functions and serve diverse roles in signal transduction.

120 Explain the intrinsic and extrinsic regulation of myocardial performance.

☐ The heart maintains adequate perfusion of noncardiac tissues by mechanisms that are inherent to the cardiac muscle (intrinsic regulation) and by mechanisms that do not pertain to the myocardium (extrinsic regulation involving neurohormonal mechanisms). Examples of intrinsic regulation of myocardial performance include the Frank-Starling relationship, frequency-induced modulation of myocardial contractility, and postextrasystolic potentiation of cardiac contraction. The Frank-Starling relationship predicts that an increase in myocardial fiber length preceding contraction (such as with an increase in ventricular end-diastolic volume) augments the force of the subsequent contraction. Frequency-induced modulation describes the increasing force of contraction observed with decreasing intervals between cardiac systoles (i.e., increasing heart rate). Postextrasystolic potentiation describes an augmentation of the force of contraction that follows a premature ventricular contraction. Because the latter produces a low stroke volume, the following more forceful postextrasystolic beat helps to secure an effective emptying of the cardiac chamber. Examples of extrinsic regulation of myocardial performance include nervous and hormonal mechanisms. Sympathetic nerve stimulation increases atrial and ventricular contractility. Parasympathetic stimulation has inhibitory effects on firing rate of the cardiac pacemaker, conduction of AV node, and contractility of atrial and ventricular myocardium. The most important humoral factors involved in extrinsic regulation of heart function are the catecholamines, but thyroid hormones and insulin might also augment myocardial contractility. Catecholamines and thyroid hormones increase heart rate (chronotropic effect) in addition to their inotropic action.

121 What are the major areas/centers within the central nervous system (CNS) that control the circulation (heart and peripheral vessels)?

☐ CNS control of the heart and caliber of blood vessels is largely performed by an area known as the vasomotor center that comprises the following three major pools of neurons: (1) the cardiovascular excitatory center (also called pressor area or vasoconstrictor area), bilaterally located in the anterolateral area of the upper portion of the medulla, whose neurons modulate the activity of other nerve cells distributed throughout the spinal cord and transmit excitatory influences responsible for the vasoconstrictor effects of stimulation of the sympathetic nervous system; (2) the cardiovascular inhibitory center (also called depressor area or vasodilator area), bilaterally located in the anterolateral area of the lower portion of the medulla, whose neurons have nerve endings that directly inhibit those of the cardiovascular excitatory center causing vasodilation; and (3) a "sensory area" that receives afferent signals from the vagus and glossopharyngeal nerves and is bilaterally located in the posterolateral area of the lower pons and medulla, in close contact with the pressor and depressor areas. The neurons of this sensory area, also referred to as tractus solitarius, participate in cardiovascular reflexes, baroreceptor function, and control of arterial pressure. This "sensory area" of the vasomotor center is also in close proximity with the dorsal motor nucleus of the vagus nerve. The control of heart function by the vasomotor center includes: (1) stimulatory influences originated in the lateral portion of this center, which are transmitted through sympathetic pathways; and (2) inhibitory influences originated in the medial portion of this center (these neurons are in close contact with the dorsal motor nucleus of the vagus nerve), which are transmitted through parasympathetic pathways.

---

122 What are the main nervous influences or systems that participate in the control of cardiac function?

☐ The nervous control of cardiac function involves the sympathetic and parasympathetic systems. Sympathetic nerve endings (which synthesize and release norepinephrine) reach the entire atria and ventricles as well as the SA and AV nodes. Parasympathetic nerve endings (which synthesize and release acetylcholine) arising from the vagal nerves (tenth cranial nerve) predominantly innervate the atrial musculature and SA and AV nodes. Parasympathetic nerve endings also reach the ventricles where, on activation, they modestly decrease contractility.

---

123   Further characterize the nervous influences on cardiac function.

□ In general, the effects of sympathetic stimulation are opposite to those observed with parasympathetic stimulation. Activation of the sympathetic nervous system augments heart rate, increases atrial and ventricular contractility, and speeds excitation through the AV node and to a lesser degree, through the ventricles. Vagal parasympathetic stimulation slows the intrinsic rate of the sinus node (normal cardiac pacemaker) in the resting state to about 70 beats/min or further in response to exercise training (resting bradycardia of athletes). The nervous influences or systems that control cardiac function participate as major pathways of responses that originate in the carotid sinus and aortic stretch receptors (carotid and aortic baroreceptors, respectively). When stretching of carotid sinus decreases (such as with arterial hypotension), a reflex response occurs, which elicits sympathetic stimulation that augments the following: atrial and ventricular contractility, venous return (due to venoconstriction), and peripheral vascular resistance. Consequently, arterial pressure rises toward its normal level. By contrast, increased stretch of the carotid sinus as might occur with arterial hypertension produces effects that are opposite to those described for decreased stretch of the carotid sinus.

---

124   Describe the main autonomic (sympathetic and parasympathetic) centers involved in the control of heart function.

□ The sympathetic and parasympathetic systems have two types of neurons, known as preganglionic and postganglionic neurons. The cell body of preganglionic neurons that control heart function are located in the intermediolateral columns of the upper 5 to 6 thoracic and lower 1 to 2 cervical segments of the spinal cord. The preganglionic sympathetic fibers that exit from these neurons synapse largely with postganglionic neurons located in the stellate and middle cervical ganglia (components of the two paravertebral sympathetic chains of ganglia). The preganglionic parasympathetic fibers originate in the medulla oblongata (dorsal motor nucleus of the vagus nerve) and synapse with postganglionic cells located on the epicardial surface or within the walls of the heart itself.

---

125 Delineate the afferent pathways of the neural control of cardiac function.

□ Sensory receptors located in the heart and peripheral vessels collect information sent through afferent pathways that include the vagus nerve (supraspinal reflex arc) and the posterior roots of spinal nerves (spinal reflex arc). The corresponding afferent pathways that originate in the carotid sinus (baroreceptors and chemoreceptors) travel toward the brain through the IX nerve. The first synapse for the afferent pathway in the supraspinal arc is at the nucleus tractus solitarius (NTS) located in the medulla ("sensory area" of the vasomotor center). This area is close to the dorsal motor nucleus of the vagus and the "pressor" and "depressor" areas of the vasomotor center. Higher centers located in the forebrain including the hypothalamus, thalamus, and cortex receive information through the fasciculus of tractus solitarius (that departs in the NTS, which represents the "sensory area" of the vasomotor center).

---

126 Outline the efferent pathways of the neural control of cardiovascular function.

□ The efferent pathways that mediate the neural control of cardiovascular function include the sympathetic and parasympathetic systems. The outflow of the two components of the autonomic nervous system is modulated by major influences originating in the forebrain, especially the hypothalamus. The sympathetic efferent pathways start on neurons located in the medulla (below the NTS) and the thoracic spinal cord (intermediolateral column) that send axons or preganglionic sympathetic efferent fibers to the corresponding sympathetic ganglia located throughout the body (two paravertebral sympathetic chains of ganglia, as well as the two prevertebral ganglia named celiac and hypogastric plexus) and the adrenal glands. The postganglionic sympathetic efferent fibers reach the heart and arteries and veins throughout the body. The parasympathetic efferent pathways start on neurons located in the medulla including the dorsal motor nucleus of the vagus, the external cuneate nucleus, the midline raphe nuclei, and neurons located between the NTS and nucleus ambiguous. All these neurons represent preganglionic parasympathetic nerve cells that, through one or more intermediate synapses at a variety of sites (this concept also applies to the corresponding sympathetic outflow pathways), reach the parasympathetic ganglia throughout the body. The axons of neurons located in these ganglia innervate the various components of the circulatory system.

---

127 Elaborate further on the neural modulation of cardiac function by the various areas of the CNS.

☐ The cardiovascular centers located in the brain medulla, operating independently of higher structures, are capable of regulating heart rate and contractility, arterial blood pressure, and regional blood flow distribution. Yet, the activity of medullary centers is modulated under normal conditions by higher centers including the cerebral cortex, the hypothalamus, and the reticular substance in the mesencephalon/pons. The medullary cardiovascular-excitatory center displays tonic activity (vasomotor tone) that is constantly inhibited by afferent impulses from the cardiovascular mechanoreceptors (carotid sinus and aortic high-pressure receptors, and the low-pressure receptors located in the atria, ventricles, and pulmonary vessels). If the traffic of afferent impulses that arise from the cardiovascular mechanoreceptors is higher than normal, a reflex increase in efferent vagal discharges as well as a decrease in efferent sympathetic tone develop. Consequently, depression of the vasomotor tone acting on resistance and capacitance vessels as well as on the heart produces a lower blood pressure, diminished venous return, reduced cardiac output, and bradycardia. Conversely, a lower than normal traffic of afferent impulses from cardiovascular mechanoreceptors produces augmentation of vasomotor tone and therefore opposite effects including tachycardia, increased cardiac output, and systemic vasoconstriction. A similar response might be observed with emotional stress, wakefulness, mental and muscular effort, and stress, due to effects of these stimuli acting on the medullary vasomotor center. The latter center also receives input from receptors located in the special senses, viscera, skeletal muscle, and skin, and their interaction with the vasomotor center allows for further adjustments of the circulatory system to metabolic demands of tissues.

---

128 How do autonomic pathways control heart rate?

☐ The heart rate is controlled by the combined influence of the sympathetic and parasympathetic divisions of the autonomic nervous system through their nerve endings on the main cardiac pacemaker, the SA node. Sympathetic stimulation increases the heart rate, whereas parasympathetic stimulation decreases it. Changes in the heart rate usually involve reciprocal actions of these two divisions of the autonomic nervous system. For example, an increased heart rate is usually due to a combination of augmented sympathetic activity and decreased parasympathetic activity. A decreased heart rate is usually achieved by opposite processes. Complete suppression of parasympathetic influences increases heart rate substantially, whereas removal of all sympathetic influences decreases heart rate only slightly. When both divisions of the autonomic nervous system are blocked or abolished, heart rate of adults increases from a normal resting value of 70 beats/min to about 100 beats/min, the latter commonly referred to as the intrinsic heart rate. Consequently, parasympathetic tone ordinarily prevails in healthy individuals at rest.

---

129 What "higher" centers of the CNS might modify heart rate?

☐ The thalamus, hypothalamus, and cerebral cortex might alter the frequency of cardiac contractions (heart rate). Stimulation of the thalamus might induce tachycardia (e.g., response to somatic pain). Changes in temperature of blood perfusing the hypothalamus alters both heart rate and peripheral resistance. The cardiac reactions to excitement, anxiety, and other emotional states are initiated in multiple brain centers including cortical areas in the frontal lobe, orbital cortex, premotor and motor cortex, anterior part of the temporal lobe, insula, and cingulate gyrus.

---

130 What are the consequences of stimulation and inhibition of carotid and aortic baroreceptors on heart rate?

☐ Stimulation of arterial or high-pressure baroreceptors located in the carotid sinus (at the bifurcation of the primary carotid into its internal and external branches) and aortic arch due to stretching of the vessel wall (e.g., hypertension, external massage of the carotid sinus) decreases heart rate as well as cardiac output and blood pressure. Inhibition of arterial baroreceptors due to a reduction of vessel wall tension (e.g., hypotension) increases heart rate as well as cardiac output and blood pressure. The baroreceptor nerve terminals in the vessel walls increase their firing with greater stretching of the vessel wall while reduced stretching causes decreased firing. The decreased heart rate elicited by stimulation of baroreceptors is due to a combination of decreased sympathetic and increased parasympathetic activity. Conversely, the increased heart rate elicited by inhibition of baroreceptors is due to changes in the activity of the two components of the autonomic nervous system that are opposite to those described for baroreceptor stimulation. It should be apparent that the function of baroreceptors (through changes in cardiac output and vascular resistance) is of critical importance in the maintenance of normal blood pressure because they continuously monitor this cardiovascular function and promote circulatory responses that return blood pressure toward the normal level.

---

131 Describe the effects of arterial chemoreceptors on heart rate.

☐ The response of heart rate to stimulation (e.g., hypoxemia) of arterial chemoreceptors (carotid and aortic) is a combination of primary and secondary effects. The primary effect of carotid chemoreceptor stimulation on the SA node is inhibitory and leads to slowing of the heart rate (bradycardia). This response can be demonstrated if pulmonary ventilation is inhibited as occurs when diving under water (protective mechanism that prevents water entry into the lungs) in human beings and other animals (ducks, crocodiles). On the other hand, if ventilation is not inhibited, activation of chemoreceptors elicits secondary effects leading to increased pulmonary ventilation as well as increased heart rate. The complete (primary and secondary effects) cardiovascular and pulmonary response to hypoxia mediated by arterial chemoreceptors is aimed at achieving optimal pulmonary oxygen uptake by stimulating ventilation and circulation. Hypoxia that occurs when the animal or human being is under water triggers reflex mechanisms by the chemoreceptors that are aimed at reducing tissue oxygen demand (reduction of heart rate and cardiac output) because in this circumstance oxygen uptake by the lungs cannot be sustained (i.e., respiratory arrest is present). The chemoreceptor-induced changes in heart rate are generally accompanied by parallel changes in cardiac output.

---

132   What is the Bainbridge reflex?

☐ The Bainbridge reflex is the change in heart rate that occurs in response to stimulation of atrial stretch receptors induced by changes in atrial volume. Distention of the atria elicits an increased heart rate as well as stronger atrial contractions. This response promotes the forward movement of blood and prevents venous pooling in the systemic and pulmonary circulations (i.e., in the right and left atria, respectively). The afferent pathway (from stretch receptors of the atria to the brain) travels in the vagus nerve(s) to the brain medulla and the efferent pathway (from the brain to the heart) is routed through both the vagal and sympathetic nerves. It should be apparent that the main task of the Bainbridge reflex is to promote the forward movement of blood but not the control of blood pressure. The latter is the main task of the arterial baroreceptors.

---

133   Describe reflexes arising from ventricular receptors.

☐ Cardiac depression might arise from activation of reflexes initiated by sensory receptors located near the endocardial surfaces of ventricular walls. These receptors respond to stretching of the ventricles in a fashion similar to that of the arterial baroreceptors described previously. Increases in ventricular pressure stimulate receptor firing rate and lead to a decreased heart rate. The pathways involved in this reflex are the parasympathetic and sympathetic nervous systems as described for the arterial baroreceptors. Bradycardia (decreased heart rate) elicited by this reflex represents a self-preservation mechanism for the myocardium that allows for reduced oxygen consumption (heart rate is a major determinant of myocardial oxygen consumption) in states of exceedingly high work load demand. It must be recognized that increased preload and afterload generally lead to increased oxygen consumption by the ventricles due to the increased ventricular work load. Activation of ventricular receptor reflexes might prevent exhaustion of the ventricles when the imposed work load is overwhelming, but occasionally leads to cardiac syncope (i.e., circulatory arrest).

134   What types of adrenergic receptors regulate heart function?

☐ The heart contains α- and β-adrenergic receptors that play a major role in the control of cardiac function. β-adrenergic receptors are of two subtypes, β_1 and β_2. Stimulation of α receptors activates phospholipase C (but has no effects on cyclic AMP levels) and starts a chain reaction that induces Ca^{++} release from the SR that leads to increased myocardial contractility. On the other hand, β receptor agonists increase intracellular cyclic AMP, which is thought to mediate the cardiac stimulation observed with these compounds.

135   Further characterize the α- and β-adrenergic receptors in the heart.

☐ The inotropic effects of β-agonists are mediated by activation of the β_1 subtype receptors located on effector cells near adrenergic neural synapses. This characteristic location is important because β_1 receptors respond primarily to norepinephrine released by neurons. β_1 receptors are the exclusive β subtype present in the cardiac ventricles and account for the majority of β receptors present in the heart. β_2 receptors, which mediate relaxation of vascular and bronchial smooth muscle, account for about 25% of atrial receptors. The atrial receptors are located within the SA node and presumably mediate the chronotropic (increased heart rate) effects of catecholamines. In addition, β_2 receptors are located far from the adrenergic synapses (in contrast to the proximity of β_1 receptors) and respond preferentially to circulating epinephrine secreted by the adrenal medulla (inner portion of the adrenal gland). α-adrenergic receptors (most likely α_1 subtype) located in the heart respond to circulating catecholamines. Activation of those α receptors located in the presynaptic membrane inhibits the release of norepinephrine, whereas activation of presynaptic β receptors stimulates the release of norepinephrine.

---

136 Describe the origin and final disposal of norepinephrine present in the heart.

□ Norepinephrine present in the heart is synthesized, stored, and eventually released in the sympathetic nerve endings. These nerve endings are interposed between muscle bundles forming a perimuscular or perimysial plexus that is in close contact with the myocardial cells. The sympathetic endings contain neurosecretory granules that migrate to the cell membrane of neural axons for their discharge, in response to an increase in axonal cytosolic $[Ca^{++}]$ triggered by depolarization of the neuron. The final disposal of released norepinephrine occurs by: (1) reuptake by the neurons (about 75% of total) into neurosecretory granules, and thereafter it becomes available for subsequent release; (2) reuptake by the neurons and local degradation of norepinephrine by monoamine oxidase (MAO); and (3) escape of norepinephrine into the circulation followed by peripheral degradation by the action of MAO and catechol-O-methyltransferase (COMT).

---

137 What are the major elements of the β-adrenergic signaling system in the heart?

□ Sympathomimetic amines (e.g., the catecholamines epinephrine and norepinephrine) interact with β receptors on the cell membrane of cardiac myocytes (cardiocytes). This interaction activates adenylate cyclase that catalyzes the production of cyclic AMP from ATP in the presence of Ca^{++}. The activity of adenylate cyclase is modulated by G proteins, characterized by their guanine nucleotide-binding properties, that can have either stimulatory (G_s proteins) or inhibitory (G_i proteins) effects on this enzyme. Adenylate cyclase in the presence of G_s proteins converts ATP to cyclic AMP. The latter acting via a protein kinase enhances phosphorylation of the cell membrane Ca^{++} channel allowing for a greater cellular entry of Ca^{++}. The effects of G_s and G_i are mediated by stimulation and suppression, respectively, of the catalytic unit of adenylate cyclase that promotes the formation of cyclic AMP from $ATP-Mg^{++}$.

---

138   Does sympathetic stimulation alter ventricular relaxation in diastole?

☐ Yes. Sympathetic stimulation causes more rapid relaxation of the ventricular muscle in diastole in addition to producing a more forceful and faster contraction (systole). The faster diastolic relaxation augments rapid ventricular filling and lowers diastolic pressure, allowing a larger ventricular diastolic volume. The combination of a more vigorous relaxation and contraction increases stroke volume. The term diastolic suction describes increased ventricular filling due to enhanced ventricular relaxation. Negative diastolic pressures during ventricular filling have been documented within the left ventricle in early diastole during strenuous exercise and after clamping of the ventricle during rapid filling. Thus, suction in the full meaning of the term occurs during ventricular diastole, and it is stimulated by sympathetic activation.

---

139   What drugs or conditions lead to increased responsiveness to norepinephrine by the cardiovascular system and other organs?

☐ The administration of cocaine (all uses but especially illicit or recreational use) and of tricyclic antidepressants, as well as surgical denervation, inhibit the neuronal uptake of norepinephrine. This phenomenon makes a larger quantity of norepinephrine available at the receptor sites, augmenting the response to this neurotransmitter. In addition, hyperresponsiveness to circulating catecholamines may be observed.

Consequently, the use of these drugs might produce manifestations of intense sympathetic activation (e.g., tachycardia, hypertension, tissue ischemia).

---

140   Delineate the cascade for cell signal transduction of α- and β-adrenergic agonists.

☐ Adrenergic agents interact with two general classes of receptors on the cell surface called α and β receptors. Stimulation of the α-adrenergic receptor causes G protein-mediated activation of phospholipase C, an enzyme that hydrolyses phosphatidylinositol-4,5-bisphosphate (PIP_2) to yield inositol-1,4,5-triphosphate (IP_3) and diacylglycerol (DAG). IP_3 releases Ca^{++} from intracellular stores, whereas DAG activates plasma membrane Ca^{++} channels to allow for Ca^{++} influx. β-Adrenergic stimulation causes G protein-mediated activation of adenylate cyclase to form cyclic AMP as well as direct activation of plasma membrane Ca^{++} channels to cause cellular Ca^{++} influx. Stimulation of the α and β receptors generally increases cardiac contractility due to increased cytosolic $[Ca^{++}]$ in myocardial cells. The β-adrenergic agonists have a more prominent effect on heart function than do α-adrenergic agonists whose most important cardiovascular effect is on the vascular smooth muscle to cause vasoconstriction.

---

141   Outline the two main classes of receptors that mediate the pharmacologic effects of acetylcholine (cholinergic receptors).

☐ The two main classes of cholinergic receptors are the muscarinic and the nicotinic receptors. The names given to the cholinergic receptors derive from their specific response to plant alkaloids obtained from either *Amanita muscaria* (muscarinic) and *Nicotiana tabacum* (nicotinic). The muscarinic receptors belong to the class of G protein-coupled receptors; the nicotinic receptors are ligand-gated ion channels. The response of muscarinic receptors might be either excitatory or inhibitory and is relatively slow. By contrast, the response of the nicotinic receptors is fast and always leads to excitation caused by an increase in ion permeability that leads to membrane depolarization. The tissue distribution of each of these receptors differs because the heart, smooth muscle, and secretory glands contain muscarinic receptors, whereas the neuromuscular junction, autonomic ganglia, adrenal medulla, and central nervous system contain nicotinic receptors.

---

142   Describe the cascade for cell signal transduction of acetylcholine.

☐ Acetylcholine binds to muscarinic receptors on the cell membrane, which causes a G protein-mediated activation of plasma membrane K^+ channels as well as inhibition of adenylate cyclase. Activation of cell membrane K^+ channels increases the rate of K^+ exit causing hyperpolarization of the membrane potential and slowing of pacemaker activity. An inhibitory G protein mediated effect also decreases cellular entry of Na^+ and Ca^{++} contributing to cell membrane hyperpolarization and to the decrease in pacemaker activity. Inhibition of adenylate cyclase activity decreases cellular cyclic AMP concentration, which further reduces cellular Na^+ and Ca^{++} entry. Stimulation as well as inhibition of muscarinic receptors in the heart alter spontaneous depolarization, conduction velocity, and contractile force of cardiac tissue as described in greater detail in the answer to the next question.

---

143   What is the cardiac response to stimulation of cholinergic receptors?

☐ Cholinergic receptors modulate heart function at the SA node, atrium, AV node, and ventricle. Stimulation of cholinergic receptors located at each of these regions of the heart produces the following responses: (1) on the SA node, a decreased pacemaker activity, slowing spontaneous depolarization and producing hyperpolarization of the cell membrane; (2) on the atrium, decreased contractility and shortened duration of the action potential; (3) on the AV node, a partial or complete blockade of impulse conduction between atria and ventricles because of a decreased conduction velocity in this tissue; and (4) on the ventricle, a slight decrease in contractility. The pharmacologic inhibition of cholinergic heart receptors produces responses that are opposite to those described above.

144 Outline the cascade for cell signal transduction of angiotensin II within the heart.

☐ Angiotensin II interaction with its receptor activates phospholipase C, which hydrolyses PIP_2 to IP_3 and DAG as described for the α-adrenergic agonists (see question 140). Intracellular $[Ca^{++}]$ is increased by a combination of IP_3-induced release of Ca^{++} from intracellular stores and by stimulation of Ca^{++} influx through plasma membrane Ca^{++} channels mediated by DAG. The effect of angiotensin II on the heart is similar to that of α-adrenergic agonists (causing a mild increase in contractility). The most important cardiovascular effect of angiotensin II occurs in the vasculature causing arteriolar constriction (resembling α-adrenergic stimulation).

145 What are the major regulatory influences on glycolysis of myocardial cells?

☐ The major regulatory influences on myocardial glycolysis are: (1) the cardiac stores of ATP or coenzymes of the oxidative energy-producing pathway; and (2) neurohormonal influences. Low ATP levels stimulate glycolysis; high cellular ATP stores inhibit it. This influence is exerted through phosphofructokinase, a key glycolytic enzyme. The level of reduced nicotinamide adenine dinucleotide (NADH), coenzyme of the oxidative energy-producing pathway, exerts a major effect on glycolysis. Under anaerobic conditions, the myocardial cell becomes less able to oxidize NADH to NAD^+, the latter being essential for the action of the glycolytic enzyme glyceraldehyde-3-phosphate dehydrogenase. Thus, NADH levels increase, causing inhibition of this enzyme and thereby depression of glycolysis. The neurohormonal influences include the blood and tissue levels of catecholamines (epinephrine and norepinephrine), which increase energy utilization by the heart while simultaneously promoting the breakdown of hepatic glycogen to glucose. Therefore, catecholamines simultaneously increase myocardial work and provide additional substrate for energy production. In summary, influences arising from both inside and outside the heart modulate glycolysis in myocardial cells.

146 Explain the respective roles of oxidative phosphorylation and glycolysis in providing energy for cardiac function.

☐ Oxidative phosphorylation provides most of the energy for normal cardiac function. The role of glycolysis under normal circumstances is quantitatively small. During hypoxia or ischemia, however, aerobic metabolism (oxidative phosphorylation) does not occur and glycolysis becomes the exclusive energy source. Under these circumstances the rate of glycolysis is substantially increased. Both processes produce ATP, which is hydrolyzed to yield energy for use by the myocardial cell. Aerobic metabolism (oxidative phosphorylation) is much more efficient than the anaerobic process (glycolysis), producing more ATP molecules for each glucose molecule used by the myocardium.

PATHOPHYSIOLOGY OF HEART FAILURE

---

147   What is heart failure?

☐ Heart failure is the condition in which, in the presence of adequate venous return, a cardiac abnormality makes this organ unable to pump blood at a rate that satisfies the metabolic needs of tissues. Heart failure is also present if adequate rate of blood pumping can be accomplished only with abnormally elevated filling pressure. It is also called cardiac failure.

---

148   Do the terms heart failure and circulatory failure describe the same process?

☐ No. Circulatory failure describes a broader concept because it refers to inability of the cardiovascular system to perform its basic function to provide nutrition to and remove wastes from tissues. An abnormality in any component of the circulatory system including the heart (heart failure), vessels (decreased venous return, vasodilation), and blood (decreased blood volume) might produce circulatory failure. Other conditions such as oxygen deprivation might also cause this syndrome.

---

149   Contrast the conceptual meaning of circulatory failure, heart failure, and myocardial failure.

☐ Circulatory failure denotes an abnormal blood flow through the cardiovascular circuitry that compromises tissue function with or without abnormal heart function. Examples of circulatory failure in which heart function might be normal include volume overload and tissue congestion due to renal failure, sepsis-induced vasodilation, and polycythemia-induced hyperviscosity, all causing reduced tissue perfusion. Heart failure refers to abnormal cardiac pumping of blood with or without an abnormal heart muscle (i.e., presence or absence of myocardial failure). An example of heart failure without myocardial failure is valvular heart disease. Myocardial failure denotes abnormal cardiac pumping of blood due to a defective heart muscle. It should be apparent that myocardial failure is a subset of heart failure, which is in turn a subset of circulatory failure. Furthermore, some patients have only one of these abnormalities at a given time or, on the contrary, might have all of them. Circulatory failure without heart failure or myocardial failure is typically present in the early phase of a severe bleeding episode (e.g., major blood loss due to gastrointestinal hemorrhage) causing shock secondary to hypovolemia. All three disorders are present in patients with congestive heart failure due to ischemic heart disease because myocardial failure due to reduced coronary blood flow is responsible for the heart failure and tissue underperfusion.

---

150   What are the major types of heart failure?

☐ The major types of heart failure are: (1) forward and backward; (2) left-sided and right-sided; (3) acute and chronic; (4) systolic and diastolic; and (5) low output and high output.

---

151   Describe forward and backward heart failure.

☐ Forward failure refers to decreased tissue perfusion due to reduced cardiac output leading to dysfunction of organs such as the brain (e.g., mental confusion), skeletal muscle (e.g., weakness), and kidney (e.g., salt and water retention, edema). Backward failure refers to tissue congestion due to abnormally elevated venous pressure, which leads to tissue dysfunction (e.g., arterial hypoxemia and jaundice due to pulmonary and hepatic congestion, respectively). Most patients with heart failure have evidence of both forward and backward failure.

---

152   Describe left-sided and right-sided heart failure.

☐ Left heart failure refers to abnormal function of the left cardiac chambers. Likewise, right heart failure refers to abnormal function of the right cardiac chambers. Left and right heart failure can manifest signs and symptoms of forward or backward failure of their respective chambers. Most commonly, the initial manifestations of heart failure (e.g., due to hypertension, ischemic heart failure, aortic and mitral valve disease) are those of left-sided heart failure such as weakness and shortness of breath. Thereafter, right heart failure leading to hepatic congestion and effusion in body cavities commonly ensues.

---

153 Describe acute and chronic heart failure.

☐ Acute heart failure is the unfolding of cardiac failure in minutes, hours, or only a few days; its time of onset is usually detectable with precision. By contrast, chronic heart failure gradually evolves over months to years such that establishing its time of onset is more difficult.

---

154 Describe systolic and diastolic heart failure.

☐ Systolic heart failure describes a condition in which the major abnormality is weakened ventricular contraction during systole. This process causes a decreased stroke volume, inadequate emptying of heart chambers, and cardiomegaly. Diastolic heart failure refers to a condition wherein the principal abnormality is increased resistance to filling of one or both cardiac ventricles, most commonly due to impaired myocardial relaxation during diastole. This process leads to increased filling pressures and venous congestion at a ventricular diastolic volume within normal limits. Cardiac dilatation might be present in diastolic heart failure but, in this instance, ventricular diastolic pressure is characteristically high for the ventricular volume. The main factors responsible for increased left/right ventricular diastolic pressure in diastolic heart failure (diastolic dysfunction) are: (1) increased passive stiffness of cardiac chamber (e.g., due to hypertrophy or disorganization of myocytes, fibrosis); and (2) decreased myocardial relaxation (e.g., due to hypertrophy, asynchrony of relaxation in diastolic phase, ischemia, abnormalities in ventricular loading, defects in Ca^{++} kinetics). Most patients with diastolic dysfunction have a combination of these two mechanisms causing the increased resistance to ventricular filling.

155 Compare the main features of ventricular systolic and diastolic dysfunction.

☐ Systolic dysfunction is characterized by decreases in stroke volume and ejection fraction and by increases in end-systolic volume, end-diastolic volume, and end-diastolic pressure. Patients with pure diastolic dysfunction have a normal stroke volume and ejection fraction. In addition, diastolic dysfunction is characterized by normal or decreased end-systolic volume and end-diastolic volume, accompanied by increases in filling pressures (end-diastolic pressure and mean diastolic pressure). Ejection fraction might be "supernormal," as high as 60% to 80%, in middle-aged and elderly patients with diastolic dysfunction secondary to concentric left ventricular hypertrophy associated with systemic hypertension. The "supernormal" ejection fraction observed in some patients with diastolic dysfunction might simply be due to the altered anatomy of the left ventricle. This alteration (due to the increased thickness of the ventricular wall and reduced diastolic and systolic cavity size observed with concentric hypertrophy) reduces end-diastolic blood volume but preserves stroke volume such that the increased ejection fraction is not indicative of increased myocardial contractility.

156 How common is diastolic dysfunction of the left ventricle in patients with heart failure? Name two conditions wherein treatment with specific drugs might help correct diastolic dysfunction.

☐ Diastolic dysfunction of variable degree is most likely present in all patients with heart failure who have systolic dysfunction. The signs and symptoms of heart failure in patients with systolic dysfunction are due primarily to a decreased ejection fraction (abnormal systolic function) and the diastolic dysfunction might play only a minor role. Currently available medication for congestive heart failure is most effective for systolic dysfunction (e.g., digitalis, nonglycoside inotropic agents) but has limited benefit in the management of diastolic dysfunction. Patients with heart disease who have predominantly diastolic dysfunction include those with myocardial deposition of amyloid, hemosiderin, or fibrosis. Two important conditions with a partially reversible component of diastolic dysfunction are the severe forms of hypertrophic cardiomyopathy and hypertensive cardiac hypertrophy. Calcium channel blocker therapy (especially some new Ca^{++} antagonists, discussed in another section) can be useful in the management of diastolic dysfunction because it increases left ventricular volume at a given end-diastolic pressure in patients with severe hypertrophic cardiomyopathy. Similarly, angiotensin-converting enzyme (ACE) inhibitors (e.g., captopril, enalapril), as well as α-adrenergic blockers (e.g., prazosin), used in patients with severe hypertensive hypertrophy that restricts ventricular filling, might promote regression of the cardiac hypertrophy, thereby reducing diastolic dysfunction. β Blockers (e.g., metoprolol) might increase myocardial relaxation and therefore potentially have a useful role in patients with diastolic dysfunction. The latter class of drugs must be used with caution in patients with heart failure, however, because β blockade can depress myocardial contractility. On the other hand, digitalis and other positive inotropic drugs generally have deleterious effects in patients with diastolic dysfunction.

---

157 Is systolic dysfunction universally observed in patients with symptomatic heart failure?

☐ No. As many as 40% of patients with clinically evident heart failure might have normal systolic function so that they have pure diastolic heart failure. Furthermore, most patients with symptomatic heart failure have some degree of diastolic dysfunction. Systolic and diastolic heart failure are simultaneously present in the majority of patients with cardiac hypertrophy and dilatation in whom the ventricle(s) fill and empty abnormally.

---

158 What is low output heart failure?

☐ Low output heart failure is the condition in which this organ pumps blood at rest or during exertion at a rate that is below physiologic range, causing abnormal widening of the arterial-mixed venous oxygen difference (normal is 3.5 to 5.0 mL/dL in the basal state). The abnormally large difference in the oxygen content between arterial and venous blood (while the arterial level is normal, the venous level of oxygen is diminished) is due to a relatively preserved oxygen uptake by tissues that received a diminished blood flow. The low cardiac output state might cause narrowing of the pulse pressure in severe cases as well as cold, pale, and cyanotic extremities. The physiologic range of cardiac output is wide (2.3 to 3.9 L/min/m^2) and some patients with low output heart failure might have cardiac outputs that are within the low-normal range. Causes of low output heart failure include ischemic heart disease, hypertension, cardiomyopathy, and valvular/pericardial disease.

---

159   What is high output heart failure?

☐ High output heart failure is the condition wherein this organ pumps blood at rest or during exertion at a rate that is above the physiologic range so that arterial-mixed venous oxygen difference is either normal or low despite the presence of signs of cardiac failure. The increased cardiac output might be associated with decreased resistance to ventricular emptying due to peripheral vasodilation (thyrotoxicosis, anemia), blood shunting (patent ductus arteriosus, arteriovenous fistula), reduced blood viscosity (anemia), and other factors. The decreased resistance to ventricular emptying is accompanied by increased venous return that participates as a determinant of the increased cardiac output. In addition, augmented tissue oxygen demands might activate the cardiovascular system leading to further increase in cardiac output. Warm and flushed extremities and normal-to-wide pulse pressure might be observed. Cardiac output in these patients might be in the upper limits of the normal range. Low output and high output heart failure cannot always be readily distinguished in clinical practice.

---

160   What is the normal range of cardiac output in adults at rest?

☐ The normal cardiac output at rest in adults is 2.3 to 3.9 L/min/m^2 body surface area. Expression of cardiac output per unit of body surface area is known as cardiac index. This parameter allows for a meaningful evaluation of hemodynamic status in a given individual and its comparison with the individual's expected normal levels (i.e., the cardiac index for a dwarf and a giant are similar but their cardiac outputs are dramatically different). Lower levels of cardiac index are generally observed in low output heart failure and higher ones are present in high cardiac output states (hyperdynamic or hyperkinetic conditions).

---

161   What levels of cardiac index satisfy tissue demands in conditions of reduced, normal, and vigorous activity?

☐ The approximate levels of cardiac index are 2, 4, and 10 L/min/m^2 in conditions of reduced physical activity, normal activity, and vigorous muscle exercise, respectively. The obligatory metabolic demands of body tissues are satisfied with about 2 L/min/m^2, the level of cardiac performance attained with reduced physical activity. Thus, the failing heart might adequately satisfy tissue oxygen demands of vital organs (brain, heart, kidney) by reducing the blood flow to other tissues such as the skeletal muscle.

---

162   What levels of stroke index (stroke volume corrected for body surface area) are required in conditions of normal and reduced physical activity?

☐ The levels of stroke index are 30 to 65 mL/m^2 and 25 mL/m^2 in conditions of normal and reduced physical activity, respectively. The decreased stroke index in heart failure limits the level of activity patients might tolerate. The obligatory metabolic demands of body tissues are satisfied with a stroke index of about 25 mL/m^2. Normal young individuals might increase stroke index up to 100 mL/m^2 during vigorous activity. The cardiac index attained at any level of physical activity also depends on heart rate because cardiac index is equal to stroke index multiplied by heart rate. Thus, cardiac index might be maintained by a higher stroke index when heart rate is low (longer duration of ventricular filling during diastole). By contrast, stroke index tends to diminish at high heart rate, thereby limiting the maximum cardiac index.

163   What left ventricular end-diastolic pressure (LVEDP) values are observed at increasing levels of physical activity in normal individuals compared to patients with symptomatic backward heart failure?

☐ The values of LVEDP are about 4, 10, and 20 mm Hg, in conditions of reduced physical activity, normal activity, and strenuous muscle exercise in normal individuals. Symptoms of pulmonary congestion generally develop when LVEDP reaches 20 mm Hg. Patients with symptomatic backward heart failure generally have LVEDP values of 20 to 30 mm Hg despite a reduced physical activity and have decreased cardiac index and stroke index (i.e., lower than 2 L/min/m² and 25 mL/m², respectively).

164   Is it possible to have signs and symptoms of "full blown" heart failure, known as congestive heart failure, when cardiac function is normal?

☐ Yes. Circulatory overload or congestion due to abnormal salt and water retention (e.g., renal failure, intravenous infusion of large amounts of saline) can produce signs and symptoms that closely resemble those of congestive heart failure in the presence of normal cardiac function. Management of this condition should not aim at improving heart function but to correct fluid overload.

165   What disease states produce overt salt and water retention?

☐ Congestive heart failure, hepatic cirrhosis, and nephrotic syndrome are the most important conditions characterized by generalized fluid retention. Distribution of the fluid excess differs in each disorder. Generalized venous congestion (manifested by neck vein distention) and fluid accumulation in body cavities and dependent areas are observed in congestive heart failure. By contrast, the venous congestion is restricted to the splanchnic region (portal hypertension and venous distention in the periumbilical area) and fluid accumulation is most evident in the abdominal cavity (ascites) in hepatic cirrhosis. Venous congestion is most frequently absent in patients with nephrotic syndrome, yet edema is generalized including the face and upper extremities.

166 Name the hormonal systems that control Na^+ excretion.

□ Natriuretic and antinatriuretic hormones modulate Na^+ excretion. The renin-angiotensin-aldosterone system promotes antinatriuresis, whereas natriuresis is induced by the following three hormonal systems: (1) atrial natriuretic peptide, (2) renal prostaglandin system, and (3) renal kallikrein and kinin system.

167 What are the major properties of the kidney that result from the renin-angiotensin-aldosterone system?

□ The renin-angiotensin-aldosterone system enables the kidney to exert major effects on arterial blood pressure, blood/ECF volume, and body electrolyte content. These effects are mediated by angiotensin II/III that modify vascular tone, aldosterone secretion, and glomerular/tubular function.

168 Which are the active components of the circulating renin-angiotensin system?

□ Active renin, a glycoprotein enzyme mostly produced by the juxtaglomerular cells (less important sites of production are brain, adrenal cortex, large vessels, and uterus during pregnancy), cleaves angiotensinogen, a circulating α_2 globulin made in the liver, producing angiotensin I. The latter two substances have no effects on vascular tone or on the adrenal gland. Converting enzyme transforms angiotensin I, a decapeptide, to the octapeptide angiotensin II, an active messenger that stimulates arteriolar smooth muscle contraction and adrenal secretion of aldosterone. The nonapeptide angiotensin III, produced by aminopeptidases from angiotensin II, is also an active messenger that stimulates aldosterone secretion. Angiotensinases rapidly destroy angiotensin II and III, which have half-lives of about 1 minute, and the liver clears renin whose half-life is 10 to 20 minutes.

169   How does the renin-angiotensin-aldosterone system decrease natriuresis in response to ECF volume depletion?

☐ ECF volume depletion stimulates renin secretion, which acts on angiotensinogen producing angiotensin I; the latter is converted to angiotensin II by the converting enzyme. High levels of angiotensin II promote increased renal Na^+ reabsorption (decreased natriuresis) by: (1) stimulating aldosterone secretion in the adrenal gland (zona glomerulosa); (2) increasing renal vascular resistance and thereby decreasing renal interstitial pressure; (3) decreasing renal medullary blood flow; and (4) directly stimulating Na^+ reabsorption by the renal tubules. The renin-angiotensin-aldosterone system is the most important humoral mechanism responsible for the control of NaCl excretion.

170   What are the roles of aldosterone?

☐ The major roles of aldosterone include: (1) regulation of ECF volume; (2) control of body stores and plasma levels of K^+; and (3) modulation of renal net acid excretion. It should be noted that aldosterone is the major mineralocorticoid hormone.

171   What factors control aldosterone secretion?

☐ Aldosterone secretion is controlled as follows: (1) renin-angiotensin system, whereby angiotensin II and III promote the adrenal secretion of aldosterone; (2) plasma K^+ concentration ($[K^+]_p$) directly modifies aldosterone secretion independently of the renin-angiotensin system, with small increments in $[K^+]_p$ (of only 0.1 to 0.2 mEq/L) inducing significant rises in aldosterone secretion, which in turn promotes kaliuresis and normalizes $[K^+]_p$; (3) pituitary hormones including ACTH (adrenocorticotrophic hormone also called corticotropin) and growth hormone stimulate secretion and have a permissive effect that enhances aldosterone production and release, respectively; and (4) neurotransmitters (e.g., dopamine) and humoral factors (e.g., atrial natriuretic peptide, ouabain-like factors) inhibit aldosterone release. Hyponatremia might also stimulate aldosterone secretion, yet the associated changes in effective blood volume usually override the direct effects of $[Na^+]_p$ on the adrenal gland. Although aldosterone secretion is increased in a patient with hyponatremia and volume depletion, its secretion is reduced in hyponatremia with volume expansion.

---

172 What changes in electrolyte composition of urine and stool are observed in patients with primary (e.g., adrenal adenoma) and secondary (e.g., congestive heart failure) hyperaldosteronism?

☐ Increased Na^+ reabsorption and K^+ secretion by the renal tubule and colon in response to aldosterone decreases the $[Na^+]/[K^+]$ ratio in urine and feces in patients with primary and secondary hyperaldosteronism.

---

173 How does aldosterone control urinary Na^+ excretion?

☐ The renal effects of aldosterone occur within the distal nephron, mostly on the collecting tubules. Aldosterone actions on the renal collecting duct include: (1) increasing the permeability of the apical (luminal) membrane to Na^+; (2) stimulating the Na^+,K^+-ATPase located in the basolateral (contraluminal) membrane; and (3) augmenting intracellular ATP levels, thereby providing energy for Na^+ transport. A current hypothesis proposes that the primary effect of aldosterone is on the apical membrane permeability to Na^+, and that stimulation of Na^+,K^+-ATPase is secondary to the increment in intracellular $[Na^+]$ due to higher cellular entry of Na^+ across the apical membrane. The aldosterone-induced enhancement of Na^+ reabsorption might account for the concomitantly increased K^+ and H^+ secretion in the collecting duct (see answer to previous question). In addition, aldosterone stimulates H^+ secretion in the collecting duct by a direct action on the transport of this ion.

---

174 Are the effects of aldosterone on the renal tubules limited to Na^+ and K^+ transport?

☐ No. Aldosterone has a permissive effect on antidiuretic hormone (ADH)-induced water permeability of the collecting duct. In addition, aldosterone stimulates H^+ secretion acting in the outer medullary collecting duct as described in the answer to the previous question. Sodium reabsorption and K^+ secretion in the collecting duct are the most important actions of this hormone on the renal tubules.

---

175   What are the afferent and efferent mechanisms involved in the regulation of ECF volume?

☐ The afferent or sensor limbs of the control mechanisms of ECF volume include: (1) renal receptors such as the juxtaglomerular cells and those from the macula densa; (2) stretch receptors such as the arterial baroreceptors (high-pressure receptors) and those located in cardiac atria (low-pressure receptors); and (3) interstitial volume/pressure receptors whose nature and location are still undefined. The efferent limbs of the control mechanisms of ECF volume include: (1) changes in sympathetic outflow to the heart (altering cardiac output), vascular smooth muscle (modifying peripheral resistance), and the kidneys (modulating renin secretion, renal hemodynamics, and salt/water reabsorption); and (2) hormonal secretions (e.g., atrial natriuretic peptide, ADH, renal prostaglandins) that modify salt/water excretion. The integration of afferent and efferent pathways occurs in distinct areas of the brain including the medulla oblongata, hypothalamus, and neurohypophysis.

---

176   Outline the physiologic mechanisms responsible for maintaining ECF volume relatively constant.

☐ An increment in ECF volume acting on "volume receptors" (most probably "stretch" receptors) distributed throughout the body (i.e., left atrium, pulmonary vasculature, splanchnic circulation) triggers an increase in the renal excretion of Na^+ salts. This augmented natriuresis will in turn contract the ECF volume, restoring its normal size. In a comparable manner, a decreased ECF volume stimulates volume receptors, which will activate renal conservation of Na^+ salts. Consequently, ECF volume will be expanded and the decreased ECF volume will be corrected. ECF volume is maintained relatively constant by physiologic mechanisms that control the amount of Na⁺ salts (main solute in this compartment) in ECF.

177 Is K⁺ the major determinant of ICF volume in a manner comparable to that of Na⁺ for the ECF volume?

☐ Yes. The volume of ICF depends on the cellular content of solutes, and K⁺ is a major solute that balances the electric charge of most intracellular anions. When total body K⁺ depletion occurs, physiologic mechanisms that control cell volume are recruited which reestablish ICF volume by incorporating Na⁺ into the cells as a substitute for K⁺. Consequently, the total electrolyte content of ICF tends to remain constant to preserve the volume and shape of all body cells.

178 Describe the changes in volume and tonicity of body fluids that follow an increased NaCl intake.

☐ Because NaCl is mostly restricted to ECF, positive salt balance causes an osmotic shift of water from ICF to ECF. The tonicity of body fluids increases (because total body osmoles increase, whereas total body water remains constant) and stimulates thirst and vasopressin (ADH) inducing an increased intake and reduced excretion of water. Consequently, positive water balance occurs and restoration of a normal osmolality of body fluids is achieved. The expansion of ECF (due to water shift from ICF and positive external water balance) promotes the renal excretion of the NaCl load, correcting the initial disorder. It should be recognized that an increased NaCl intake does not lead to a sustained elevation of plasma osmolality (P_{osm}) and $[Na^+]_p$, if physiologic mechanisms that control water balance are intact (thirst, ADH release, renal effects of ADH).

179 How is an expanded ECF volume perceived by mechanisms that control NaCl excretion?

☐ ECF expansion stimulates volume receptors (most likely "stretch" receptors) located in strategic areas of the circulation, which modulate renal NaCl excretion. These volume receptors include: (1) high pressure or arterial; (2) low pressure or intrathoracic; (3) hepatic; and (4) intracranial. The volume receptors perceive changes in the "effective circulating blood volume" and trigger increased natriuresis in response to volume expansion and antinatriuresis (renal conservation of Na⁺) in response to volume contraction.

180 Explain further the perception of ECF volume changes due to alterations in "effective circulating blood volume."

☐ The "fullness" of body fluid compartments should be viewed as determined by the relationship between the volume of body fluids and the holding capacity of body tissues. Volume receptors perceive the "fullness" of ECF volume (intravascular and interstitial), which is determined by the dynamic interrelationship of fluid volume and the compliance/capacity of the vascular bed (arterial, capillary, and venous components) and that of the interstitial space.

181 Where are high-pressure/volume receptors located and how do they alter renal excretion of NaCl?

☐ High-pressure/volume receptors are located in the carotid sinus (at the bifurcation of the common carotid artery in its internal and external branches) and in the kidney (juxtaglomerular apparatus). These high-pressure receptors monitor the "fullness" of the arterial circulation. The carotid sinus receptors are instrumental for water regulation and less important for ECF volume regulation because of their important effect on ADH release (and therefore on water excretion) and small or no effect on Na⁺ excretion. In contrast with the carotid volume receptors, the intrarenal receptors play a dominant role in the control of renal Na⁺ excretion by releasing renin in states of volume depletion and suppressing renin release with ECF expansion. Changes in renin secretion modify plasma aldosterone levels, which in turn modulate renal Na⁺ and Cl⁻ excretion.

182 Where are low-pressure/volume receptors located and how do they alter renal excretion of NaCl?

☐ Low-pressure/volume receptors are located within the thorax, and more specifically, in the heart (left and right atria). Whereas high-pressure/volume receptors respond to changes in "fullness" of systemic arterial circulation, low-pressure/volume receptors respond to similar changes in pulmonary circulation. Distention of both atria (the left one seems to be more important than the right one) releases atrial natriuretic peptide, which acts on the kidney to increase NaCl excretion. In some pathologic conditions such as congestive heart failure, the expected increased natriuresis due to intrathoracic vascular congestion fails to develop because of incompletely understood mechanisms.

183 Explain the role of hepatic volume receptors.

☐ The hepatic volume receptors respond to changes in the "fullness" of the low-pressure splanchnic circulation. Because salt and water intake occur normally by the oral route, their absorption through the gastrointestinal tract mandates an obligatory passage through the hepatic (portal) circulation. Consequently, hepatic volume receptors are strategically positioned to detect any addition of salt and water to body fluids and to send neurohormonal messages to the kidney to adjust excretion, achieving body fluid homeostasis. The precise location of hepatic volume receptors and the pathways that mediate their effects on salt and water excretion remain poorly defined.

184 Explain the role of intracranial volume receptors.

☐ Because substantial changes in brain ionic and water content can cause severe or fatal injury, the CNS possesses receptors that monitor the volume of this vital organ. Changes in volume of whole body ICF and ECF tend to induce parallel alterations in brain volume. Detection of volume expansion by intracranial receptors triggers increased renal NaCl excretion, whereas intracranial volume depletion induces renal salt retention. The importance of intracranial volume receptors in NaCl homeostasis remains incompletely understood.

---

185   What are the pathways for increased NaCl excretion in ECF expansion?

☐ A decreased renal secretion of renin (and secondary reduction in the adrenal production of aldosterone), depressed renal sympathetic nerve activity, increased secretion of renal prostaglandins responsible for renal vasodilation, increased secretion of atrial natriuretic peptide, and other mechanisms of renal vasodilation are critical determinants of the increased NaCl excretion in response to ECF volume expansion.

---

186   How does the message to increase NaCl excretion following an excessive NaCl intake reach the kidney?

☐ The ECF expansion resulting from excessive NaCl intake is the signal for enhanced natriuresis (increased urinary Na^+ excretion). Such ECF expansion induces an increase in the "effective circulating blood volume," which plays the dominant role in eliciting the increased Na^+ excretion. Additionally, decreased plasma oncotic pressure (dilution of plasma proteins) due to ECF expansion promotes natriuresis by diminishing NaCl reabsorption in the renal tubules.

---

187   Does ECF expansion always induce an increased renal excretion of salt?

☐ No. ECF expansion fails to enhance renal NaCl excretion if "effective circulating blood volume" is not transiently increased. Examples of this condition are patients with congestive heart failure, cirrhosis of the liver, and nephrotic syndrome, all characterized by a decreased "effective circulating blood volume." The latter does not consistently increase after a NaCl load in these patients and salt is therefore retained.

188 What is the "third factor" that modulates NaCl excretion in response to ECF volume changes?

☐ Atrial natriuretic hormone, increased papillary blood flow, and changes in peritubular capillary hemodynamics predominantly acting on the proximal nephron are the major components of the "third factor." This "third factor" participates in the control of Na^+ excretion, in addition to the well-established "first factor" (glomerular filtration rate and the filtered load of Na^+) and "second factor" (decreased aldosterone secretion during volume expansion).

189 How does atrial natriuretic peptide increase natriuresis in response to ECF volume expansion?

☐ Atrial natriuretic peptide, stored in atrial cardiocytes from left and right heart chambers, is released into the circulation in response to stretch (volume receptors) of these structures and promotes increased natriuresis by hemodynamic and hormonal mechanisms. The hemodynamic effects include increased glomerular filtration rate (the increased Na^+ filtered load might promote enhanced natriuresis) and increased medullary blood flow (Na^+ reabsorption in the renal tubules is depressed and urinary Na^+ excretion increases). The hormonal effects include direct depression of aldosterone secretion and of renin release (and subsequent depression of angiotensin levels) by the high plasma levels of atrial natriuretic peptide. These hormonal changes decrease Na^+ reabsorption and promote urine Na^+ excretion. Conversely, diminution of ECF volume and of vascular volume provides negative feedback that suppresses release of atrial natriuretic peptide leading to renal Na^+ retention.

190 Describe the role and pathways of the sympathetic nervous system in modulating renal NaCl excretion.

☐ The sympathetic system is activated by ECF volume depletion (mediated by low- and high-pressure baroreceptors), inducing a decrease in renal NaCl excretion. Hemodynamic and hormonal mechanisms mediate this effect by increasing renal NaCl reabsorption. The hemodynamic mechanisms consist of a reduction in renal interstitial pressure (due to increased vascular resistance) and medullary blood flow, factors that increase renal salt reabsorption. The hormonal mechanisms include stimulation of renin release and subsequent generation of angiotensin II, which in turn: (1) augments renal vascular resistance and thereby decreases interstitial hydrostatic pressure, (2) directly acts on the renal tubules, and (3) stimulates adrenal secretion of aldosterone. These hormonal mechanisms act in concert to increase Na^+ reabsorption leading to diminished urinary excretion.

---

191   What effect does efferent renal nerve activity have on urinary salt and water excretion?

☐ Adrenergic and dopaminergic fibers are involved in urinary salt and water excretion. Augmented renal nerve activity plays a significant role in the Na^+ retention observed in several diseases states (e.g., congestive heart failure, circulatory collapse) and in conditions of low salt intake.

---

192   What are the direct effects of angiotensin, parathyroid hormone (PTH), calcitonin, and glucagon on NaCl and water transport by the renal tubules?

☐ Angiotensin stimulates Na^+ and H_2O absorption in the proximal tubule, whereas PTH inhibits this process. The effects of calcitonin are limited to the thick ascending limb of Henle's loop, distal tubule, and cortical collecting duct, where it stimulates NaCl absorption. Glucagon acts on the thick ascending limb of Henle's loop, where it increases NaCl absorption.

---

193   What effect does head-out water immersion have on Na^+ excretion and solute-free water clearance?

☐ Water immersion to the level of the neck produces a prompt and potent central hypervolemia due to increased venous return caused by compression ("squeezing out") of blood stored in the subcutaneous venous plexus (i.e., redistribution of blood volume toward the heart and pulmonary circulation). This maneuver augments cardiac output, reduces renal vascular resistance, and induces a marked Na^+ and water diuresis. These events occur in normal subjects, in patients with liver cirrhosis, and in those with other conditions (e.g., nephrotic syndrome and some patients with heart failure). Thus, head-out water immersion might improve the deranged salt and water homeostasis in various disease states. The effects are only transient because they generally vanish shortly after termination of water immersion (e.g., the subject sits in the study tank immersed in water, kept at a constant temperature of about 35°C for about 4 hours). A transient increment in glomerular filtration rate during water immersion also occurs in patients with decompensated cirrhosis.

---

194 How does increased blood pressure augment renal NaCl excretion? Explain this phenomenon.

☐ Increased blood pressure augments salt excretion by diminishing renal NaCl reabsorption. Hemodynamic and hormonal mechanisms mediate this effect on NaCl reabsorption. Hemodynamic mechanisms include higher renal interstitial pressure (due to diminished renal vascular resistance) and medullary blood flow induced by renal hyperperfusion. Hormonal mechanisms include inhibition (e.g., renin release) and stimulation (e.g., prostaglandins, kallikrein, and kinins secretion) of renal humoral factors controlling NaCl excretion. The inhibition of renin release depresses the renin-angiotensin-aldosterone axis, increasing salt excretion.

---

195 Describe the concept and importance of "pressure-natriuresis/diuresis" in the control of fluid volume and blood pressure.

☐ "Pressure natriuresis/diuresis" refers to the increased Na^+ (mostly as NaCl) and water excretion leading to decreased blood volume, cardiac output, and blood pressure in response to higher arterial blood pressure. These physiologic responses restore blood pressure to its normal value. "Pressure natriuresis/diuresis" also includes the reduction in Na^+ and water excretion leading to increased blood volume, cardiac output, and blood pressure in response to decreases in arterial pressure. These physiologic responses restore blood pressure to its normal value. The importance of "pressure natriuresis/diuresis" in the long-term control of body fluid volume and arterial pressure has not been established with certainty.

---

196   What is the importance of "pressure-induced natriuresis" in the "escape phenomenon"?

☐ Prevention of the increased renal perfusion pressure observed in response to aldosterone infusion causes persistent salt and water retention (absence of "escape phenomenon"). Thus, pressure-induced natriuresis has a major role in the "escape phenomenon" of mineralocorticoid excess. Although limited and transient salt and water retention occurs in animals receiving long-term mineralocorticoid therapy, using a device that maintains renal perfusion pressure constant during aldosterone infusion produces massive fluid retention and severe hypertension. Consequently, pressure-induced natriuresis is a major determinant of the "mineralocorticoid escape."

---

197   Why does underfilling of the arterial compartment promote renal salt and water retention?

☐ Underfilling of the arterial compartment promotes positive salt and water balance because it decreases renal filtration of salt and water (due to decreased glomerular filtration rate) and increases NaCl and water reclamation (due to stimulated reabsorption in the proximal tubule and other segments of the nephron). The decreased glomerular filtration rate is associated with depressed renal blood flow. The increased salt and water reabsorption in the proximal tubule is accounted for by decreased renal perfusion pressure and increased α-adrenergic and angiotensin II activity.

---

198   What is the most significant renal response to heart failure?

☐ Salt and water retention is the most significant renal response to heart failure. The determinants of salt and water retention in congestive heart failure are a decreased cardiac output ("forward" failure) and right-sided venous congestion ("backward" failure). The importance of each of these mechanisms varies widely and partly depends on the etiology of heart failure and its severity.

---

199   What are the major effects of a decreased cardiac output on the renal circulation?

☐ A decreased cardiac output reduces systemic perfusion pressure leading to an "underfilled" arterial tree. Although renal blood flow is decreased in the early stage of heart failure, glomerular filtration rate is preserved because of preferential constriction of the postglomerular vessels (more intense constriction of the efferent than the afferent arteriole), which in turn favors increased proximal reabsorption of filtrate. In addition, redistribution of renal blood flow away from the cortical glomeruli and toward the juxtamedullary glomeruli (which have longer loops of Henle with greater Na^+ reabsorptive capacity) promotes further fluid retention. In more advanced stages of heart failure, glomerular filtration rate decreases because of more intense constriction of preglomerular arterioles (afferent arterioles). Consequently, patients develop prerenal azotemia with a blood urea nitrogen: creatinine ratio that exceeds 10:1 and they retain waste products and fluid. Patients with severe forward failure (e.g., cardiogenic shock) might develop acute renal failure with all the signs and symptoms of acute tubular necrosis.

---

200   Contrast how salt and water retention modifies heart function in the early ("compensated") compared to late ("decompensated") phases of heart failure.

☐ Salt and water retention expands plasma volume and increases venous return to the heart. Consequently, diastolic volume and pressure increase in response to the progressive salt and water retention. In the initial phase of this process, sarcomere lengths are optimal because there is maximal overlapping of thick and thin filaments. At this early "compensated" phase of volume overload, the mild distention of cardiac chambers helps to maintain normal (or near normal) stroke volume. As volume overload and ventricular dilation develop, end-diastolic pressure as well as wall tension and myocardial oxygen consumption concomitantly increase. In addition, the myocardial capillary network does not increase in proportion to the increase in myocardial mass, further straining the balance between energy supply and demand. There is also less overlap between thick and thin filaments, reducing the force of contraction. At this late or "decompensated" phase, a further increase in salt and water retention does not increase cardiac output but dramatically increases end-diastolic pressure leading to venous congestion in the pulmonary and systemic circulations. This late phase of "decompensated" heart failure is characterized by compromised tissue perfusion in association with expansion of ECF volume throughout body tissues (congestive heart failure).

---

201   How does neurohormonal activation occur in heart failure? What are its renal effects?

☐ The decreased effective arterial volume acting on high-pressure baroreceptors leads to increased sympathetic activity, stimulation of the renin-angiotensin-aldosterone system, and increased vasopressin release. The increased sympathetic tone promotes fluid reabsorption in the proximal nephron by its action on the renal circulation and by direct stimulation of renal tubular solute reabsorption. In addition, sympathetic activation and reduced renal perfusion pressure stimulate renin release from juxtaglomerular cells, which leads to angiotensin generation and subsequent stimulation of aldosterone secretion. Aldosterone increases NaCl reabsorption in the distal nephron (i.e., cortical collecting duct). Furthermore, angiotensin contributes to salt retention through its vasoconstrictor effect and by direct action on proximal tubular cells. Renal unresponsiveness to atrial natriuretic factor is also partly responsible for edema formation in heart failure. Enhanced vasopressin release contributes to water as well as to salt retention in heart failure. Patients with heart failure have abnormal action of vasodilatory hormones including the prostaglandins, dopaminergic system, the kinin-kallikrein system, and atrial natriuretic hormones, but its full importance in edema formation remains unclear.

202 How might "backward" heart failure promote renal retention of salt and water?

☐ The increased venous pressure characteristic of "backward" heart failure favors the exit of fluid from the intravascular to the interstitial space of pulmonary or systemic tissues by increasing the transcapillary hydraulic pressure gradient. In addition, venous hypertension reduces lymphatic return by increasing hydrostatic pressure at the thoracic duct ostium, thereby contributing to expansion of tissue interstitial fluid volume. The overall reduction of intravascular volume due to the two mechanisms previously mentioned contributes to diminished effective arterial blood volume characteristic of heart failure and thereby promotes Na^+ retention by the kidney. Furthermore, renal vein hypertension decreases renal blood flow and glomerular filtration rate, contributing to renal retention of salt. Finally, venous hypertension stimulates release of atrial natriuretic factor, which might augment capillary hydraulic permeability, increasing interstitial fluid volume and further decreasing effective arterial blood volume.

203 How is edema classified?

☐ Edema is classified according to the primary process. Thus, edema might be due to: (1) renal failure, in which there is a primary reduction in renal salt excretion due to acute glomerulonephritis, tubular necrosis, or other types of renal disease; (2) heart failure, low and high output forms, in which reduced effective arterial blood volume causes renal retention of salt and water; (3) damage to the capillary endothelium, localized or generalized, because of chemical, bacterial, thermal, or mechanical injury; and (4) diminished colloid-osmotic pressure such as in severe nutritional deficiency, hypercatabolic states, protein-losing enteropathy, chronic liver disease, and nephrotic syndrome. Although edema is initiated by abnormal Starling forces across the capillaries (e.g., heart failure, venous obstruction, hypoalbuminemia), salt retention must be present to replete the intravascular volume loss. The absence of such salt and water retention by the kidney would reequilibrate Starling forces, preventing further edema formation. It should be recognized that in all forms of edema except that occurring in renal disease, salt and water retention by the kidney is a secondary defect.

---

204 How can edema be classified according to the renal mechanisms responsible for its development?

☐ Primary and secondary edema are the two general forms of fluid accumulation based on differences in the role played by the kidney in the development of these conditions. In primary edema, renal retention of salt and water is the initial event that leads to expansion of plasma and ECF volume (e.g., acute glomerulonephritis, some forms of nephrotic syndrome, renal diseases with severe reduction of glomerular filtration rate). In secondary edema, also called "underfill edema," renal hypoperfusion, due to decreased "effective circulating blood volume," initiates salt and water retention by the kidney (e.g., congestive heart failure, some forms of nephrotic syndrome). Thus, the kidney is always involved in the development of positive salt and water balance that leads to generalized edema, yet the renal action might be due to abnormalities initiated within it (primary edema) or in response to "effective" intravascular volume depletion (secondary edema).

---

205 Provide examples of edema formation accompanied by a preceding interval of fluid accumulation.

☐ Patients with congestive heart failure and those with nephrotic syndrome have altered Starling forces in the capillaries leading to edema formation in all tissues. The preceding interval of positive fluid balance allows extravasation of fluid into the interstitial fluid of all tissues (this is more evident in some tissues than in others) without a concomitant reduction in the fluid content of other tissues. Consequently, physical examination of these patients reveals generalized swelling (accompanied by pitting edema in dependent areas) instead of the fluid accumulation limited to a body region (localized swelling), that might be observed in the absence of a previous interval of positive fluid balance.

206   Provide examples of edema formation not accompanied by a preceding interval of fluid accumulation.

☐ If trauma limited to a body region (e.g., a lower extremity) is inflicted on a normal individual, fluid accumulates in the area of trauma within minutes. This fluid is diverted from other tissues that have been forced to lose fluid. A comparable situation develops if multiple bee stings occur simultaneously (e.g., on an upper extremity while collecting honey), inducing swelling that is limited to the injured extremity. Another prominent example is that of a previously normal individual who suddenly develops a large myocardial infarction leading to forward and backward heart failure. This patient would manifest severe shortness of breath within minutes due to pulmonary edema but would not exhibit any evidence of peripheral edema (i.e., absence of pitting edema in dependent areas such as ankles and feet) at this early stage.

207   What is the major determinant of renal salt and water retention in congestive heart failure, cirrhosis of the liver, and nephrotic syndrome?

☐ The major anasarca syndromes have a common mechanism responsible for the positive salt and water balance. The ECF expansion in these diseases occurs in response to underfilling of the arterial compartment (diminished effective arterial blood volume), which produces excessive renal salt and water retention. Arterial underfilling is due to: (1) a decreased cardiac output in heart failure (e.g., congestive heart failure due to incomplete ventricular emptying known as systolic dysfunction or inadequate ventricular relaxation known as diastolic dysfunction); (2) peripheral arterial vasodilation (e.g., high output heart failure due to anemia, cirrhosis of the liver); and (3) diminished plasma colloid osmotic pressure leading to contraction of intravascular volume in nephrotic syndrome.

208   Are plasma volume and hormonal levels altered in heart failure?

☐ Yes. In a manner comparable to liver cirrhosis, a progressive decline in cardiac index (cardiac output corrected for body surface area) in patients with low output cardiac failure is accompanied by a progressive rise in plasma volume and hormonal levels (norepinephrine, ADH, renin, aldosterone). Thus, in end-stage heart failure, the severe reduction in cardiac index is accompanied by significant plasma volume expansion and high plasma levels of norepinephrine, ADH, renin, and aldosterone. It should be noted that aldosterone is a major factor in the NaCl retention of hepatic cirrhosis but plays a less significant role in the salt retention of heart failure.

---

209   What are the main causes of generalized edema and normal/near-normal serum albumin?

☐ Salt and water retention due to primary renal disease and congestive heart failure are the main causes of this syndrome. Absence of proteinuria (protein in the urine) argues against renal disease as the primary cause of fluid retention. Patients with heart failure usually have either minimal or mild urinary protein excretion (1+ or 2+ on dipstick determination), whereas those with renal disease including nephrotic syndrome have, as a rule, severe proteinuria (3+ or 4+ by dipstick). It is common for physicians to incorrectly diagnose congestive heart failure on the basis of shortness of breath and bilateral lower extremity edema, without realizing that a similar syndrome is observed in patients with salt and water retention due to a primary renal disease.

---

210   What level of net filtration pressure (difference between forces favoring filtration and those opposing filtration) is necessary for fluid accumulation (edema) in the interstitial compartment?

☐ Experimental and clinical studies have demonstrated that a net filtration pressure of 10 to 15 mmHg is required for the development of significant interstitial fluid accumulation (edema). The relatively large net pressure gradient required is due to a secondary increment in hydrostatic pressure in the interstitium that promotes a higher lymphatic flow, which in turn protects against tissue fluid excess. When these protective mechanisms against fluid accumulation are overwhelmed, edema develops.

211   Does a net filtration pressure of 10 to 15 mmHg always lead to generalized edema?

☐   No. A preceding interval of fluid accumulation (positive salt and water balance) is necessary for the development of generalized edema so that an expansion of all body fluids must be present. In the absence of previous fluid accumulation, edema formation in one or more tissues is necessarily accompanied by a reduced fluid content in other tissues.

212   Describe Starling's law of fluid exchange across capillary walls.

☐   Osmotic forces contribute to the distribution of water across capillary walls, yet the high permeability of these membranes to Na^+ salts and glucose makes these solutes ineffective determinants of intravascular volume. By contrast, plasma proteins are effective osmoles in the vascular space because these large molecules do not significantly cross the capillary walls. The transfer of fluid across the capillary walls is determined by the difference between forces that favor filtration and forces that favor reabsorption. Starling's law can be generally expressed as follows:

Net fluid transfer = Permeability of the capillaries ×

(Filtration forces – Reabsorption forces)

213   Provide a more detailed explanation of the various components of Starling's law of capillary-interstitial fluid exchange.

☐   Starling's law can be described using the general formula of fluid transfer by convection as follows:

$$J_v = (\Delta P + \Delta \pi) \times A \times L_p$$

where J_v is net fluid transfer or net volume flux; ΔP is hydrostatic pressure gradient; $\Delta \pi$ is osmotic pressure gradient; A is membrane area for volume flow; and L_p is hydraulic permeability of the membrane. The ΔP is calculated as follows:

$$\Delta P = P_{cap} - P_{ISF}$$

where P_{cap} is capillary hydrostatic pressure and P_{ISF} is interstitial fluid hydrostatic pressure. The $\Delta\pi$ is calculated as follows:

$$\Delta\pi = \pi_{cap} - \pi_{ISF}$$

where π_{cap} is capillary oncotic pressure and π_{ISF} is interstitial oncotic pressure (due to filtered plasma proteins and interstitial mucopolysaccharides).

The term K_f (filtration coefficient or net permeability of capillary membrane) is most frequently used in the Starling equation to replace the terms $A \times L_p$ (surface area available for fluid transfer multiplied by hydraulic permeability of the capillary wall) because the composite value expressed as K_f can be quantified precisely, whereas the individual components cannot be measured with accuracy.

---

214   How would you classify the mechanisms of edema formation based on Starling's law of fluid exchange?

☐   Starling's law indicates the existence of two general mechanisms of edema, commonly referred to as "increased pressure" and "increased permeability" edema. The former type includes cases in which edema is caused by altered hydrostatic or colloid-osmotic pressure gradients in the capillaries. The latter type is due to increased capillary permeability, leading to the formation of edema fluid that is characteristically rich in proteins (i.e., protein concentration of edema fluid is greater than 70% of plasma level).

---

215   Are all capillaries of the circulatory system continuously perfused with blood?

☐   No. Most of the capillaries in some dominant tissues (e.g., skeletal muscle) are collapsed and without any blood flow in the basal or resting state. The release of vasodilator metabolites, hormones, and neural influences that accompany activation of a particular tissue induces relaxation of arterioles and precapillary sphincters, which in turn increase intracapillary pressure, establishing a blood flow.

216   Describe the mechanisms involved in the control of hydrostatic pressure within the capillaries.

□ The resistance of arterioles and precapillary sphincters determines the degree to which the systemic arterial pressure is transmitted to the capillaries. The hydrostatic pressure within the capillaries is not uniform along their course. The mean capillary hydrostatic pressure of about 25 mmHg derives from a higher level (about 32 mmHg) at their arterial end and a lower level (about 15 mmHg) at the venous end. Consequently, forces favoring net fluid exit from the capillaries are present at the arterial end, whereas net fluid uptake by the capillaries is facilitated at the venous end. An increased mean hydrostatic pressure within the capillaries develops if arterioles and precapillary sphincters dilate; the opposite occurs when these structures constrict.

217   Describe other major mechanisms that alter net fluid transfer across the capillaries.

□ Because hydrostatic and oncotic pressures are the major physiologic determinants of net fluid transfer across the capillaries, changes in any of these variables can significantly alter fluid exchange in body tissues. Consequently, an increased capillary hydrostatic pressure due to increased venous pressure (e.g., congestive heart failure) or a decreased colloid osmotic pressure (e.g., low serum albumin concentration due to protein malnutrition, liver cirrhosis, or nephrotic syndrome) favor fluid accumulation in peripheral tissues. Increased capillary permeability is the third major mechanism (first and second mechanisms being increased filtration pressure and decreased colloid osmotic pressure gradient, respectively) that enhances fluid exit from the intravascular compartment. Histamine, kinins, and substance P are some of the humoral factors that increase capillary permeability.

218   Is the interstitial fluid pressure approximately equal among body tissues?

□ No. Large differences in interstitial fluid pressure are found among the various tissues, the lowest being the lung (about −2 mmHg) and the highest the brain (about +6 mmHg). Intermediate levels are found in subcutaneous tissue, liver, and kidney. A subatmospheric level, about −1 mmHg, is found in the first of these tissues, whereas supra-atmospheric levels are in the last two organs (about +2 to 4 mmHg).

---

219 What are the values of Starling forces across the capillaries of the systemic circulation?

☐ The ΔP is approximately 20 mmHg because P_{cap} is about 24 mmHg and P_{ISF} is about 4 mmHg. The $\Delta \pi$ is about 20 mmHg because π_{cap} is about 25 mmHg and π_{ISF} is about 5 mmHg. Thus, forces favoring filtration (volume flux leaving the capillaries) are identical to forces favoring reabsorption (volume flux entering the capillaries). The aforementioned values change in response to physiologic conditions. It should be recognized that forces favoring filtration can exceed those favoring reabsorption of fluid by a small margin (i.e., about 0.5 mmHg) leading to a net fluid loss from the capillary bed that returns to the circulation by way of the lymphatic flow. During nutrient absorption within the alimentary tract, a pressure gradient develops between opposing forces, accounting for the formation of lymphatic fluid.

---

220 What are the values of Starling forces across the capillaries of the pulmonary circulation?

☐ The ΔP is about 16 mmHg because P_{cap} is 14 mmHg and P_{ISF} is −2 mmHg. The $\Delta \pi$ is about 16 mmHg because π_{cap} is 25 mmHg and π_{ISF} is 9 mmHg. Thus, forces favoring fluid reabsorption (volume flux entering the capillaries) are identical to forces favoring filtration (volume flux leaving the capillaries). Consequently, the pulmonary alveoli remain "dry," allowing an optimal gas exchange. These values of Starling forces in the pulmonary capillaries represent composite levels of all pulmonary zones. Zone 1 (comprising the apical areas) has a lower vascular than alveolar pressure, whereas in zone 3 (comprising the basal areas) the vascular is higher than the alveolar pressure.

221   Describe the three pulmonary zones that result from the gravity-dependent, apex-to-base distribution of pulmonary blood flow in upright lungs (e.g., standing or sitting position).

☐ The three pulmonary zones, known as 1, 2, and 3, comprise approximately the upper, middle, and lower third of the lungs, respectively. In zone 1 or apical area, the pulmonary capillaries are almost bloodless because their internal pressure is less (or about the same) than the external or alveolar pressure, making blood flow either very low or absent. In theory, zone 1 should not have any capillary perfusion because the relationship among pressures is as follows: $P_A > P_a > P_v$ (alveolar, arterial, and venous pressures, respectively).   In zone 2 or middle area, the pulmonary blood flow is intermediate between the very low one observed in zone 1 and the larger capillary flow found in zone 3.   Capillary pressure at the arterial side in zone 2 exceeds alveolar pressure, the latter in turn exceeds capillary pressure at the venous side (thus $P_a > P_A > P_v$).   In zone 3 or basal area, the capillary vessels are constantly distended (as opposed to the collapse of capillaries at their venous end in zone 2) and have the highest blood flow because the internal pressure in the capillaries at the arterial and venous ends are higher than the alveolar pressure (thus $P_a > P_v > P_A$).

222   What is vascular redistribution of pulmonary blood perfusion?

☐ In normal human beings in the upright position, blood perfusion is greater in the pulmonary bases than in the apical areas.   Any deviation from this gravity-dependent pattern of pulmonary blood perfusion is known as vascular redistribution.   Thus, an increase in apical perfusion in association with a reduction in the perfusion of the bases is present in vascular redistribution of pulmonary blood flow.   This phenomenon occurs because of compression of capillaries at the lung bases due to pulmonary edema and to hypoxia-induced constriction of pulmonary arterioles in this area.   Vascular redistribution is diagnosed by radiologic examination (i.e., chest x-ray) and is not an early sign of pulmonary edema because it occurs after the onset of alveolar edema, when auscultatory findings are already present.

223 Why does pulmonary edema first appear at the lung bases as opposed to the lung apices?

☐ The gravity-dependent distribution of pulmonary edema is due to the greater effects of gravity on blood flow of different lung zones in comparison with its effects on airway flow/pressures. The effective perfusion pressure in the pulmonary capillaries increases by about 1 cm H_2O/cm vertical distance from apex to base, whereas pleural pressures increase by only about 0.25 cm H_2O/cm vertical distance. However, alveolar pressure does not differ in the pulmonary base as compared to its apex. Consequently, gravity has no effect on alveolar pressure, a small effect on pleural pressure, and a large effect on capillary perfusion pressure. These differences explain why pulmonary edema is first evident at the lung bases (see also answers to other related questions for additional explanation of the concept). Thus, the higher hydrostatic pressure within the pulmonary capillaries at the basilar compared to the apical areas is the main reason for detection of alveolar rales first at the lung bases of patients with pulmonary edema.

224 What lung zones are examined in the course of hemodynamic evaluations aimed at assessing pulmonary vascular resistance or pulmonary capillary wedge pressure?

☐ Zone 3 is considered to be the exclusive area for a meaningful measurement of pulmonary capillary wedge pressure or calculation of pulmonary vascular resistance. In zone 3, increases in pulmonary arterial pressure in the apex-to-base direction are offset by nearly identical increases in venous pressure so that gravity-dependent effects on the pulmonary circulation are minimized as compared to areas 1 and 2 of the lung.

225 What factors protect the lung against edema?

☐ The lung possesses several mechanisms that prevent the development of edema including: (1) an effective lymphatic system; (2) low hydraulic permeability of the pulmonary capillaries; (3) very low diffusibility of proteins across the capillary walls; and (4) very low electrolyte conductance of the epithelial barrier.

---

226 Explain the role of lung lymphatic vessels in the pathogenesis of pulmonary edema.

☐ The lymphatics play a critical role in removing fluid from the interstitial space (ISF). The rate of fluid accumulation in the lung can be theoretically estimated as the difference between the net fluid flow from the pulmonary capillaries to the interstitium $[\dot{Q}(pc \rightarrow ISF)]$ and the lymphatic flow ($\dot{Q}$ lymph) from the pulmonary tissue to the systemic circulation as follows:

$$\text{Rate of fluid accumulation} = \dot{Q}(pc \rightarrow ISF) - \dot{Q} \text{ lymph}$$

The pulmonary lymphatic flow in a normal man at rest is about 20 mL/h and can increase up to tenfold on stimulation (e.g., pulmonary hypertension, lung inflammatory process). Consequently, the large lymphatic reserve plays a major role in protecting the lung from developing pulmonary edema. The lymphatic flow is facilitated by the additive effects of active contraction of lymphatic capillaries that have valves, which allow unidirectional fluid transport, and compression of lymphatic vessels secondary to respiratory movements and vascular pulsations. The pulmonary lymph drains into the thoracic duct, which empties into the systemic venous system. Consequently, increased systemic venous pressure secondary to right-sided heart failure opposes lymph drainage and facilitates the development of pulmonary edema.

---

227 Provide a classification of pulmonary edema according to its pathogenesis.

☐ Pulmonary edema might be caused by: (1) an imbalance of Starling forces (e.g., increased pulmonary capillary pressure as in heart failure or decreased oncotic pressure as in hepatic failure with hypoalbuminemia); (2) increased alveolar-capillary membrane permeability as in acute respiratory distress syndrome (ARDS); and (3) insufficiency of pulmo–

nary lymphatic drainage as might be observed after lung transplant, lymphangitis carcinomatosis, or in fibrosing lymphangitis. Pulmonary edema caused by heart failure can occur with myocardial failure (e.g., cardiomyopathy) or without it (e.g., mitral stenosis). It should be recognized that pulmonary edema can be initiated or exacerbated in individuals with a mild or moderate increase in pulmonary capillary pressure (e.g., heart failure) who concomitantly have decreased plasma oncotic pressure (hypoalbuminemia due to hepatic failure or nephrotic syndrome), "leaky" alveolar-capillary membranes, or pulmonary lymphatic insufficiency.

---

228   Can hypoalbuminemia in the absence of other cofactors cause pulmonary edema?

□ No. Although hypoalbuminemia favors the exit of fluid from the vascular into the perivascular space of all body capillaries (pulmonary as well as systemic) due to decreased intravascular colloid osmotic pressure, it does not cause pulmonary edema in the absence of other cofactors. The increased rate of fluid loss from pulmonary capillaries augments the net amount of fluid collected by pulmonary lymphatics for return to the systemic circulation. Unless other factors intervene, significant pulmonary fluid accumulation does not occur. Factors that might have additive effects to hypoalbuminemia to cause pulmonary edema include increased pulmonary capillary hydrostatic pressure as well as conditions, such as infections, that cause "leaky" alveolar-capillary membranes.

---

229   Name conditions that might cause pulmonary edema due to increased permeability of the alveolar-capillary membrane.

□ Pulmonary edema due to increased permeability of the alveolar-capillary membrane (also called noncardiogenic pulmonary edema) might be caused by: (1) infections (e.g., bacterial, viral, etc.); (2) inhaled irritants (e.g., aspiration of gastric contents, toxic substances contained in inspired air such as phosgene); (3) blood-borne endogenous or exogenous substances (e.g., histamine, bacterial endotoxins, snake venoms); (4) exogenous physical factors (e.g., trauma, radiation pneumonitis); (5) blood disorders (e.g., disseminated intravascular coagulation), (6) hypersensitivity-immunologic reactions, and (7) circulatory catastrophes (e.g., shock lung, acute hemorrhagic pancreatitis). Despite the variety of underlying causes, the clinical and pathophysiological sequence of events is remarkably similar among most patients, producing a condition known as adult respiratory distress syndrome.

230 Describe the three stages of fluid accumulation in the lung leading to pulmonary edema (cardiogenic and noncardiogenic types).

☐ Stage 1 of pulmonary edema is an exaggeration of the normal physiologic process of fluid leaving the pulmonary capillaries and entering the pulmonary interstitial space. This fluid subsequently returns to the vascular compartment by way of pulmonary lymphatics. The exaggerated fluid flow observed in stage 1 might be due either to an imbalance of Starling forces favoring exit of fluid from capillaries (increased hydrostatic pressure or decreased oncotic pressure within pulmonary capillaries) or to damage of alveolar/capillary membranes. The augmented fluid traffic of stage 1 prevents significant fluid accumulation in the interstitial space. In stage 2, the traffic of fluid and proteins exceeds the maximum rate of lymphatic drainage, causing expansion of the interstitial space. Because the negative pressure and compliance of the peribronchial and perivascular interstitial space are larger than those of the interstitial space surrounding alveoli, fluid accumulation (edema) around bronchi and small blood vessels precedes that developing around alveoli. This fluid accumulation causes compression of small airways and blood vessels in the lung. Stage 3 is the state of alveolar flooding that might occur: (1) directly from the surrounding alveolar interstitial space and caused by high pressures that disrupt the alveolar membrane, or (2) indirectly due to overflow of fluid from the peribronchiolar/perivascular space into alveoli with intact structure of their walls (i.e., normal alveolar/capillary barrier). It must be recognized that the indirect mechanism is the most common in clinical practice (e.g., pulmonary edema due to heart failure or fluid overload). When alveolar flooding occurs with intact alveolar membranes as with the indirect mechanism, reversal of pulmonary edema might be achieved more promptly and completely.

---

231   What is the so-called high-altitude pulmonary edema?

☐ High-altitude pulmonary edema is a syndrome that might develop shortly after rapid ascent to altitudes in excess of 2700 m. It occurs mostly in adolescents and young adults who engage in demanding physical activity before they become acclimatized to high altitude. Symptoms include cough, dyspnea, chest pain, and tachycardia that usually develop within a day of ascent. Physical examination reveals cyanosis, bilateral pulmonary rales, and patchy infiltrates scattered throughout both lung fields on chest x-ray. Administration of high oxygen concentration or returning the patient to a lower altitude reverses the syndrome within 1 or 2 days. Preventive measures include avoidance of vigorous exercise for the first 2 or 3 days at high altitude and gradual ascent if possible. The pathogenesis of this syndrome is still unknown. Hemodynamic evaluation of patients with high-altitude pulmonary edema reveals pulmonary artery hypertension and near-normal pulmonary capillary wedge pressure.

---

232   What is neurogenic pulmonary edema?

☐ Neurogenic pulmonary edema refers to a form of lung edema that occurs in patients with major neurologic disorders such as head trauma or grand mal seizures in the absence of other common causes of pulmonary edema. The pathogenesis of this entity includes both an imbalance of Starling forces in the pulmonary capillaries and increased permeability of these vessels. The intense and sustained sympathetic discharge observed in these neurologic disorders might be responsible for the pulmonary edema according to the following mechanisms: (1) constriction of arterioles and veins in the systemic circulation that produces hypertension with left ventricular afterload and shifts of blood from the systemic to the pulmonary circulation, thereby increasing hydrostatic pressure in the pulmonary capillaries and favoring exit of fluid from the vasculature due to abnormal Starling forces; and (2) increased permeability of the capillaries due to direct effects or constriction of vessels including the veins in the pulmonary circulation. In experimental models of this disorder, the pulmonary edema that follows severe CNS injury can be completely prevented by sympathectomy. Thus, it appears that neurogenic pulmonary edema is caused by a combination of a neurally mediated increase in both the hydrostatic pressure and permeability of pulmonary capillaries.

---

233 Describe the acute pulmonary edema secondary to overdose of narcotics.

☐ Overdose of heroin, morphine, methadone, and dextropropoxyphene can cause pulmonary edema by mechanisms incompletely understood. Increased permeability of pulmonary capillaries due to narcotic-induced release of histamine has been proposed because pulmonary capillary pressure is normal and edema fluid is rich in protein.

---

234 Compare the pathogenesis of acute pulmonary edema due to pulmonary embolism with large thrombi (massive) to that observed with multiple small emboli (microemboli).

☐ Acute pulmonary edema in patients with massive pulmonary embolism is due to backward failure of the left ventricle secondary to encroachment of its cavity by the interventricular septum (displaced because of distention of the right ventricle) as well as due to myocardial depression resulting from associated profound hypoxemia. Examples of this form of pulmonary embolism include those secondary to displacement of thrombi originating in the lower extremities, pelvic veins, renal veins, and right atrium. A different pathogenesis has been proposed for the pulmonary edema secondary to microemboli. In this case, intravascular coagulation generates thrombin, which causes platelet aggregation, complement activation, degradation of fibrinogen and fibrin, which eventually leads to pulmonary edema secondary to increased permeability of the alveolar-capillary membrane. An example of microemboli-induced pulmonary edema is that present in patients with endocarditis involving the right side of the heart (e.g., tricuspid endocarditis).

235   What are the mechanisms responsible for the acute pulmonary edema observed in eclampsia?

    ☐ The massive sympathetic discharge and hypervolemia observed in eclampsia are implicated in the acute systemic hypertension, which leads to left ventricular failure and secondary pulmonary edema. Hypoalbuminemia due to renal losses also contributes to fluid accumulation in the lungs and elsewhere. In addition, disseminated intravascular coagulation might play a pathogenetic role in the pulmonary edema of eclampsia.

236   What is the pathogenesis of pulmonary edema observed following general anesthesia?

    ☐ A large positive fluid balance (fluid administration significantly exceeds urine output and other fluid losses) in the course of general anesthesia, especially in patients with heart disease, might precipitate pulmonary edema. Reduction of pulmonary lymphatic drainage due to general anesthesia might explain the development of pulmonary edema when fluid overload and left ventricular dysfunction are absent.

237   What is the pathogenesis of pulmonary edema after cardioversion?

    ☐ Several mechanisms have been implicated in the pathogenesis of pulmonary edema after cardioversion. Possible determinants include ineffective left atrial function immediately following cardioversion (i.e., patients with atrial fibrillation), left ventricular dysfunction, and activation of neural pathways in a manner comparable to that occurring in neurogenic pulmonary edema.

238   Explain the mechanisms responsible for pulmonary edema observed with the use of cardiopulmonary bypass.

    ☐ Possible pathogenetic mechanisms for this type of pulmonary edema include anaphylactic reactions to the infusion of fresh frozen plasma, loss of alveolar surfactant due to pro–

longed lung collapse during the procedure, and barotrauma with high negative intrapleural pressure to reverse lung collapse.

---

239 Is the demonstration of a normal cardiac output (e.g., in the intensive care unit, cardiac catheterization laboratory) in the resting state evidence of normal cardiac function?

☐ No. Many patients with cardiac diseases leading to low output heart failure, particularly at early stages, develop effective compensatory mechanisms such that cardiac outputs in the resting (basal) state are normal. The expanded plasma volume due to salt and water retention augments ventricular end-diastolic pressure, allowing for preservation of near-normal stroke volume and cardiac output. Nevertheless, this failing heart produces less cardiac output for a given ventricular end-diastolic volume. In other words, the cardiac output is kept at the normal level due to increased end-diastolic ventricular volume and pressure. Furthermore, the failing heart is less able to increase cardiac output in response to exercise, even if its output is normal at rest.

---

240 Is the circulation time (e.g., arm to tongue) a sensitive test for the diagnosis of heart failure?

☐ No. The circulation time is not a sensitive test but remains as a useful tool (unfortunately, it is rarely performed in some institutions) for the diagnosis of heart failure. This simple test helps to differentiate high output from low output heart failure, and pulmonary from cardiac dyspnea. The prolonged circulation time observed in patients with low output cardiac failure is due to reduced velocity of blood flow and to dilution of the test substance (3 to 5 mL of 20% dehydrocholic acid or Decholin) by the increased blood volume within the congested venous systems in the systemic and pulmonary circulations.

---

241 What is the Valsalva maneuver?

☐ The Valsalva maneuver is a forced expiration against a resistance (e.g., closed glottis, column of water, manometer) so that intrathoracic pressure rises, producing characteristic hemodynamic effects. This test has been standardized and is useful in the diagnosis of heart failure.

---

242   How is the standardized Valsalva maneuver performed and what are its hemodynamic effects in normal individuals?

□ The patient is asked to forcefully expire (blow) against a resistance of 40 mmHg (aneroid manometer) for 30 seconds. Intrathoracic pressure rises during the Valsalva maneuver, decreasing systemic venous return to the heart and leading to reduced stroke volume and increased systemic venous pressure. The following changes in blood pressure and heart rate occur. (1) Arterial pressure immediately rises with initiation of the expiration effort due to transmission of the increased intrathoracic pressure. (2) Thereafter, arterial pressure decreases (systolic, diastolic, and pulse pressure levels) due to diminished systemic venous return during sustained expiration; the arterial hypotension characteristic of this phase produces reflex tachycardia mediated by depressed activity of arterial baroreceptors. (3) Subsequently, blood pressure decreases further on release of expiration effort due to transmission of the fall in intrathoracic pressure. (4) Finally, arterial pressure and pulse pressure abruptly increase accompanied by reflex bradycardia on discontinuation of the expiratory effort; the increase in systemic venous return observed during this phase produces the rise in blood pressure, which in turn acts on arterial baroreceptors (stimulation) to produce reflex bradycardia. Thus, changes in blood pressure during phases 1 and 3 (initiation and interruption of expiratory effort) of the Valsalva maneuver result from transmission of changes in intrathoracic pressure and, thereby, are independent of hemodynamic responses. Consequently, only phases 2 and 4 of the Valsalva maneuver evaluate cardiovascular function.

---

243   What are the hemodynamic effects of the Valsalva maneuver in patients with heart failure?

□ Patients with heart failure exhibit neither the decreased arterial pressure with tachycardia of phase 2 (sustained expiration) nor the increased arterial pressure with bradycardia of phase 4 (recovery phase postexpiration) that are characteristic of normal individuals. The lack of changes in arterial pressure during phases 2 and 4 of patients with heart failure is due to the constancy of their stroke volume throughout the course of this maneuver. The absence of reflex tachycardia and bradycardia of phases 2 and 4, respectively, are due to the lack of inhibition and stimulation, respectively, of arterial baroreceptors, leading to a constant arterial pressure during these phases. Careful examination of the arterial pulse during the Valsalva maneuver allows recognition of the changes in heart rate observed in normal individuals and their absence in heart failure. A more rigorous evaluation of all the hemodynamic effects of the Valsalva maneuver requires insertion of an indwelling needle/catheter connected to a blood pressure transducer and a recorder for examination of the tracing. Changes in intra-arterial pressure during the Valsalva maneuver in normal individuals can be summarized as follows: increase, decrease, further decrease, and recovery, for phases 1, 2, 3, and 4, respectively. Because the increased (phase 1) and decreased (phase 3) blood pressure that accompany initiation and termination of respiratory effort are also present in patients with heart failure, while blood pressure changes of phases 2 and 4 are absent, the tracing in cardiac failure resembles a "square wave." That is, blood pressure increases on initiation of the maneuver and remains elevated as long as the expiratory effort is sustained and decreases on discontinuation of forced expiration in patients with heart failure.

---

244 Provide a classification of heart failure according to its pathogenesis.

☐ Heart failure might be caused by: (1) increased preload (e.g., mitral insufficiency, aortic insufficiency, arteriovenous shunt and other forms of high-output cardiac failure); (2) increased afterload (e.g., hypertension, aortic stenosis, and coarctation of the aorta produce left-sided heart failure; pulmonic stenosis, embolism, or hypertension of the pulmonary circuit produce right-sided heart failure); and (3) structural (e.g., congenital and acquired defects) and functional (e.g., depression of myocardial contractility) cardiac abnormalities. Diseases of the myocardial fibers that might lead to diminished contractility can be further classified into primary and secondary ones. Primary abnormalities include cardiomyopathy (e.g., idiopathic, alcoholic, amyloidosis) and myocarditis. The most prominent secondary abnormality of the myocardial fibers is ischemic heart disease. Causes of heart failure due to structural abnormalities of the heart other than the myocardial fibers (myocytes) include valvular diseases, congenital defects, pericardial abnormalities, and ventricular aneurysm.

---

245   How might the causes of circulatory failure be classified?

☐ Circulatory failure might result from abnormalities in heart function (see previous question on causes of heart failure according to pathogenesis), the circulating fluid (volume or viscosity of blood/plasma), or the blood vessels (resistance or permeability). Examples of decreased intravascular volume and increased fluid viscosity that might lead to circulatory failure are gastrointestinal hemorrhage and polycythemia/ hyperproteinemia, respectively. Examples of decreased vascular resistance and increased vessel permeability that might cause circulatory failure are sepsis-induced vasodilation and anaphylactic shock, respectively.

---

246   What are the two general pathogenetic mechanisms that might lead to myocardial failure?

☐ Myocardial failure occurs because of either a quantitative or a qualitative defect in the myocardium. A quantitative defect is due to a reduction in the number of functioning myofibers and is exemplified by heart failure secondary to a large myocardial infarction. A qualitative defect is characterized by a generalized abnormality in myocardial performance without a reduction in the number of functioning myocytes. A representative example of a qualitative abnormality is idiopathic cardiomyopathy.

247   What are the precise mechanisms of cellular dysfunction in myocardial failure?

☐ Substantial controversy remains as to the specific cellular defects leading to myocardial failure. Proposed mechanisms include: (1) a reduction of myosin ATPase activity; (2) a defective SR with diminished ability to retrieve Ca^{++} released during contraction; (3) a reduction in coronary blood flow and cardiac oxygen consumption per unit of tissue plus mitochondrial dysfunction; (4) decreased cardiac norepinephrine stores reducing the efficacy of compensatory mechanisms for heart failure; and (5) diastolic dysfunction due to myocardial hypertrophy and excess collagen deposition. It is likely that more than one mechanism is operative in any given case of myocardial failure. Furthermore, the specific defect might depend on the cause (e.g., ischemic heart disease, myocarditis, etc.) of heart failure.

248   Compare the normal Frank-Starling curve with that of myocardial failure.

☐ Because initial muscle length determines the force of contraction, the increased end-diastolic volume (or preload) in myocardial failure improves ventricular output. Yet, the higher end-diastolic pressure required to maintain cardiac output increases hydrostatic pressure in pulmonary capillaries and might aggravate dyspnea and even precipitate pulmonary edema. In addition, for any given increase in end-diastolic volume and pressure, patients with heart failure respond with a smaller stroke volume (i.e., amount of blood pumped forward by a single contraction of the ventricle). It is apparent that the Starling curve in myocardial failure is displaced to the right on the horizontal axis (e.g., increased ventricular end-diastolic volume) and has a diminished height on the vertical axis (e.g., decreased systolic work of the ventricle).

249   What are the major causes of right-sided heart failure?

☐ The major causes of right-sided heart failure are: (1) chronic left-sided congestive heart failure such as that due to ischemic or valvular heart disease; (2) mitral stenosis with pulmonary hypertension; (3) cor pulmonale due to chronic obstructive pulmonary disease (COPD); (4) pulmonary hypertension due either to an unknown cause (primary form), congenital heart abnormalities, or collagen vascular diseases; (5) valvular diseases of the right ventricle including pulmonic stenosis, tricuspid stenosis and regurgitation; and (6) myocardial diseases of the right ventricle such as infarction and dysplasia involving this chamber.

---

250   What pathophysiologic mechanism is commonly present in high cardiac output states (hyperdynamic or hyperkinetic circulation)?

☐ A decreased systemic vascular resistance is generally found in high cardiac output states. Such reduction in vascular resistance (e.g., arteriovenous fistula, anemia) tends to decrease mean arterial pressure (it lowers cardiac afterload) and increase mean venous pressure (it augments cardiac preload) because of greater transmission of pressure from the arterial to the venous compartment. Consequently, increased venous return participates in maintenance of the hyperdynamic circulation. Sympathetic activation might also produce a high cardiac output state in which heart stimulation might be intense. A practical classification of hyperdynamic conditions based on the dominant defect include: (1) increased preload, observed in states of enlarged blood volume and reduced venous compliance; (2) decreased afterload, observed when systemic vascular resistance is diminished due to anatomic (e.g., systemic arteriovenous fistulae), functional (e.g., pregnancy, sepsis, thyrotoxicosis), pharmacologic (e.g., hydralazine, captopril, enalapril), and rheologic (e.g., anemia) factors; (3) cardiovascular activation secondary to neurogenic (e.g., β_1-sympathetic stimulation), humoral (e.g., serotonin), and pharmacologic (e.g., isoproterenol, terbutaline, amrinone) influences.

---

251   What are the most common causes of a hyperkinetic circulation (hyperdynamic state at rest)? Name other causes of high cardiac output state and their roles in causing heart failure.

☐ The most common causes of a hyperdynamic circulation at rest are emotional excitement, fever, and pregnancy. Except for these causes that are observed daily by the practicing physician/nurse, the conditions most frequently encountered as determinants of a high cardiac output state include liver disease, severe anemia, and thyrotoxicosis. Other causes of high cardiac output state include: (1) central shunting of blood (e.g., patent ductus arteriosus); (2) peripheral shunting of blood (e.g., systemic arteriovenous fistulae); (3) vasodilation of peripheral circulation (e.g., thyrotoxicosis); and (4) reduced blood viscosity (e.g. anemia). Not unusually, two or more of these mechanisms are superimposed in a patient and their combined effects play a role the development of high output. It must be recognized that high cardiac output states by themselves are seldom responsible for heart failure in the absence of underlying heart disease (e.g., ischemic heart disease, hypertension). However, a hyperkinetic state commonly precipitates cardiac failure when superimposed on an abnormal heart.

---

252   Does renal salt and water retention occur in high output cardiac failure?

☐ Yes. Salt and water are retained in both low and high output heart failure (e.g., thyrotoxicosis, vitamin B_1 deficiency known as beriberi). Underfilling of the arterial compartment is present in both types of heart failure but is due to different mechanisms. A reduced entry of blood to the arterial compartment (and normal exit) occurs in low cardiac output failure, whereas an increased exit/run-off of blood (and normal entry) due to arteriolar vasodilation develops in high cardiac output failure. Thus, a reduced effective arterial blood volume is present in low and high cardiac output failure.

---

253   Compare the intensity of cardiac stress to altered ventricular loading in mitral versus aortic regurgitation and ventricular septal defect versus patent ductus arteriosus.

☐ For an equivalent stroke volume (total and effective, referring to forward plus backward volume in the former, and net forward volume in the latter) mitral regurgitation imposes lesser cardiac stress with lower end-diastolic volume and pressure than aortic regurgitation. Although increased preload is observed in these two conditions, ejection and subsequent return of regurgitant volume from the low-pressure left atrium (mitral defect) produces a milder cardiac stress than ejection and subsequent return of regurgitant volume from the high-pressure aorta (aortic defect). In a comparable manner, for an equivalent left-to-right shunt, ventricular septal defect imposes lesser cardiac stress (the shunted blood is ejected in the low-pressure right ventricle) than patent ductus arteriosus. Left ventricular ejection is facilitated in mitral regurgitation and ventricular septal defect (because blood leaves the left ventricle in early systole) and the afterload reduction diminishes myocardial oxygen consumption. On the other hand, the impedance to ventricular ejection is not facilitated in aortic regurgitation and patent ductus arteriosus.

---

254   Is the natural history of heart failure generally characterized by a steady progressive downward course or by abrupt steps of deterioration of cardiac function?

☐ Bouts of acute worsening of heart function rather than a slow smooth downward course characterize the natural history of heart failure. Consequently, measures should be taken to prevent the precipitating causes of heart failure (e.g., systemic anticoagulation as a prophylactic measure of pulmonary embolism in some patients with myocardiopathies and atrial fibrillation) as well as promptly and effectively treating all causes of cardiac decompensation. This approach might lead to stabilization of heart failure for months or even years. Nevertheless, some patients with asymptomatic heart failure might have stable cardiac function for many years, whereas other patients might experience a gradual (as opposed to abrupt) decline of their heart condition over time.

---

255   Describe the concept of precipitating causes of heart failure.

☐ Precipitating causes of heart failure are those conditions that might prompt symptoms of heart failure in patients with clinically silent heart disease or worsen the syndrome in patients known to have this condition. Proper recognition of precipitating causes is important because adequate management of this new insult might return the patient's clinical condition to baseline status.

---

256   What are the most important precipitating causes of heart failure?

☐   Major precipitating causes of heart failure include: (1) cardiac conditions such as arrhythmias, myocardial ischemia, endocarditis, and pericarditis; (2) noncardiac diseases such as systemic infection and pulmonary embolism; (3) fluid overload and hypertension due to excessive salt intake or renal insufficiency (functional or structural); (4) high cardiac output states, including pregnancy, anemia, hyperthyroidism; (5) cardiac depressant drugs (e.g., β-adrenergic blockers); and (6) lack of compliance to an effective drug regimen.   Often more than one precipitating cause worsens signs and symptoms of heart failure in a given patient.

---

257   How might cardiac arrhythmias precipitate heart failure?

☐   Cardiac arrhythmias might precipitate heart failure because of marked changes in heart rate, loss of effective atrial contraction, or loss of normal synchronicity of ventricular systole.   Marked changes in heart rate include tachyarrhythmias originating in the atria (i.e., atrial fibrillation, atrial flutter, multifocal atrial tachycardia) or the ventricles (i.e., ventricular tachycardia) and marked bradycardia.   Tachyarrhythmias might shorten diastole, thereby reducing ventricular filling.   These fast rhythms also increase myocardial oxygen demand possibly leading to worsening myocardial ischemia, which in turn impairs cardiac contraction and relaxation. Marked bradycardia can depress cardiac output because stroke volume might not increase enough to completely compensate for the decreased heart rate.   Loss of effective atrial contraction (i.e., atrial fibrillation/flutter, junctional rhythms) decreases ventricular filling, and as a consequence, reduces cardiac output and increases atrial pressure.   Loss of the atrial "kick" might greatly reduce ventricular filling in patients with rigid hearts (e.g., severe diastolic dysfunction observed in patients with concentric cardiac hypertrophy including aortic stenosis, systemic hypertension, and hypertrophic cardiomyopathy). Loss of normal synchronicity of ventricular systole might occur in patients with abnormal intraventricular conduction (e.g., bundle branch block). Arrhythmias might be lethal in patients with heart failure.

---

258 What are the major factors that predispose to cardiac arrhythmias and sudden death in patients with heart failure? What effects might angiotensin-converting enzyme (ACE) inhibitors have on cardiac arrhythmias?

☐ Major factors that predispose to arrhythmias include: (1) positive inotropic agents (e.g., digitalis, nonglycoside inotropic agents); (2) proarrhythmogenic effects of antiarrhythmic drugs (e.g., quinidine); (3) electrolyte disturbances (e.g., hypokalemia, hypomagnesemia, hyponatremia); (4) high plasma catecholamines and sympathetic activation; (5) coronary artery disease and all forms of myocardial ischemia; (6) hypotension of any cause; and (7) cardiac enlargement and myocardial stretching. A close interrelationship exists between the renin-angiotensin system and the sympathetic nervous system such that activation of either of these mechanisms exerts stimulatory effects on the other. This interrelationship explains the depressor effects of ACE inhibitors as well as that of β blockers on both the renin-angiotensin and the sympathetic nervous system activation. Furthermore, inhibition of the neurohormonal pathways involved in the so-called compensatory (yet they are truly deleterious in the long term) mechanisms of heart failure with β blockers and ACE inhibitors can partly explain the salutary effects of these drugs. ACE inhibitors might reduce premature ventricular complexes by mechanisms that include an increase in body stores and serum level of potassium, a decrease in myocardial oxygen consumption, reduction of sympathetic tone, as well as unloading of the left ventricle, which reduces chamber size and stretch-induced arrhythmias.

259 What electrolyte abnormalities might play a pathogenetic role as determinants of ventricular arrhythmias and sudden death in patients with heart failure?

☐ Potassium and Mg^{++} depletion due to increased urinary losses caused by loop and thiazide diuretics as well as from secondary hyperaldosteronism might lead to ventricular arrhythmias and sudden death. In addition, K^+ and Mg^{++} depletion increases the risk for digitalis toxicity, which might cause ventricular arrhythmias and sudden death. Consequently, depletion of these electrolytes must be avoided in the management of patients with congestive heart failure. Although hyponatremia is associated with an increased risk of cardiac arrhythmias (possibly due to the concomitant activation of the sympathetic and angiotensin-aldosterone systems), this electrolyte disturbance most likely does not play a direct role as a determinant of cardiac arrhythmias.

260 Might physical, emotional, and environmental factors precipitate heart failure in susceptible individuals?

☐ Yes. Physical activity of unusually high intensity or prolonged duration might precipitate cardiac decompensation. Similarly, intense emotions might trigger episodes of heart failure. Additionally, a hot and humid environment might initiate clinical manifestations of heart failure because of the hemodynamic strain on the heart due to generalized skin vasodilation (aimed at dissipation of heat).

261 What cardioinhibitory substances or drugs might precipitate heart failure?

☐ Excessive alcohol intake can precipitate heart failure in patients with compensated cardiac disease. Many drugs including β-adrenoreceptor blocking agents (e.g., propranolol), calcium channel blockers (e.g., verapamil), antiarrhythmic agents (e.g., quinidine), and antineoplastic drugs (e.g., doxorubicin, cyclophosphamide) have cardioinhibitory properties and therefore are potential causes of cardiac decompensation that might lead to heart failure. It should be recognized that these agents might be safely used in many patients with heart disease despite the potential risk of inducing heart failure.

---

262   How might myocarditis and endocarditis precipitate heart failure?

☐ Depression of myocardial function due to myocarditis (e.g., acute rheumatic fever, viral myocardial infections) or bacterial endocarditis (e.g., acute infective endocarditis due to staphylococci, subacute bacterial endocarditis due to streptococci) might precipitate heart failure. Valvular damage due to bacterial endocarditis further aggravates the concomitant myocardial depression. Fever, anemia, and tachycardia accompany myocarditis and pericarditis, worsening the syndrome of heart failure.

---

263   How might pulmonary embolism precipitate heart failure? What are its manifestations and the factors that predispose to the development of this complication?

☐ Pulmonary embolism obstructs the arterial circulation within the lung and increases its pressure, thereby inducing systolic overload of the right ventricle. Common manifestations include tachycardia, tachypnea, cyanosis, and fever. Bed confinement is a major predisposing factor for the development of pulmonary embolism because the venous stasis that accompanies immobilization promotes blood clot formation in major veins of the pelvic cavity and lower extremities.

---

264   Can noncardiac diseases precipitate heart failure?

☐ Yes. Noncardiac diseases might precipitate heart failure in patients with compensated cardiac disease. A febrile syndrome independent of its cause, anemia, as well as fluid retention due to noncardiac mechanisms (e.g., renal disease) are some of the noncardiac conditions that might produce heart decompensation. Fluid accumulation that precipitates heart failure might be due to blood transfusions, administration of drugs (e.g., estrogens, androgens, corticosteroids, and nonsteroidal anti-inflammatory agents), development of an un-related salt-retaining renal or hepatic disease, and obstructive uropathy (e.g., prostatic enlargement).

---

265 What endocrine disorder should be considered among the possible precipitating causes of heart failure?

☐ Thyrotoxicosis might precipitate heart failure because this condition imposes an increased work load on the heart to sat-isfy the abnormally high oxygen demand of peripheral tissues. Correction of thyrotoxicosis rapidly reverses the heart failure. Elderly individuals are at increased risk of thyrotoxicosis-in-duced heart failure because of the concomitant presence of organic heart disease (e.g., ischemic myocardiopathy). Failu-re to diagnose thyrotoxicosis is responsible for treatment failure in a small but clinically important group of patients with heart failure.

---

266 Describe the adaptive responses to an acute reduction in cardiac output.

☐ The major adaptive responses to an acute reduction in cardiac output are vasoconstriction and salt and water retention. Vasoconstriction is primarily due to activation of the neurohormonal systems leading to increased secretion of catecholamines, stimulation of the renin-angiotensin system, and increased production of arginine vasopressin. Norepinephrine, angiotensin, and vasopressin induce constriction of vascular smooth muscle of resistance vessels, helping to sustain arterial pressure. Consequently, perfusion of major organs including the brain and heart is restored. Salt and water retention by the kidney occurs because of decreased renal perfusion and stimulation of the neurohormonal mechanisms acting on renal tubules. The resulting expansion of plasma volume increases ventricular end-diastolic volume and thereby restores the diminished cardiac output. The adaptive responses to acute reduction in cardiac output are similar to those induced by acute hemorrhage. The short-term effects of these homeostatic mechanisms are salutary. Nevertheless, when these mechanisms are chronically sustained, they might be detrimental for long-term survival.

267   What factors stimulate and which ones depress myocardial contractility in the intact organism?

☐ Myocardial contractility at any given ventricular end-diastolic volume is stimulated by the following major factors: (1) sympathetic nerve activity; (2) circulating catecholamines derived from the adrenal medulla and carried by the blood stream to the myocardium; (3) inotropic effect of a higher heart rate; and (4) exogenous inotropic agents (e.g., cardiac glycosides, sympathomimetic agents, caffeine, theophylline, amrinone). In a comparable manner, myocardial contractility at any given ventricular end-diastolic volume is depressed by the following major factors: (1) myocardial anoxia, ischemia, and acidosis; (2) drugs including calcium antagonists, β-adrenoreceptor blocking agents, norepinephrine-depleting drugs (e.g., barbiturates, local anesthetics, most general anesthetics); (3) parasympathetic or vagal nerve activity; (4) intrinsic myocardial depression (e.g., primary myocardiopathies); and (5) loss of contractile mass (e.g., myocardial infarction).

268   Is tachycardia (increased heart rate) a compensatory mechanism recruited in heart failure?

☐ Yes. Tachycardia is a compensatory mechanism that might allow the heart to maintain cardiac output when stroke volume is reduced. The increased heart rate, however, increases cardiac oxygen consumption, which might in turn produce myocardial ischemia, possibly aggravating the patient's condition.

269   Describe the compensatory mechanisms enlisted in heart failure.

☐ Compensatory mechanisms are recruited to improve pumping ability in cases of myocardial failure or increased ventricular work load (e.g., hypertension, aortic valve disease). Short-term compensatory mechanisms include those dependent on the initial length-force of contraction relationship defined by Frank-Starling and the activation of neurohormonal systems (i.e., sympathetic nervous system, renin-angiotensin-aldosterone system, and ADH). The neurohormonal activation may persist for long periods and have nonsalutary effects. Long-term compensatory mechanisms also include two different patterns of ventricular hypertrophy (i.e., concentric hypertrophy in response to pressure overload and eccentric hypertrophy in response to volume overload). Presumably, the substantial increase in wall thickness and relatively small volume of chamber cavity in a chronically pressure-overloaded ventricle (e.g., concentric left ventricular hypertrophy in systemic hypertension) is due to augmented systolic pressure within this chamber and thereby a higher systolic wall stress that leads to parallel addition of new myofibrils (i.e., wall thickening). On the other hand, the mild increase in wall thickness and relatively large volume of chamber cavity in a volume-overloaded ventricle (e.g., eccentric left ventricular hypertrophy in arteriovenous fistula) is due to augmented diastolic pressure within this chamber and thereby a higher diastolic wall stress that leads to addition of new sarcomeres in series (i.e., enlargement of ventricular chamber). Signals for cardiac growth due to higher stress (i.e., increased preload, increased afterload, primary loss of myocytes, primary depression of contractility) alter gene expression producing the so-called compensatory cardiac hypertrophy.

270 How do the compensatory mechanisms of heart failure relate to the clinical manifestations of this condition?

☐ The compensatory mechanisms of heart failure allow maintenance of cardiac output in the setting of compromised heart function. Thus, these compensatory mechanisms delay the appearance of signs and symptoms of heart failure. Eventually, cardiac dysfunction progresses to point at which compensatory mechanisms are unable to maintain a satisfactory cardiac output and the clinical syndrome of heart failure becomes clinically evident.

271 Compare the relative contribution of each neurohormonal compensatory mechanism to the vasoconstriction observed in congestive heart failure.

☐ Several neurohormonal factors are progressively activated in heart failure as the severity of this condition increases.

Such neurohormonal responses, which are aimed at maintaining arterial pressure in states of decreased cardiac output, include the following factors arranged in order of importance with respect to their relative vasoconstrictor effects: (1) sympathetic stimulation and increased plasma catecholamine levels; (2) activation of renin-angiotensin-aldosterone system; (3) increased secretion of arginine vasopressin (ADH); and (4) augmented levels of atrial natriuretic factors. The relative importance of each mechanism can be assessed with the use of specific antagonists that counteract the vasoconstriction produced by a given neurohormonal factor. Because atrial natriuretic substances are virtually free of constrictor effects, they are positioned at the end of the listed factors. Infusion of an arginine vasopressin antagonist produces only minimal vasodilation in patients with heart failure. By contrast, ACE inhibitors such as captopril produce significant vasodilation accompanied by an increase in cardiac output and a reduction in ventricular filling pressure. The greatest hypotensive effect occurs in response to α-adrenergic blockers (e.g., phentolamine) that antagonize the peripheral vasoconstrictor action of the sympathetic system and circulating catecholamines. Consequently, α-adrenergic blockers can produce the largest increase in cardiac output and the greatest reduction in diastolic filling pressure.

272   Explain the mechanisms that maintain near-normal levels of renal blood flow and glomerular filtration rate in congestive heart failure, liver cirrhosis, and nephrosis (nephrotic syndrome).

☐ Increased renal production of vasodilatory prostaglandins induced by decreased effective arterial blood volume maintains near-normal renal function in patients with congestive heart failure, liver cirrhosis, and nephrotic syndrome. The importance of vasodilatory prostaglandins is supported by the development of acute renal failure in patients with these diseases who receive prostaglandin inhibitors such as nonsteroidal anti-inflammatory drugs (NSAIDs).

---

273 What are the possible adverse effects of NSAIDs on renal function and on salt, water, and potassium balance?

☐ NSAIDs are characterized by their property to inhibit prostaglandin synthesis and are used in the treatment of common aches and pains, as well as rheumatologic diseases. If NSAIDs are administered to patients with volume depletion, hypotension, renal ischemia, or edematous states (e.g., congestive heart failure, cirrhosis of the liver, nephrotic syndrome), the following major drug-related adverse effects can develop: acute renal failure, hypertension, hyperkalemia, Na^+ retention, and water retention leading to hyponatremia. The adverse renal effects of NSAIDs are more likely to occur in the disease states previously mentioned because increased synthesis of renal prostaglandins contributes to the compensatory mechanisms that help to maintain renal function in these conditions.

---

274 What are the major abnormalities in the peripheral circulation and their respective salutary effects (compensatory mechanisms) in patients with heart failure?

☐ The major abnormalities in the peripheral circulation and their corresponding salutary effects (compensatory mechanisms) in patients with heart failure include: (1) venoconstriction that mobilizes blood from the capacitance system, increasing cardiac preload, thereby improving cardiac performance by the Frank-Starling mechanism; (2) arteriolar constriction that helps to restore tissue perfusion by augmenting mean arterial pressure; (3) altered regional blood flow that allows preservation of coronary and cerebral blood flow due to redistribution of cardiac output; (4) decreased peripheral vasodilation in response to normal stimuli, thereby preventing a major decrease in blood flow to vital organs (i.e., myocardium, brain) that would develop if the increased demand for blood flow by nonvital organs (i.e., skeletal muscle) were to be satisfied; and (5) blunting of baroreceptor reflexes that might prevent a critical reduction of blood flow to already underperfused tissues (e.g., kidneys) on activation of baroreceptors (e.g., by assuming a standing position). It should be recognized that the above-mentioned abnormalities of the peripheral circulation might also have deleterious effects that are described in the answer to a subsequent question. Another abnormality of patients with heart failure is the extremely low concentration of norepinephrine in both atrial and ventricular myocardium (norepinephrine levels correlate directly with ejection fraction and inversely with plasma norepinephrine concentration).

---

275 What are the compensatory mechanisms in chronic pulmonary edema that diminish the intensity of clinical manifestations as compared with those of acute pulmonary edema?

☐ These compensatory mechanisms include: (1) increased precapillary (arteriolar) vascular resistance, which reduces the transmission of arterial pressure to the pulmonary capillaries so that fluid transudation from the capillaries to the alveolar space is reduced; this "compensatory" response aggravates pulmonary hypertension and leads to chronic cor pulmonale; (2) thickening of alveoli walls and septa due to chronic passive congestion that inhibits fluid transudation into pulmonary alveoli secondary to imbalance of Starling forces; (3) desensitization of "j" receptors in the pulmonary interstitium so that the threshold for dyspnea is increased; and (4) reduction of physical activity leading many of these patients to bed confinement; in this way cardiac output is maintained at a basal level so that blood pressure in all areas of the pulmonary circulation is at its lowest value.

---

276 Do compensatory mechanisms of heart failure have effects on cardiac function that might be not beneficial or even harmful?

☐ Yes. Activation of neurohormonal systems in heart failure including sympathetic stimulation and increased release of renin and vasopressin promote salt and water retention and increase systemic vascular resistance. These compensatory mechanisms of heart failure might increase afterload of the left ventricle, reduce stroke volume, and worsen congestion in the pulmonary and systemic circulations. Sympathetic stimulation increases heart rate and might precipitate myocardial ischemia and arrhythmias. Thus, compensatory mechanisms of heart failure might be salutary or harmful depending on multiple factors such as severity of the disease, intensity of adaptive mechanisms, and cardiac and noncardiac responses to these compensatory mechanisms.

---

277 What is the so-called vicious cycle in the pathophysiology of congestive heart failure?

☐ Depression of left ventricular function in patients with congestive heart failure reduces cardiac output. Short-term compensatory responses to the diminution of forward blood flow include vasoconstriction, and salt plus water retention due to the combined activation of the sympathetic nervous system, the renin-angiotensin-aldosterone system, and increased levels of arginine vasopressin (AVP or ADH). Counterregulatory responses that partially offset the previously mentioned compensatory responses (i.e., vasoconstriction and volume expansion) include increased levels of certain prostaglandins, atrial natriuretic peptide, and dopamine, all of which have vasodilatory and natriuretic effects. Because the compensatory responses are of greater intensity than the counterregulatory responses, increased vascular resistance and excessive salt retention augment impedance (afterload) to left ventricular ejection. The higher afterload further reduces left ventricular performance leading to an even lower cardiac output, so that a new cycle of deteriorated cardiac function is initiated (vicious cycle).

---

278 Explain how the compensatory mechanisms of heart failure might produce deleterious hemodynamic effects in patients with this condition.

☐ Mild to moderate sympathetic activation and increased catecholamine levels might produce salutary effects (e.g., stimulation of myocardial contractility that increase cardiac output), yet excessive activation of this neurohormonal system might be counterproductive (e.g., excessive tachycardia that critically shortens the time for diastolic filling, increased myocardial oxygen demand leading to cardiac ischemic damage and higher risk for arrhythmias). Activation of the renin-angiotensin-aldosterone system in heart failure due to decreased renal perfusion (in turn caused by a reduction in both cardiac output and arterial pressure) might help to increase stroke volume by the Frank-Starling mechanism due to augmented cardiac preload mediated by the renal retention of salt and water (ECF volume expansion) and restoration of normal blood pressure (mild systemic vasoconstriction). Nevertheless, an overshoot of this compensatory mechanism might cause excessive fluid retention (e.g., producing pulmonary edema) and a harmful increase in left ventricular afterload (due to a substantial rise in systemic vascular resistance that occurs with arteriolar constriction) that have deleterious hemodynamic effects. High levels of vasopressin might help to maintain blood pressure in heart failure (due to arteriolar vasoconstriction), yet it might lead to excessive water retention and hypotonic hyponatremia (antidiuretic effect). Consequently, activation of neurohormonal mechanisms in heart failure might be either beneficial or counterproductive depending on the intensity of the effects and the overall condition of the patient.

---

279   What are the major abnormalities in the peripheral circulation and their respective deleterious effects (of the so-called compensatory mechanisms) in patients with heart failure?

☐ The major abnormalities in the peripheral circulation and their corresponding deleterious effects (of the so-called compensatory mechanisms) in patients with heart failure include: (1) venoconstriction, which shifts blood from the systemic circulation to the pulmonary circuit producing congestion or edema in the respiratory tract and alveoli; (2) arteriolar constriction, which increases systemic vascular resistance, augmenting left ventricular afterload; (3) altered regional blood flows, which might seriously compromise renal function due to severe underperfusion of the kidney; (4) decreased peripheral vasodilation to normal physiologic stimuli, which impairs the circulatory adaptation to exercise because of excessive sympathetic tone and plasma norepinephrine levels at low work loads; and (5) blunting of baroreceptor reflexes that account for the lack of change in plasma norepinephrine level that normally occurs in response to assuming an upright position in patients with congestive heart failure. The mechanism responsible for the abnormal baroreceptor response in heart failure remains undefined. As previously explained, this baroreceptor abnormality can be clinically demonstrated with the Valsalva maneuver.

---

280 Summarize the mechanisms wherein persistent neurohormonal stimulation observed in low cardiac output states might be detrimental to heart function.

☐ Persistent neurohormonal stimulation adversely affects cardiac performance by multiple mechanisms including: (1) elevation of systemic vascular resistance (thereby increasing afterload) and (2) remodeling the cardiac chambers so that a less efficient contraction (relatively high oxygen consumption per liter of cardiac output) develops. The increased systemic vascular resistance is due to the additive effects of functional (contraction of vascular smooth muscle of arterioles) and structural (thickening of vascular walls due to hypertrophy and proliferation of smooth muscle and other components of blood vessels) changes. In addition, persistent neurohormonal stimulation desensitizes myocardial catecholamine receptors, further reducing ventricular contractility. Pharmacologic intervention (e.g., α blockers, β blockers, ACE inhibitors, AVP antagonists, vasodilators, diuretics, dopaminergic receptor agonists, atrial natriuretic peptide) helps to counterbalance the negative cardiovascular effects of persistent neurohormonal stimulation.

---

281 Recapitulate the main salutary and nonsalutary effects of the compensatory mechanisms of heart failure.

☐ Salutary and nonsalutary effects of compensatory mechanisms of heart failure include: (1) the compensatory increase in end-diastolic volume and pressure increases myocardial contractile force through the Frank-Starling mechanism (salutary action); yet when end-diastolic pressure reaches high levels, pulmonary and peripheral congestion and edema develop (nonsalutary action); (2) the compensatory increase in sympathetic tone augments myocardial contractility and helps maintain tissue perfusion pressure (salutary action); yet when sympathetic activation is intense, tachycardia and peripheral vasoconstriction (increased afterload) lead to a substantial increase in myocardial oxygen consumption (nonsalutary action); (3) the compensatory stimulation of the renin-angiotensin-aldosterone system increases diastolic filling pressure due to renal retention of salt and water as well as helps to maintain tissue perfusion pressure due to vasoconstrictor effects (salutary actions); yet, when these effects are excessive, systemic and venous pulmonary congestion occur and increased cardiac afterload develops, leading to a rise in myocardial oxygen consumption (nonsalutary action); and (4) the compensatory ventricular hypertrophy provides more contractile elements increasing myocardial systolic function (salutary action); yet, this ventricular hypertropy might lead to substantial heart enlargement with abnormal diastolic relaxation leading to systemic and pulmonary congestion as well as excessive myocardial oxygen consumption (nonsalutary action).

---

282   Is the reduced caliber of small arteries and arterioles in patients with heart failure exclusively due to functional changes? What is the effect of increased constrictor tone?

□ No. The reduced caliber of small arteries and arterioles in heart failure is due to a combination of structural alterations in the vascular wall and to increased vasoconstrictor tone. Structural changes in the vasculature might include a smaller lumen size due to vascular smooth muscle growth, remodeling of the vascular smooth muscle, or an increase in the Na^+ and water content of the arterial/arteriolar wall. The increased vasoconstrictor tone in heart failure is due to: (1) activation of the sympathetic nervous system and transient elevation of norepinephrine concentration; (2) increased levels of angiotension II due to stimulation of the renin-angiotensin system; (3) augmented secretion of arginine vasopressin, a potent circulating vasoconstrictor; (4) high endothelin (an endothelium-derived constrictor substance) levels; and (5) reduced endogenous release of nitric oxide, also known as endothelium-derived relaxing factor. Constriction of small arteries and arterioles has effects on peripheral tissues (further reduction in blood perfusion), blood pressure (increases its level, thereby helping to restore tissue perfusion), and on the heart (augmented impedance to left ventricular outflow or afterload). The constrictor influences are also determinants of the increased tone of the venous vasculature (or capacitance vessels) in heart failure. The enhanced tone in capacitance vessels increases cardiac preload, facilitates formation of peripheral edema by increasing pressure in systemic capillaries, reduces peripheral storage capacity of the venous system, and shifts blood toward the cardiac chambers and pulmonary circulation.

283 How might angiotensin II affect patients with heart failure?

□ Angiotensin II has multiple biologic effects including: (1) arteriolar vasoconstriction; (2) enhancement of sympathetic nervous system activity (e.g., it activates presynaptic neuronal receptors that increase release of norepinephrine); (3) stimulation of aldosterone release from the adrenal gland; (4) vessel hypertrophy with proliferation of smooth muscle cells; (5) myocardial hypertrophy due to direct actions on cardiocytes; (6) increased thirst, by activating the CNS to promote water drinking; (7) renal mesangial contraction that reduces the glomerular filtration rate and increases filtration fraction; (8) constriction of renal efferent arterioles, leading to intraglomerular hypertension; (9) renal Na^+ retention due to direct stimulation of reabsorption by the renal tubules; and (10) stimulation of AVP release by the posterior pituitary gland. These multiple actions of angiotensin II are intensified in patients with severe congestive heart failure.

284 Compare the systemic, circulating, or classic renin-angiotensin system with the local, noncirculating, or tissue renin-angiotensin system.

⊓ The systemic, circulating, or classic renin-angiotensin system includes renin (protease released by the kidney) that cleaves four amino acids from angiotensinogen (α_2 globulin synthetized by the liver) to form angiotensin I. The latter substance is in turn transformed by the carboxypeptidase ACE into angiotensin II, mostly in the pulmonary circulation. Angiotensin II is the active component of the renin-angiotensin system and exerts diverse effects including stimulation of the adrenal gland to secrete aldosterone. The classic renin-angiotensin system has messengers that are transported throughout the body by the circulatory system and allow communication among different organs (e.g., kidney, adrenal gland). The local, noncirculating, or tissue renin-angiotensin system is a physiologic network that acts independently of the classic system and plays an important role in cardiovascular regulation and in the pathogenesis of heart failure. Locally produced angiotensin II within the heart and the vascular wall regulates cardiac contractility, vascular tone, and normal/abnormal growth of myocytes that might lead to hypertrophic changes. All the necessary elements for the local production of angiotensin II (including renin-like activity, angiotensinogen, and ACE) are present in some tissues such as the heart, vascular wall, and brain. Furthermore, activation of the local renin-angiotensin system might increase systemic vascular resistance despite normalcy of the classic system.

---

285   What is the clinical importance of the local, noncirculating, or tissue renin-angiotensin system in patients with heart failure?

☐ Because ACE inhibitors (e.g., captopril, enalapril) exert effects on the tissue and systemic renin-angiotensin systems of patients with heart failure, the salutary effects of these drugs might be mediated in part by their direct action on the local system within the myocardium and the vessel walls. Indeed, the renal and hemodynamic effects of ACE inhibitors in heart failure correlate better with the activity of tissue renin-angiotensin system than with systemic renin-angiotensin. Furthermore, the impact of ACE inhibitors in the management of heart failure and hypertension cannot be adequately explained by their effects on the systemic renin-angiotensin system because salutary actions are commonly observed in patients with normal or even depressed classic renin-angiotensin system. Activation of tissue renin-angiotensin system within the vascular wall might produce smooth muscle constriction, stimulate Na^+ and Ca^{++} transport in smooth muscle, facilitate transmission of sympathetic signals, decrease vascular compliance, and promote abnormal growth of one or more elements of the vascular wall.

286 What are the deleterious effects of a persistently elevated angiotensin II level in patients with heart failure?

☐ A sustained increase in angiotensin II might have nonsalutary effects in heart failure due to: (1) its potent vasoconstrictor action that contributes to the abnormally high systemic vascular resistance; (2) stimulation of sympathetic outflow, which is additive to the preexisting sympathetic stimulation mediated by independent mechanisms; (3) excessive salt and water retention that might compromise alveolar gas exchange producing hypoxemia and thereby exacerbating cardiac dyspnea; and (4) mechanisms incompletely understood that lead to increased mortality.

287 What is the effect of afterload-reducing agents on the Frank-Starling curve of heart failure?

☐ Afterload-reducing agents diminish the forces that oppose ventricular emptying during systole. Thus, these agents allow for a larger stroke volume per systole and secondarily reduce end-diastolic volume and pressure. Consequently, these agents displace the abnormal Frank-Starling curve of heart failure to the left on the horizontal axis (i.e., lower diastolic volume and pressure) and upward along the vertical axis (i.e., higher systolic stroke volume for a given end-diastolic volume) at a given level of ventricular filling. It should be apparent that the effects of afterload-reducing agents in heart failure are additive to those due to positive inotropic agents/maneuvers.

288 What are the effects of diuretics on the Frank Starling curve of heart failure?

☐ Diuretics cause negative fluid balance and thereby reduce end-diastolic volume and pressure in patients with cardiac failure. This effect of diuretics shifts the Frank-Starling curve to the left along the horizontal axis. Although diuretics have their major pharmacologic effect on the kidney rather than on the heart, their effects on body electrolyte composition might secondarily modify cardiac function and myocardial contractility. Diuretic-induced K^+ depletion increases cytosolic

[Ca^{++}]. This change might augment myocardial contractility, displacing the Frank-Starling curve upward along the vertical axis in a fashion comparable to that for positive inotropic agents. The effects of diuretics on cardiac output in patients with heart failure might also be counterproductive because a critical reduction in intravascular volume induced by these agents might drastically reduce end-diastolic pressure, leading to severe forward failure. The latter situation is due to the dependence of cardiac output on high end-diastolic pressure in patients with heart failure.

---

289   What are the effects of positive inotropic agents/maneuvers on the Frank-Starling curve of heart failure?

□ Successful treatment of heart failure with these agents or maneuvers shifts the Starling curve upward and to the left so that a higher stroke volume occurs at lower levels of diastolic volume and pressure. Drugs and conditions that produce this salutary effect on the Starling curve include positive inotropic agents (e.g., digitalis, circulating catecholamines, and drugs that resemble their effects), sympathetic nerve stimulation, any condition that increases the contractile state of the myocardium, and the high frequency-induced stimulation in contractility.

CLINICAL PICTURE OF HEART FAILURE

290 What are the most common causes of congestive heart failure in the general population?

☐ Coronary artery disease is the most common underlying cause of heart failure and accounts for 50% to 75% of patients with this condition. Although hypertension is a contributing factor in some patients with heart failure, the importance of hypertension is substantially smaller than that of coronary artery disease (all clinical forms including myocardial infarction). Cardiomyopathy, including all etiologies, is the next most common cause. Valvular heart disease, especially mitral regurgitation and aortic stenosis, remains as a common cause of heart failure despite the major decline in rheumatic heart disease in developed countries. Congenital heart disease, a leading cause of heart failure in infants and children, represents a small fraction of all patients with heart failure.

291 Provide a practical approach to the causes of heart failure in broad categories that are useful for clinicians evaluating and caring for these patients.

☐ The causes of heart failure can be classified in terms of: (1) structural abnormalities responsible for the heart dysfunction (e.g., congenital defects, acquired heart diseases involving the cardiac valves or the myocardium), also known as underlying causes; (2) functional abnormalities that produce the syndrome of heart failure (e.g., increased preload, increased afterload, reduced oxygen delivery to the myocardium, primary depression of myocardial contractility, diastolic dysfunction), also known as fundamental causes; and (3) precipitating causes that include the specific conditions that initiate/aggravate heart dysfunction leading to overt heart failure. Precipitating causes may be recognized in 50% to 90% of episodes of heart failure. Whenever a clinician confronts a patient with heart failure, the patient's disease should be considered in terms of all three categories previously outlined.

292 Why is it important for clinicians to consider in each patient with heart failure the causes of this illness in terms of structural abnormalities, functional abnormalities, and precipitating causes?

☐ The importance of identifying the structural and functional abnormalities, as well as precipitating causes of heart failure, relates to patient management. Adequate knowledge or understanding of the underlying structural abnormalities, functional abnormalities, and precipitating causes allows the clinician to select therapeutic strategies designed to correct or alleviate each of the three defects responsible for the syndrome of heart failure. Management of a structural abnormality might involve surgery in patients with valvular heart disease (e.g., valve replacement) or severe coronary artery disease (e.g., coronary artery bypass). Therapy of functional abnormalities in these same patients might require the administration of afterload-reducing agents or a digitalis preparation. In addition, such patients might require measures to prevent or treat precipitating causes of heart failure such as the administration of heparin/coumadin (e.g., recurrent pulmonary thromboembolism).

293 Provide a classification of heart disease based on the intensity of physical activity that elicits symptoms.

☐ A widely used functional classification of heart disease is that proposed by the New York Heart Association (NYHA). Patients are classified into the following four groups:

Class I: No limitation of physical activity. Absence of dyspnea, fatigue, and palpitations with ordinary physical activity.

Class II: Slight limitation of physical activity. Ordinary physical activity produces dyspnea, fatigue, or palpitations, but patients are comfortable at rest.

Class III: Marked limitation of physical activity. Symptoms present in class II develop with less than ordinary physical activity, yet patients are comfortable at rest.

Class IV: Symptoms mentioned for other classes are present at rest and their intensity is augmented by any physical activity.

It should be recognized that individuals with normal heart function or incipient heart disease belong to class I. As heart function deteriorates, symptoms develop so that patients move to classes I through III. End-stage heart failure or the more severe forms of the disease produce symptoms in patients at rest (class IV).

---

294 What is the practical value of the NYHA functional classification of heart disease?

☐ The NYHA classification of heart disease, based on subjective manifestations obtained in the clinical history, is useful to compare individuals and groups of patients, to follow the course of their heart failure, and to assess the results of therapy.

---

295 How common is heart failure? What age group is most often affected?

☐ Approximately 400,000 individuals each year develop heart failure in the United States, and this country has about 3 million patients with this disease. Heart failure is most commonly observed in the elderly and shortens life expectancy. Because the fraction of the population that is elderly is growing throughout the world, the importance of heart failure as a determinant of disability and mortality is unfortunately increasing. Consequently, new efforts are under way to prevent this disease as well as improve its diagnosis and treatment.

---

296 What are the Framingham criteria for the diagnosis of congestive heart failure?

☐ The Framingham study on the natural history of congestive heart failure, completed in the early 1970s, defined major and minor criteria for the diagnosis of this condition. These criteria are useful guidelines because the signs and symptoms of heart failure are neither specific for this condition nor constant in all patients. Major criteria include: acute pulmonary edema, paroxysmal nocturnal dyspnea or orthopnea, neck vein distention, venous pressure higher than 16 cm H_2O, hepato-jugular reflux, pulmonary rales, S_3 gallop, cardiomegaly, and elbow-to-tongue circulation time longer than 25 seconds. Minor criteria include: dyspnea on exertion, heart rate at rest higher than 120 beats/min, night cough, ankle edema, hepatomegaly, pleural effusion, and reduced vital capacity by one third from maximum value. A criterion considered major or minor is weight loss greater than 4.5 kg in response to 5 days of treatment.

---

297   Describe the general appearance of patients with heart failure.

☐ The general appearance of patients varies greatly from a normal one to that of a cachectic individual in a terminal state. A normal appearance might be seen in patients who have mild or moderate heart failure and are free of any distress after a few minutes of rest. Patients with more advanced heart failure might be asymptomatic at rest but might develop dyspnea, tachycardia, and palpitations if they are requested to perform physical activity, occasionally an activity as light as undressing or walking around the physician's office. A patient who was asymptomatic while sitting or standing might become dyspneic after being requested by the examiner to lie flat for a few minutes. Patients with recently developed heart failure are usually well nourished. By contrast, patients with chronic heart failure of severe degree might be malnourished and even cachectic. The latter group of patients might also manifest a malar flush, cyanosis, and jaundice. In addition, these patients might have an abnormal arterial pulse (see answer of a subsequent question).

---

298   What are the most important factors responsible for differences among patients in the clinical manifestations of heart failure?

☐ Important factors responsible for differences in the signs and symptoms of heart failure include the specific ventricle initially involved, the etiology of the heart disease, age of the patient, and precipitating causes of heart failure. In addition, whether the manifestations are present or not as well as their severity depend on the degree of impairment of cardiac function. When heart dysfunction is mild, clinical manifestations are evident only during marked stress. With severe heart failure, symptoms and signs are present even at rest.

---

299 Do patients commonly present with "pure" forms of either forward or backward heart failure?

☐ No. Both forms are present in the majority of patients with chronic heart failure. By contrast, relatively pure forms of either type might occur in acute heart failure, an entity less common than the chronic one. Relatively pure forward heart failure occurs in patients with massive pulmonary embolism that prevents adequate left ventricular filling, thereby syncope develops due to forward failure of the left ventricle that fails to pump blood. Although jugular vein distention might be evident due to backward failure of the right ventricle, the dominant clinical manifestations are those of left ventricular forward failure. In contrast with the previous condition, relatively pure backward heart failure is evident in patients with slowly developing cardiac compression due to pericardial effusion whose major manifestations are congestion in systemic veins, peripheral edema, and fluid accumulation in major body cavities (pleural effusion, ascites).

---

300 What are the main characteristics of edema in patients with heart failure?

☐ Edema of cardiac origin usually develops first in the feet or ankles of ambulatory patients and might resolve after a night's rest. It is symmetrical and pitting in early stages of the disease. Long-standing peripheral edema, however, produces induration of the skin, especially in the pretibial areas and dorsum of the feet, accompanied by reddening and dark pigmentation. Because cardiac edema occurs first in the dependent portions of the body where venous pressure is highest, in bedridden patients edema is most commonly found over the sacrum. In advanced heart failure, edema might become generalized and massive (anasarca) involving all extremities, thoracic and abdominal walls, genital areas, and body cavities (ascites, pleural effusion, pericardial effusion).

---

301 Does fluid retention manifested as peripheral edema correlate with cardiac output and systemic venous pressure?

☐ No. Fluid retention might be absent in patients with a major reduction in cardiac output (e.g., heart failure of recent onset due to acute myocardial infarction leading to forward circulatory failure). On the other hand, anasarca might be present in patients with normal or even high cardiac output at rest (e.g., cor pulmonale with all the manifestations of right-sided heart failure). In addition, significant peripheral edema might be present in association with only a small elevation in systemic venous pressure (e.g., many patients with chronic left ventricular failure). Consequently, cardinal manifestations of heart failure such as peripheral edema might be either present or absent depending on multiple factors including, among others, duration of disease, heart chambers involved, and therapy (e.g., usage of diuretic agents).

---

302 What are pitting edema and anasarca?

☐ Edema is a localized or generalized expansion of interstitial fluid volume. Pitting edema is the persistent skin indentation due to applied pressure by the examiner (i.e., physician) or spontaneously (e.g., clothing). Anasarca refers to massive generalized edema.

---

303 How is pitting edema demonstrated?

☐ To demonstrate pitting edema, a common finding in the physical diagnosis of salt-retaining disorders, the examiner firmly presses a thumb into the patient's soft tissues for at least 10 seconds. A persistent skin depression establishes the presence of pitting edema. It is most important to evaluate this physical finding in all body regions (e.g., ankles, thighs, sacrum, flanks, upper extremities, face) to establish whether pitting edema involves only a body region or is generalized and to estimate the magnitude of total fluid retention in the patient.

---

304 What are the differences among pitting, nonpitting, and brawny edema?

☐ Increased interstitial fluid in peripheral tissues is present in the three forms of edema. Yet, the tissues are noncompressible or unyielding in brawny edema (e.g., myxedema observed in hypothyroidism), whereas they are compressible in pitting (e.g., congestive heart failure, nephrotic syndrome) and nonpitting (e.g., lymphedema) edema. The relatively high protein concentration in the interstitial fluid in patients with lymphedema decreases fluid mobility so that a rubbery consistency is found with nonpitting edema. The tissue induration of brawny edema is due to an increased mucopolysaccharide content that makes the extracellular matrix noncompressible.

---

305 Name causes of localized and generalized edema.

☐ Common causes of localized edema are insect bites, trauma, and venous or lymphatic obstruction (e.g., thrombophlebitis, lymphangitis, resection of regional lymph nodes). Generalized edema is observed in congestive heart failure, cirrhosis of the liver, nephrotic syndrome, acute and chronic renal failure, toxemia of pregnancy, and idiopathic (cyclic) edema. Malnutrition and protein-losing enteropathy are also important causes of generalized edema in children.

---

306 Does the distribution of edema offer any insight as to its cause?

☐ Yes. The distribution of edema might offer some clues as to its cause in localized and in generalized edema. Unilateral edema can be observed with neurologic conditions that impair the innervation of both skeletal muscle (paralysis reduces venous and lymphatic drainage) and vasculature of one side of the body. Alternatively, unilateral edema can be observed in patients with generalized edema who remained in a lateral decubitus position (dependent edema) for many hours. Edema most evident in the face and eyelids and especially pronounced in the morning (due to bed rest at night) is observed in generalized hypoproteinemia. Patients with edema caused by heart failure have fluid accumulation more evident in the presacral region if they have been confined to bed or in the legs (accentuated in the evening) if they are ambulatory. Facial edema is commonly observed with allergic reactions, tooth/mouth infections, myxedema, and parasitic infections (e.g., trichinosis, Chagas' disease). Edema involving one leg or one/or both arms is commonly due to venous or lymphatic obstruction. The combination of edema involving the face, neck, and upper extremities is characteristic of obstruction of the superior vena cava. Fluid collection localized to the pleural space or abdominal cavity might be due to inflammatory (e.g., pleuritis, peritonitis) or neoplastic diseases (e.g., lung, pleura, peritoneum).

---

307   What other physical findings are helpful in diagnosing localized edema?

☐   Examination of the skin, including color, temperature, presence/absence of pain, and thickness or induration, provides relevant data to establish the mechanism (pathogenesis) of localized edema. A bluish violet color (cyanosis) or distended local veins indicate venous obstruction, whereas a red area (erythema) suggests inflammatory edema (e.g., local infection, insect bites, or noninfectious dermatitis). An area of thickened, indurated, and often dark red skin is commonly observed when edema is of long duration or after repeated bouts of localized edema in the same area. Increased temperature, in comparison with surrounding or contralateral areas, accompanied by pain or tenderness, is characteristic of inflammatory edema.

---

308   How does examination of the fluid help to evaluate localized or generalized edema?

☐   The physical and chemical characteristics of the fluid might help to establish the cause of localized or generalized edema. Thin-needle aspiration of the fluid (e.g., local abscess or phlegmon in an extremity, joint effusion, ascites, or pleural fluid accumulation) must be considered only if this procedure can be done safely. The fluid color might be red or brown if extravasated blood is present, yellowish and creamy in lymph accumulation or empyema, and yellow or pink in noninflammatory edema. Fluid accumulation due to noninflammatory causes including venous obstruction, congestive heart failure, liver cirrhosis, or nephrosis is called a transudate; a fluid collection due to inflammatory causes is known as exudate. Main differences between transudates and exudates are: (1) protein concentration in fluid and ratio of fluid protein to that of serum are lower in transudates (less than 3 and 0.5 g/dL, respectively) than in exudates (greater than 3 and 0.5 g/dL, respectively); (2) lactate dehydrogenase (LDH) and the ratio of its fluid concentration to that in serum are lower in transudates (less than 200 and 0.6 IU/L, respectively) than in exudates (greater than 200 and 0.6 IU/L, respectively). A fluid sample should be routinely sent to the bacteriology laboratory for direct microscopic examination with Gram staining and investigation for microorganism growth in culture.

---

309 How might fluid retention be clinically evaluated by measures other than assessment of the presence or severity of peripheral edema (and fluid accumulation in body cavities)?

☐ A close follow-up of the patient's weight obtained in the examination office and by the patient at home (either daily or less frequently according to prescribed regimen) is a most effective and reliable method to evaluate changes in net fluid balance.

---

310 How large must the expansion of ECF volume be in an average size adult to produce peripheral edema detectable on physical examination?

☐ The expansion of ECF volume needed to produce peripheral edema in a adult amounts to at least 5 L. Thus, evaluation of fluid accumulation on the basis of the absence or presence of peripheral edema, and in the latter instance, whether it is of minimal (+), intermediate (++), or severe (+++) degree, is a very gross estimation of fluid retention.

311   How do changes in body weight elicited by the medical history help in the diagnosis of heart failure?

☐ Increases in body weight of 10 lb (about 5 kg) or more due to abnormal salt and water retention usually precede recognition of peripheral edema. Fluid retention might be detected at the end of the day and improves or disappears with bed rest. The clinical history might also provide information about a large weight loss over a short period (e.g., 5 lb or more in 24 to 48 hours) due to diuretic therapy. Large fluctuations in body weight that occur over a few days are due to changes in fluid balance but not to alterations in body fat content. It should be recognized, however, that fluid retention might be due to noncardiac diseases (e.g., liver cirrhosis, nephrotic syndrome) and therefore is not specific for heart failure.

312   How does information about increases in abdominal girth elicited by the medical history help in the diagnosis of heart failure?

☐ The spontaneous accumulation of fluid in the peritoneal space, a process referred to as ascites, is most frequently detected by the patient as an increase in abdominal girth. Ascites might develop in patients with congestive heart failure, especially if cardiac cirrhosis is present or if the systemic venous hypertension is due to constrictive pericarditis, restrictive cardiomyopathy, or tricuspid valve disease.

313   What are the main features of ascites due to heart failure?

☐ Long-standing hypertension of the systemic veins (including the hepatic veins and those draining the peritoneum) is required for the development of ascites. Congestive hepatomegaly most frequently accompanies this fluid retention. A relatively large ascites in association with a modest degree of peripheral edema is characteristically present in patients with chronic constrictive pericarditis and organic tricuspid valve disease. Needle aspiration of ascitic fluid might demonstrate a transudate that is rich in protein and referred to as a "pseudoexudate."

314 Is oliguria a sign of heart failure?

☐ Oliguria, defined as a daily urine output below 0.4 L in average size adults, might be a sign of severe or advanced cardiac failure. The diminished diuresis is a consequence of severe reduction of cardiac output and thereby renal underperfusion in association with neurohormonal stimulation. Sympathetic stimulation as well as high levels of aldosterone and ADH contribute to the pathogenesis of oliguria in patients with advanced heart failure. It must be recognized that oliguria is also observed in patients with renal (e.g., oliguric phase of acute tubular necrosis), urologic (e.g., incomplete obstruction of urine flow due to prostatic enlargement), and other diseases (e.g., depletion of body fluids, fever), without any evidence of cardiac disease.

315 What is nocturia?

☐ Nocturia is the predominantly nighttime production and excretion of urine associated with a diminished rate of urine formation (diuresis) during the day. This symptom prevents patients from resting and sleeping. The pattern of diuresis in normal individuals is precisely the opposite to that described for patients with nocturia because urine production and excretion in health occurs mostly during the day. When patients with heart failure rest in the recumbent position at night (as opposed to the daytime upright position), intravascular blood volume is redistributed away from the lower body and increases the effective circulating blood volume so that a greater fraction of cardiac output perfuses the kidneys where vasodilation occurs. In addition, sequestered fluid in the lower extremities (i.e., peripheral edema) and in body cavities (i.e., ascites, pleural effusion) returns to the systemic circulation when resting in the recumbent position. The additive effects of increased renal perfusion and a larger availability of body fluids as circulating blood volume at nighttime produce nocturia in patients with heart failure. The decrease in renal blood flow observed in heart failure reduces the capacity for maximal urine concentration (hypostenuria) so that fluctuations in hourly urine output diminish and diuresis is more uniform over the 24-hour period. This abnormality in urine concentration also contributes to the development of nocturia in heart failure.

---

316   Is nocturia observed exclusively in congestive heart failure?

☐ No. Patients with renal failure due to many different primary diseases might experience nocturia because of a diminished ability to concentrate and dilute urine so that diuresis is relatively constant during day and night. In addition, patients with renal failure and fluid excess manifested by peripheral edema mostly in the lower extremities have a greater availability of fluid for nocturnal diuresis due to reversal of gravity-dependent effects of fluid distribution that occurs in the recumbent position.

---

317   What is the pathogenesis of fatigue and weakness observed in patients with low output heart failure?

☐ Fatigue and weakness in low cardiac output heart failure are likely due to the low perfusion of skeletal muscles. However, salt depletion due to excessive use of diuretics and therapy with β-adrenoreceptor blocking agents (e.g., propranolol) might also cause these symptoms. It should be recognized that fatigue and weakness are notoriously nonspecific symptoms that might be caused by many diseases unrelated to heart failure. In addition, not uncommonly, patients having shortness of breath mistakenly describe this symptom with the term fatigue. Thus, it is important to help patients to distinguish fatigue (arising from skeletal muscles) from dyspnea (a cardiopulmonary symptom).

---

318   What cerebral symptoms might be present in patients with heart failure?

☐ Patients with advanced heart failure might experience many symptoms indicative of cerebral dysfunction due to underperfusion or congestion of the brain and surrounding structures. The most prominent symptoms are impairment of memory and confusion. Less commonly, hallucinations, delirium, and psychosis with disorientation might occur. Other symptoms such as headache, anxiety, insommia, and night-mares are observed earlier in the disease and with a higher incidence or prevalence. Because the most severe cerebral symptoms occur predominantly in elderly patients who might have an associated brain disease (i.e., organic brain syn-drome), it is likely that the observed cerebral manifestations might be, at least in part, independent of heart failure.

---

319 Describe clinical manifestations of heart failure that are indica-tive of increased adrenergic activity.

☐ Sympathetic stimulation in heart failure is responsible for sinus tachycardia, loss of normal sinus arrhythmia (i.e., heart rate increases with inspiration and decreases with expiration), and increased diastolic blood pressure due to diffuse arteriolar vasoconstriction of the systemic circulation. Sympathetic ac-tivation produces other manifestations including diaphoresis (increased sweating) and underperfusion of fingers and toes that are cold, pale, or cyanotic.

---

320 What is the difference between the sensation of breathlessness (dyspnea) brought on by physical exercise or emotional stress in heart failure compared to that elicited in normal individuals?

☐ The main difference between the dyspnea observed in pa-tients with heart failure compared to that of normal individuals is the intensity of the physical exercise or emo-tional stress required to trigger this symptom. Whereas normal individuals, especially those engaging in regular exer-cise, require relatively intense physical or emotional stress to trigger dyspnea, those with heart failure experience this symptom in response to a milder stress. Thus, the main dis-tinction between dyspnea in normal conditions and that in patients with disease is not qualitative (manifestations of dyspnea are similar) but is quantitative (a less intense stress initiates dyspnea in cardiac disease as well as other illnesses). Because exertional dyspnea occurs in normal individuals, it is important to determine whether there has been a change in the level of exertion causing it. Patients with exertional dyspnea will usually report that a level of activity that previously did not cause breathlessness (e.g., walking to a particular location from their homes at a given pace) now does so. As heart failure worsens, the level of exercise that causes dyspnea decreases. It must be recognized that denial of dyspnea by some patients with overt heart failure is due to their sedentary life (bedridden patients or those confined indoors) such that they do not perform even low-level physical activities.

---

321 What elements help differentiation between cardiac dyspnea and noncardiac dyspnea due to either anxiety, neurosis, or to malingering intentions?

☐ Careful examination of patients with shortness of breath based on malingering (e.g., false claim of disease in an effort to obtain monetary compensation) and that due to anxiety neurosis might disclose the following distinct features that allow differentiation from dyspnea of cardiac origin including: (1) dyspnea is present at rest and its intensity is not increased with exercise; (2) patient is unable to take a deep breath; (3) a sighing pattern of breathing is commonly observed; (4) respiration is irregular or effortless during exercise testing; (5) the breathing pattern is not rapid and shallow as in cardiac dyspnea; and (6) patient does not have other objective evidence of heart failure that explains the shortness of breath.

---

322 Describe the major clinical features of cardiac dyspnea that help to differentiate it from pulmonary dyspnea.

☐ Cardiac dyspnea generally develops more suddenly and without history of smoking or pulmonary disease. Sputum production is absent, chest x-ray does not show indices of lung disease, and pulmonary function tests show a restrictive ventilatory defect. Pulmonary dyspnea tends to occur more gradually and is often associated with a history of smoking, noxious inhalants, bronchial asthma, or chronic lung disease. Sputum production frequently occurs and coughing up bronchial secretions alleviates dyspnea. Chest x-ray often shows evidence of lung disease and pulmonary function tests reveal a ventilatory defect that is obstructive (i.e., chronic bronchitis, emphysema) or restrictive (i.e., pulmonary fibrosis).

323 How can the cause of dyspnea be determined?

☐ A thorough clinical evaluation can establish the cause of dyspnea in most patients without requesting expensive or complicated laboratory determinations. The cause of dyspnea (e.g., anxiety, lung disease, cardiac disease, superimposition of heart and lung disease in a single patient) might remain undiagnosed after clinical examination so that further studies are mandatory. Differentiation between cardiac and pulmonary dyspnea in clinical practice often requires additional evaluation including pulmonary function testing or measurement of the circulation time (see question 325).

324 What elements obtained from the clinical history, physical examination, and laboratory evaluation facilitate the differential diagnosis of cardiogenic from noncardiogenic pulmonary edema?

☐ The clinical history generally provides important information with respect to a previous disease that predisposes to the development of cardiogenic (e.g., ischemic heart disease, uncontrolled hypertension) or noncardiogenic (e.g., trauma, sepsis) pulmonary edema. In addition, an acute cardiac event (e.g., atrial fibrillation) might be detected in the cardiogenic type but is absent in noncardiogenic edema. The physical examination in cardiogenic pulmonary edema might reveal poor blood perfusion of the extremities, cardiomegaly, S_3 gallop, jugular vein distention, and pulmonary wet crackles. None of the previously mentioned physical examination findings are present in patients with noncardiogenic pulmonary edema. Laboratory evaluations that help differentiate the two main forms of pulmonary edema include: (1) blood gases (that reveal small and large venous shunting in cardiac and noncardiac edema, respectively); (2) protein level in the fluid derived from the airways (e.g., ratio of protein concentration from edema fluid to that of serum is less than 0.5 in cardiogenic and more than 0.7 in noncardiogenic edema); (3) pulmonary capillary wedge pressure is greater than 18 mmHg in cardiac type and less than 18 mmHg in noncardiac type of edema; (4) chest radiographs that show perihilar distribution in cardiogenic edema and peripheral distribution in noncardiogenic edema; and (5) ECG and cardiac enzymes might be abnormal in the cardiac type but normal in the non-cardiogenic form of edema.

---

325   Describe how a bedside evaluation of circulation time helps to differentiate cardiac from pulmonary dyspnea.

☐ Cardiac dyspnea due to low cardiac output heart failure is characterized by a prolonged arm-to-tongue circulation time (more than 16 seconds). In contrast, normal values (9 to 16 seconds) are observed in patients with pulmonary dyspnea. The test is performed by rapidly injecting 3 to 5 mL Decholin (dehydrocholic acid) in a vein of the anticubital fossa and measuring the time between start of the injection and the appearance of a bitter taste sensed by the patient. This time-honored test, less commonly used now, is of special value for cases in which the etiology of dyspnea is difficult to determine. It is also of value in assessing the relative contribution of pulmonary and cardiac dyspnea in patients with both diseases. Circulation time is normal or even reduced in patients with high output heart failure.

---

326   How might the use of diuretics help to establish whether dyspnea is due to heart failure?

☐ Improvement of dyspnea after a diuretic-induced weight loss that exceeds 2 kg (about 4 lb) supports that fluid overload due to heart failure has been responsible for the respiratory symptoms. Conversely, the lack of effects of a diuretic regimen on dyspnea suggests another pathogenesis for this symptom. It should be recognized that amelioration of the shortness of breath after the administration of diuretics simply indicates that fluid overload due to any cause (e.g., heart failure, renal failure) was responsible for the symptom but is not a specific response observed in heart failure.

---

327   What are the most relevant abnormalities in pulmonary function tests of patients with heart failure?

☐ Pulmonary function testing in heart failure might reveal: (1) reduction in arterial PCO_2 and PO_2; (2) diminished vital capacity, total lung capacity, pulmonary compliance, and pulmonary diffusion capacity during exercise and frequently at rest; (3) normal residual volume and functional residual volume; and (4) moderately augmented resistance to air flow with evidence of air trapping and increased dead space. None of the abnormalities in the pulmonary function tests is specific for heart failure or constant in this disease. Thus, the results of pulmonary function tests must be interpreted considering all the clinical and laboratory information obtained from the patient.

---

328 Why is it important to differentiate cardiac from pulmonary dyspnea?

☐ Because treatment of each of these mechanisms of dyspnea is accomplished by the use of different diet regimens (i.e., low-salt diet in cardiac dyspnea, low-carbohydrate diet in pulmonary dyspnea) and drugs (i.e., digitalis and afterload-reducing agents in cardiac dyspnea, bronchodilators in pulmonary dyspnea secondary to obstructed airways), it is important to establish the pathogenesis of dyspnea in a given patient. Furthermore, patients with combined cardiac and pulmonary dyspnea for whom only one of the two components of dyspnea is recognized might remain short of breath despite successful treatment of the recognized cause of dyspnea. Failure to completely relieve the symptoms of such a patient frequently leads to the identification and treatment of the disease responsible for the previously unrecognized cause of dyspnea (cardiac or pulmonary).

---

329 What are the characteristics of cough secondary to heart failure?

☐ Cough is a common manifestation of left-sided heart failure and might be present with or without pulmonary rales on auscultation of the chest. A dry cough (i.e., without sputum production) usually appears when the patient first lies down to rest at night and might persist, inducing restlessness and inability to sleep (insomnia due to pulmonary congestion). Patients with cough due to heart failure generally have a pattern of interstitial pulmonary edema on the chest x-ray.

330   What is orthopnea?

☐ Orthopnea is dyspnea that develops in the supine (recumbent) position and improves or disappears when the thorax is elevated toward the upright position. Most patients relieve their orthopnea by adding one or more extra pillows under their head and upper body while in the recumbent position. Consequently, questions as to the number of pillows used by the patients to rest comfortably should be asked by the treating physician. Because some normal individuals prefer to lie with their head elevated by pillows (for comfort reasons rather than relief of breathlessness), it is important to determine whether a change in the degree of head elevation necessary to provide comfort (e.g., increase in number of pillows) has occurred to establish if orthopnea is present or not. The increased venous return from body regions below the heart (abdomen and all extremities) in the recumbent as compared to the upright position imposes a load on a failing heart that is beyond its pumping capability so that pulmonary venous congestion develops. By contrast, the normal heart can accept and eject the increased venous return under these circumstances. Sometimes, patients experience a nonproductive cough instead of dyspnea in the supine position (manifestation of orthopnea), and this symptom is often called a "dyspnea equivalent."

331   What is paroxysmal nocturnal dyspnea?

☐ Paroxysmal nocturnal dyspnea (commonly called PND) is an important manifestation of congestive heart failure wherein intermittent attacks of dyspnea interrupt or disturb rest or sleep; this symptom develops while the patient is in the supine position for one or more hours. Once PND occurs, the patient sits up in bed to relieve dyspnea and frequently moves to a sofa in an attempt to resume rest in a semirecumbent position. Although the term PND denotes a nighttime occurrence of the symptom, it might also occur during the day in patients who rest or sleep at this time. The one or more hour delay for the start of dyspnea in PND, a feature that distinguishes it from other forms of orthopnea (e.g., an acute asthma attack), is due to a summation of factors including: (1) slow reabsorption of

ECF accumulation (edema) from dependent areas (e.g., lower extremities) causing increased venous return to the heart and thereby pulmonary venous congestion associated with expansion of intrathoracic blood volume;   (2) increased work of breathing due to the gravity effects of abdominal viscera that displace the diaphragm and compress the lung bases; (3) exaggerated effect of the normal nocturnal suppression of respiratory drive that accompanies the decreased CNS activity associated with sleep; and   (4) decreased sympathetic tone to the heart during sleep that further impairs myocardial contractility.   Pulmonary venous congestion in PND produces fluid accumulation in the pulmonary interstitium and bronchial mucosa compressing the small bronchi.   The wheezing sounds evident on lung auscultation are due to edema of the bronchial walls and associated bronchospasm and account for the term "cardiac asthma" frequently used instead of PND.   When associated with chest pain or "heaviness," PND might represent a symptom of myocardial ischemia or so-called angina equivalent.

---

332   What is Cheyne-Stokes respiration?

□   Cheyne-Stokes, periodic, or cyclic respiration is an abnormal pattern of breathing that might be observed in patients with left-sided heart failure.   It is due to depression or decreased sensitivity of the respiratory center located in the medulla.   The decreased sensitivity of the respiratory center to normal stimuli (e.g., carbon dioxide tension) might be due to organic (e.g., cerebrovascular lesions) or functional (e.g., barbiturates, narcotics) causes.   During the apneic phase of Cheyne-Stokes respiration, oxygen tension decreases and carbon dioxide tension increases in arterial blood.   These abnormalities in blood gas composition produce, in turn, excitation of the previously depressed respiratory center causing hyperventilation with correction of the blood gases.   The corrected blood gases lead to a new cycle of depressed ventilation with apnea.   Cheyne-Stokes respiration is most evident during sleep and might awaken the patient with an episode of acute shortness of breath.

333   What signs of left-sided heart failure might be detected on cardiac examination?

☐ Physical findings that might be present in left-sided heart failure include signs of left ventricular enlargement as well as "gallop" sounds or murmurs of mitral regurgitation. Left ventricular hypertrophy or dilation (also referred to as enlargement) most commonly accompanies long-standing cardiac disease leading to left-sided heart failure. Dilatation or enlargement of the left ventricle causes a diffuse heave over the entire precordial area with displacement of the apical impulse (apex of the heart) downward and toward the left axilla (eccentric hypertrophy). Hypertrophy of the left ventricle without significant enlargement of overall chamber size produces a distinct and localized outward motion of the chest wall during ventricular systole (concentric hypertrophy). Dilatation or hypertrophy of the left ventricle can be detected by inspection and palpation of the precordium. Third and fourth heart sounds arising from the left ventricle might be evident on auscultation. These extra sounds or gallops are best heard at the apex with the patient in the left lateral decubitus position. A murmur caused by mitral regurgitation secondary to left ventricular enlargement might be present.

334   What are the clinical manifestations of acute cardiogenic pulmonary edema?

☐ Patients experiencing this syndrome have extreme breathlessness and anxiety, elevated respiratory rate, and noisy breathing with gurgling sounds during inspiration and expiration. Cough and expectoration of pink, frothy sputum are characteristically present. The intense air hunger prompts patients to sit upright or stand and accounts for the dilated nostrils and inspiratory depression of supraclavicular fossa and intercostal spaces (reflecting large negative intrapleural pressures). Cyanosis is evident, sweating is profuse, and the skin is cold and ashen due to sympathetic activation yielding poor perfusion. Auscultation of the lungs reveals rhonchi, wheezes, and crepitant rales (fine and moist). The latter appear first at the lung bases and extend upward as pulmonary edema worsens. Cardiac auscultation might disclose a third heart sound (S_3) and accentuation of the pulmonic component of the second sound (S_2). The loud respiratory sounds make cardiac auscultation difficult.

---

335 What are the principal signs and symptoms for the three stages of acute pulmonary edema?

☐ The abnormalities of stage 1 are mild and signs and symptoms are either absent or have low intensity (particularly at rest) because there is no net fluid accumulation and pulmonary gas exchange is minimally compromised. Patients with this early stage of pulmonary edema might experience a sensation of breathlessness (dyspnea) on mild to moderate exercise, a level of activity that previously did not elicit breathlessness. Because fluid accumulates in the pulmonary interstitium in stage 2, tachypnea (increased respiratory rate) is frequently seen, even at rest. This tachypnea has been attributed to activation of interstitial receptors that stimulate breathing. In this stage, breathlessness can be elicited by a lower level of exercise than in stage 1. Pulmonary gas exchange is abnormal due to perfusion of poorly ventilated lung regions. Fluid accumulation in the pulmonary interstitium in stage 2 is responsible for the development of radiologic changes on a standard chest x-ray. These alterations include loss of the normally sharp definition of pulmonary vascular markings (due to fluid accumulation in the perivascular space), haziness and poor definition of hilar shadows, and thickening of interlobular septa. Among the radiologic findings are the Kerley B lines, which are fine, dense, horizontal lines, most prominent in the lower and mid-lung areas. They are caused by thickening of interlobular septa and surrounding lymphatics secondary to fluid accumulation. With the onset of stage 3 (alveolar flooding), the patient experiences the sensation of breathlessness at rest and literally gasps for air. The oxygen tension of arterial blood decreases due to mixing of blood from poorly ventilated (lower lung) and better ventilated (upper lung) regions. A standard chest x-ray might show "fullness" of the hilar region with "fluffiness" of the lung parenchyma, often spreading from the central (hilar) regions outward in a "butterfly" pattern. Auscultation discloses rales in the lungs and "gallop" sounds (third or fourth cardiac sounds if myocardial failure is responsible for the pulmonary edema) and arrhythmias on heart examination.

---

336   What are the clinical manifestations of chronic pulmonary edema?

☐ The clinical manifestations of chronic pulmonary edema (e.g., tight mitral stenosis, severe diastolic dysfunction of the left ventricle, long-term elevation of left atrial pressure due to multiple causes) are qualitatively similar to those found in acute pulmonary edema but their intensity is greatly diminished. Thus, the difference in symptomatology between acute and chronic pulmonary edema is quantitative but not qualitative. Recruitment of multiple compensatory mechanisms explains the ameliorated intensity of clinical manifestations of chronic pulmonary edema.

---

337   What is cardiac asthma?

☐ The remarkable similarity of many clinical manifestations observed in patients having severe bronchial asthma (i.e., acute asthma attack) and those suffering acute pulmonary edema accounts for the term "cardiac asthma" applied to the latter condition. Both entities might produce extreme dyspnea that forces an upright posture, diffuse wheezes that interfere with cardiac auscultation, and pulsus paradoxicus (reduction in the amplitude of arterial pulse or disappearance with deep inspiration).

---

338   How can cardiac asthma be differentiated from severe bronchial asthma (i.e., acute asthma attack) on first encounter by the clinician?

☐ Patients with severe bronchial asthma frequently have a history of similar episodes, allergic rhinitis or sinusitus, or other evidence of atopic reactions. Sweating and cyanosis are generally absent in bronchial asthma and present in cardiac asthma. Examination of the chest in severe bronchial asthma generally reveals greater evidence of diffuse airway obstruction so that the chest is overexpanded and hyperresonant.

Furthermore, use of accessory respiratory muscles is more prominent, wheezes are high pitched and musical, and rhonchi/rales (adventitious sounds) are less evident in bronchial than in cardiac asthma. In the latter condition, the chest is often dull to percussion, and on auscultation, rhonchi and moist/bubbly rales are characteristically present. The chest x-ray findings of pulmonary edema (described in the answer to another question) are absent in severe bronchial asthma in which pulmonary hyperinflation is the most prominent abnormality.

---

339 What are the clinical manifestations of noncardiogenic pulmonary edema?

☐ An increase in respiratory rate or dyspnea accompanied by hypoxemia and hypocapnia (assessed by arterial blood gas measurement) are early signs and symptoms of noncardiogenic pulmonary edema. Thereafter, examination of the lungs might reveal dry crackles that are accompanied by tubular breath sounds in advanced stages of this condition. Laryngeal intubation and mechanical ventilation with high oxygen mixtures are generally required to manage the progressive abnormality in blood gas composition observed with severe forms of noncardiogenic pulmonary edema (e.g., ARDS). The underlying disease (e.g., trauma, sepsis) produces clinical manifestations that are additive to those caused by the pulmonary edema.

---

340 How can cardiogenic and noncardiogenic pulmonary edema be differentiated?

☐ The clinical setting in which pulmonary edema occurs is an important clue in differentiating cardiogenic from noncardiogenic causes. Patients with pulmonary edema associated with a history of heart disease or current signs and symptoms of heart failure (particularly acute) should be strongly suspected of having cardiogenic pulmonary edema. On the other hand, patients with conditions that can cause noncardiogenic pulmonary edema (e.g., septic shock, inhaled toxins, etc.) without history or evidence of heart disease should be suspected of having noncardiogenic pulmonary edema. Manifestations of left-sided heart failure including exertional dyspnea, orthopnea, paroxysmal nocturnal dyspnea, exercise intolerance, and weakness support a diagnosis of cardiogenic pulmonary edema. Elevated left heart diastolic pressures detected on invasive monitoring would be supportive of a cardiogenic etiology for the pulmonary edema, whereas normal or low filling pressures would support a noncardiogenic cause. A high oncotic pressure of bronchial secretions is evidence for a disrupted alveolar-capillary membrane and therefore supports a noncardiogenic cause for the pulmonary edema.

---

341   What is the role of pulmonary artery wedge pressure measurements in the differential diagnosis of cardiogenic and noncardiogenic pulmonary edema?

☐ Measurements of pulmonary artery wedge pressure by means of a Swan-Ganz catheter help to determine the pathogenesis of pulmonary edema. This evaluation is the most useful diagnostic aid to help resolve this common medical dilemma. Pulmonary edema might be due to an imbalance of Starling forces (cardiogenic type) or to abnormal permeability of pulmonary capillaries (noncardiogenic type of pulmonary edema). A cardiogenic origin of pulmonary edema (imbalance of Starling forces) is most likely if the pulmonary capillary wedge or pulmonary artery diastolic pressure exceeds 25 mm Hg (if previous pressure levels were normal) or 30 mm Hg (if previous pressure levels were abnormally high). The protein concentration in bronchial secretions also helps to establish the pathogenesis of pulmonary edema. Finding protein levels in these secretions that are close to those of plasma is consistent with increased capillary permeability (and therefore consistent with noncardiogenic pulmonary edema), whereas a low protein concentration in bronchial secretions is typically found in cardiogenic pulmonary edema. The two forms of pulmonary edema are not mutually exclusive because a given patient might have elements of both cardiogenic and noncardiogenic pulmonary edema contributing to the disease.

342 What chest x-ray features are useful in evaluating patients with heart failure?

☐ The size and shape of the cardiac silhouette and appearance of the pulmonary vasculature provide useful information about patients with heart failure. The area covered by the heart and the cardiothoracic ratio (maximal cardiac diameter divided by maximal internal thoracic diameter, normally less than 0.50) are useful and specific indicators of left ventricular end-diastolic volume but are relatively insensitive. The shape of the cardiac silhouette allows recognition of specific abnormalities in the size of individual cardiac chambers. Evaluation of the pulmonary vasculature allows detection of redistribution of blood flow and a gross estimation of the hydrostatic pressure in the pulmonary capillaries. The presence or absence of pulmonary edema and pleural effusion are also important findings in the evaluation of a chest roentgenogram.

343 What is the so-called vascular redistribution that can be observed on examination of a standard chest x-ray of patients with pulmonary edema?

☐ Vascular redistribution refers to an accentuation of the vascular structures in the upper regions of the lung fields in a standard posteroanterior chest x-ray that might be observed in conditions of pulmonary vascular congestion. Recognition of this important radiologic sign of pulmonary venous congestion is important in the routine care of outpatients and inpatients.

344 Recapitulate the mechanisms responsible for the vascular redistribution of blood in the pulmonary circulation in states of pulmonary venous congestion.

☐ The increased blood flow of the upper regions of the lung in individuals having "vascular redistribution" is due to the partial collapse of pulmonary blood vessels in the lower regions of the lung as a result of increased perivascular pressure due to fluid accumulation in the latter regions. Blood flow in the lower areas of the lung is higher than in the upper regions in the sitting or standing position in normal individuals as well as those with pulmonary edema. In the sitting or standing position, the gravity-related increase in hydrostatic pressure within pulmonary capillaries in the lower compared to the upper lung regions is larger than the increase in pressure of the interstitial space surrounding these capillaries. The lower pressure in the interstitial space as compared to the vascular space at the lung bases (occurring in health and disease) is due to a greater effect of the negative (subatmospheric) alveolar pressure during inspiration on the interstitium as compared to the vessels. It should be apparent that the net forces favoring exit of fluid from the pulmonary capillaries are larger in the lower compared to upper lung regions, dictating that pulmonary edema will occur first in the lower lung regions. This perivascular edema increases perivascular pressure causing collapse of blood vessels. In addition, alveolar flooding decreases oxygen tension leading to pulmonary arteriolar vasoconstriction in the lung bases.

---

345   Is vascular redistribution a specific radiologic sign indicative of actual or impending acute pulmonary edema?

☐ No. Although vascular redistribution is a typical feature of acute pulmonary edema, it is commonly found in other conditions in the absence of actual or impending pulmonary edema. Such conditions include chronic states of venocapillary pulmonary hypertension including mitral stenosis or chronic congestive heart failure. In these chronic disease states, the so-called vascular redistribution is due to a different pathogenesis than that previously explained for acute pulmonary edema. The radiologic sign of vascular redistribution in states of chronic venocapillary pulmonary hypertension (e.g., mitral stenosis) is due to interstitial fibrosis and narrowing of arteries and arterioles of the basal regions of the lungs but not to the functional redeployment of pulmonary blood flow from the lower to the upper lung regions that occurs in acute pulmonary edema.

---

346   How might chest x-ray findings in congestive heart failure correlate with pulmonary capillary pressure?

☐ The appearance of the lung fields on x-ray correlates with the levels of pulmonary capillary pressure. When capillary pressure is normal, the lung apices receive less perfusion than the bases. Equal perfusion of apical and basal areas occurs when pulmonary capillary pressure is elevated to 15 to 20 mmHg (normal values are less than 10 mmHg). With capillary pressures of 20 to 25 mmHg, upper lobe pulmonary veins are more prominent than those in the lower lobes. Fluid accumulation in the lungs such as interstitial edema, Kerley B lines, alveolar edema, and pleural effusion might be seen with capillary pressures that exceed 25 mmHg. Consequently, serial evaluation of chest x-rays in patients with heart failure allows monitoring of the severity and progression or regression of disease and results of therapy.

---

347   What are the most relevant chest x-ray findings in patients with heart failure?

☐ Examination of the chest x-ray of patients with heart failure might reveal: (1) enlarged pulmonary vessels (veins and main arteries); (2) enlarged systemic veins (superior vena cava, azygos veins); (3) lung field shadows indicative of interstitial or alveolar edema; (4) fluid accumulation in the pleural space (e.g., subpleural location, free pleural fluid effusion, interlobar fissure "thickening", pseudotumor); and (5) an enlarged cardiac silouhette (i.e., cardiothoracic ratio larger than 0.5) with possible changes in the shape and size of one or more heart chambers.

---

348   What abnormalities in the pulmonary veins and arteries might be present on chest x-ray of patients with heart failure?

☐ Prominence of the superior pulmonary veins and generalized dilatation of these vessels on an upright chest x-ray indicate pulmonary venous hypertension. Distention of the main pulmonary veins produce hilar engorgement that might be also evident on the chest x-ray. Enlargement of the main right and left pulmonary arteries caused by increased pressure in these vessels might be evident in left-sided heart failure. The increased pulmonary artery pressure observed in these patients is secondary to venocapillary pulmonary hypertension.

349   What abnormalities in the chest x-ray indicate interstitial edema and alveolar edema?

☐ Interstitial edema is the accumulation of fluid in the tissue surrounding both the pulmonary capillaries and alveoli. It might produce the following radiologic abnormalities: (1) increased linear markings in central areas of the lung fields; (2) ill-defined blotchy areas with increased density and irregular distribution ("pulmonary clouding"); and (3) haziness and loss of sharp outline of pulmonary arteries and veins. Alveolar pulmonary edema is the accumulation of fluid in the alveolar spaces. Thus, alveolar edema is a more advanced form of pulmonary fluid accumulation than interstitial edema. The radiologic findings of alveolar pulmonary edema include: (1) the "butterfly" or "bat" shadow/appearance of the chest x-ray wherein the heart and mediastinal structures make the body of the butterfly/bat and the bilateral symmetrical infiltration of lung fields due to pulmonary edema makes the wings; the shadows are more prominent in the central portions of the lungs and fade toward the periphery; the apices, bases, and lateral margins of the lungs are relatively spared (uninvolved); the butterfly or bat shadow is usually indicative of severe pulmonary edema; (2) in less severe cases, a one-winged butterfly shadow (right side is more common), ill-defined areas of increased density, or nodular/miliary infiltrates; and (3) rarely, only one lobe or the upper lung fields have shadows indicative of alveolar edema. It must be recognized that interstitial pulmonary edema and alveolar pulmonary edema might be due to noncardiac causes so that their presence is not a specific indicator of heart failure.

350   What abnormalities might be detected on macroscopic and microscopic examination of the lungs (e.g., surgical procedures, pulmonary biopsy, autopsy material) in patients with heart failure?

☐ Left ventricular failure produces enlarged lungs that are firm, dark, and filled with bloody fluid. The dark brown color of the lungs is caused by deposition of hemosiderin. Microscopic examination discloses hypertrophy of the medial layer as well as intimal hyperplasia of the pulmonary arteries and arterioles. The pulmonary capillaries are engorged, the alveolar septa are thickened, and extravasation of red cells and large mononuclear cells is evident.

---

351 What abnormalities in the arterial pulse might be present in heart failure?

☐ Tachycardia is a common finding in this condition. Amplitude of the arterial pulse in mild to moderately severe heart failure is normal at rest, whereas it might decrease during exercise. Pulse amplitude depends on pulse pressure, which is in turn largely due to the level of stroke volume. The reduced stroke volume observed in severe heart failure produces a diminished pulse pressure and a weak pulse. The ratio of pulse pressure to systolic pressure directly correlates with cardiac output. Values of this ratio less than 0.25 are generally indicative of a very low cardiac index (i.e., less than $2.0 \ L/min/m^2$). Systolic arterial pressure decreases in severe heart failure due to a major decline in cardiac output.

---

352 What is pulsus alternans?

☐ Pulsus alternans is characterized by small and large pulse waves that continuously alternate in an otherwise regular rhythm. Pulsus alternans is a clinical sign of abnormal cardiac function observed in some patients with heart failure. It is recognized by palpation of the pulse or by sphygmomanometry. The latter method might detect that systolic blood pressure in alternating heartbeats differs between 5 and 20 mmHg. Pulsus alternans is caused by the ejection of small and large stroke volumes in alternating systoles. The incomplete recovery of myocytes on every other beat accounts for the development of pulsus alternans.

---

353 How might a third heart sound (S_3) originating in the left ventricle be distinguished from one arising from the right ventricle?

☐ A third heart sound is always a low-frequency one that is heard at the end of the rapid phase of ventricular filling in early diastole (other names for this sound are protodiastolic gallop, ventricular gallop, or S_3). A left ventricular gallop is best heard over the cardiac apex immediately after inspiration, whereas a right ventricular gallop is best heard along the lower left sternal border or over the epigastrium during inspiration. Patients with heart failure might have ventricular gallops or atrial gallops (see next question).

---

354 What are the determinants of a fourth heart sound, also called S_4, atrial gallop, or presystolic gallop?

☐ An atrial gallop might develop when the ventricle (left or right) is poorly compliant (e.g., stiff wall) and atrial contraction is vigorous. A left atrial gallop is best heard over the cardiac apex; a right atrial gallop is best heart over the epigastrium or along the lower left sternal border.

---

355 Is detection of a left ventricular gallop in an adult a specific sign of left-sided heart failure?

☐ No. Conditions characterized by large ventricular diastolic volumes and stroke volumes might produce left ventricular gallops in the absence of left-sided heart failure. Examples of this combination are the high cardiac output states of pregnancy, anemia, cardiac septal defects (e.g., interatrial, interventricular), patent ductus arteriosus, mitral regurgitation, and aortic regurgitation. Consequently, the interpretation of a ventricular gallop should be made with caution. The possible role of causes other than heart failure must be always considered.

---

356 What specific cardiac diseases might preclude the development of ventricular gallops despite the presence of severe heart failure?

☐ Mitral stenosis and tricuspid stenosis, both of severe degree, preclude the development of left ventricular gallops and right ventricular gallops, respectively. The absence of a phase of rapid ventricular filling in these valvular diseases of the heart explains why the above-mentioned ventricular gallops cannot occur. Yet, a right ventricular gallop might be observed in patients with tight mitral stenosis and right-sided heart failure due to pulmonary hypertension.

357 Is it possible to have a ventricular gallop (third sound or S_3) and normal heart function?

☐ Yes. Ventricular gallops are commonly present in healthy children and young adults. These gallop sounds usually arise from the left chamber although they might occasionally originate from the right ventricle. Nevertheless, a physiologic (normal) ventricular gallop usually disappears after age 40 years so that detection of a protodiastolic gallop in older individuals is generally considered a sign of heart disease. It should be recognized, however, that cardiac diseases other than heart failure might generate a ventricular gallop. These diseases or conditions include left-to-right shunts, constrictive pericarditis, and mitral and tricuspid regurgitation.

358 What measures might help detect a ventricular gallop?

☐ Repetitive sit-ups, handgrip, or other types of exercise might help detect a ventricular gallop that was absent at rest. Palpation of the cardiac apex in the left lateral recumbent position facilitates the recognition of left ventricular gallops.

359 What pertinent findings might be disclosed on clinical examination of the eyes in patients with heart failure?

☐ A slight exophthalmos (abnormal protrusion of the eyeballs) might be present in patients with long-standing venous hypertension. In addition, jaundice due to passive liver congestion is noted in some patients. Detection of jaundice in heart failure, however, suggests centrilobular necrosis of the liver or pulmonary infarction (secondary to embolism).

360 What are the clinical manifestations of heart failure in the neonate and infant?

☐ Manifestations of heart failure in the first year of life include respiratory distress, feeding difficulties, failure to gain weight and grow normally, and excessive sweating. Repeated pulmonary infections are commonly observed and respiratory findings include grunting, flaring of the alae nasi, retraction of the ribs, and cyanosis. Facial edema, hepatomegaly, and a paradoxical pulse caused by wide variations in ventricular filling secondary to marked swings in intrathoracic pressure between inspiration and expiration are also common in infants. Radiologic examination discloses cardiomegaly and pulmonary congestion.

---

361   What is "cardiac cachexia?"

☐ Severe emaciation with a large reduction of lean body mass that is most prominent with the skeletal muscle is observed in some patients with long-standing, severe congestive heart failure. This clinical picture is known as cardiac cachexia. Its pathogenesis might include reduced caloric intake or increased energy expenditure. A diminished caloric intake results from anorexia (secondary to hepatic or intestinal congestion or digitalis intoxication), impaired intestinal absorption of fat, or protein-losing enteropathy. Severe anorexia and malabsorption are prominent with severe right-sided heart failure, the most commonly observed form of cardiac cachexia. Increased energy expenditure might be caused by excessive work of breathing (due to dysnea), high plasma levels of tumor necrosis factor with low-grade fever, and increased myocardial oxygen consumption (e.g., aortic stenosis, hypertension). The loss of lean body mass is often masked by fluid retention. Cardiac cachexia might resemble the syndrome of malignant diseases in a terminal stage with generalized metastasis of neoplastic cells.

---

362   Describe the signs and symptoms of right-sided heart failure.

☐ The signs and symptoms of right-sided heart failure are those of venous congestion in the systemic circulation. Distention of jugular veins, hepatojugular reflux, hepatomegaly, ascites, and lower extremity edema are commonly observed. Patients might complain of right upper quadrant pain caused by stretching of the hepatic capsule from liver congestion. In addition, anorexia, nausea, and abdominal bloating from venous congestion of abdominal viscera including the liver, mesentery, and spleen might be present. In the absence of left-sided heart failure pulmonary symptoms are uncommon but fatigue is a frequent complaint. Examination of the heart in patients with right-sided cardiac failure might reveal additional signs (described in the answers to subsequent questions), especially if enlargement of the right chambers is present.

---

363 What physical findings might be detected on cardiac examination in right-sided heart failure?

☐ Physical findings that might be detected in patients with right-sided heart failure include signs of right ventricular enlargement or pulmonary hypertension as well as "gallop" sounds or murmurs of tricuspid regurgitation. When right ventricular enlargement is present, a right ventricular heave may be recognized on inspection and palpation of the precordium as a diffuse lift over the lower portion of the sternum (the right ventricle is positioned behind the lower portion of the sternum). Accentuation of the pulmonary component of the second heart sound is generally evident with pulmonary hypertension. A right ventricular gallop due to a third heart sound (commonly called S_3) might be evident on cardiac auscultation. This S_3 sound is due to a rapid deceleration of blood entering the right ventricle with reduced distensibility in the filling phase of the cardiac cycle. A fourth heart sound (commonly called S_4) might also be detected immediately preceding the first heart sound (S_1) and is due to a forceful contraction of the right atrium expelling blood into a noncompliant and thickened right ventricle (hypertrophy of this chamber). Because S_3 or S_4 occur during ventricular diastole (i.e., after S_2 and before S_1), their presence along with the normal S_1 and S_2 produce a characteristic pattern of sounds that resembles a galloping horse. Thus, these extra sounds are commonly known as S_3 gallop and S_4 gallop. The gallop sounds are better auscultated with the bell (due to their low frequency) rather than the diaphragm of the stethoscope. Gallops that originate in the right ventricle are best heard at the lower sternal border and increase with inspiration. Tricuspid regurgitation due to right ventricular enlargement is present in some patients with right-sided heart failure and produces a characteristic holosystolic murmur with a systolic distention or "v" wave that may be seen and palpated in the jugular veins at the neck.

---

364   How is the clinical evaluation of systemic venous hypertension performed?

□ When patients are examined in a semirecumbent position (i.e., at a 45° angle), the jugular vein might be distended as much as 4 cm above the sternal angle in the normal state. Higher values are observed with systemic venous hypertension. Exertion decreases jugular venous pressure in normal individuals but it increases this parameter in patients with heart failure. This physical finding is known as Kussmaul's sign. Prominence of the veins in the back of the hands is a valuable sign of systemic venous congestion in infants whose short necks make detection of jugular vein distention difficult.

---

365   What abnormalities of the venous pulse might resemble the jugular vein distention observed in heart failure?

□ Prominent "a" and "v" waves of the jugular pulse might be confused with the typical jugular vein distention of heart failure on rapid examination. Enlargement of "a" wave is observed with both pulmonary hypertension and tricuspid stenosis. It is due to a more forceful right atrial contraction in the presence of higher impedance to right ventricular emptying (pulmonary hypertension) or to right ventricular filling (tricuspid stenosis). Enlargement of the "v" wave is observed with tricuspid regurgitation, a condition in which systolic distention of neck veins becomes evident because of blood backflow during ventricular systole into the right atrium and large systemic veins. The pulsatile nature of prominent "a" and "v" waves can be distinguished from the sustained jugular vein distention of congestive heart failure on careful examination.

---

366   How can systemic venous pressure be measured?

□ Venous pressure of a forearm vein might be measured after insertion of a needle or a percutaneous catheter connected to a spinal fluid manometer filled with available IV solution. The patient should remain in the recumbent position with the arm abducted. The baseline or zero level for this measurement is the estimated position of the right atrium, which is generally taken as the midaxillary line (about 5 cm below the sternal angle). Normal venous pressure is 3 to 12 cm H_2O. Patients having congestive heart failure generally exhibit higher values (above 12 cm H_2O), especially with hepatic compression by the examiner's hand or during physical exercise.

367 What chest x-ray abnormalities in the systemic veins might be recognized in patients with heart failure?

☐ Dilation of the superior vena cava and azygos veins might be present in patients with right-sided congestive heart failure. These abnormalities are due to backward failure of the right cardiac chambers, increased blood volume, and constriction of arteries and veins of the systemic circulation.

368 What are the main characteristics of the pleural effusion (hydrothorax) secondary to heart failure?

☐ Patients with heart failure who develop hydrothorax most commonly have venous hypertension of both the pulmonary and systemic circulations. The pleural effusion is usually bilateral but if unilateral it is generally located in the right hemithorax. Dyspnea intensifies as hydrothorax develops because of further reduction of pulmonary vital capacity. Some exceptions to these rules include: (1) isolated venous hypertension of either the pulmonary or the systemic circulation, if severe, might also produce pleural effusion; and (2) hydrothorax present exclusively in the left hemithorax. This unusual situation mandates that other causes of effusion including pulmonary embolism and infections be ruled out.

369 How might pleural effusions appear on a chest x-ray of patients with heart failure?

☐ The radiologic appearance of a pleural effusion in heart failure includes: (1) free pleural fluid collection, which blunts the costophrenic angle and is easily recognized in the upright position; it is located bilaterally in two thirds of patients but if unilateral it is most commonly on the right side; (2) subpleural collection in which fluid accumulates in the subpleural space, resembling either paralysis of one hemidiaphragm (elevation of one leaf) or a free pleural fluid accumulation with blunting of the costophrenic sulci; comparison of chest x-rays obtained in the upright and recumbent or Trendelenburg (head down) position allows differentiation between subpleural collections (fluid remains immobile) and free pleural collections (fluid migrates in response to gravity because it is located in the main intrapleural space); (3) interlobar fissure thickenings that are sharp linear densities located predominantly in the lower portions of the lungs; within this category are the so-called Kerley A lines that extend peripherally from the hilum in the upper and midportions of the lungs while the Kerley B lines are peripheral markings (most commonly horizontal lines) that project to the pleural space and/or over the diaphragm; and (4) pseudotumor, that consists of fluid collections located in the interlobar spaces which might simulate pneumonia, tumor, or infarction of the lung.

---

370 How does pleural effusion due to heart failure respond to successful treatment of the cardiac condition?

☐ Successful treatment of heart failure with improvement of cardiac function generally leads to reabsorption of the hydrothorax. Such reabsorption might be incomplete (partial), especially with interlobar effusions or accumulation of protein-rich pleural fluid (also called "pseudoexudate" having 2 to 3 g/dL protein). Needle aspiration might be required in such cases to drain the hydrothorax.

---

371 What is the hepatojugular reflux?

☐ Hepatojugular reflux is the development of jugular vein distention in response to compression of the right upper quadrant of the abdomen. Elicitation of hepatojugular reflux requires the combination of passive venous congestion of the liver and inability of the right side of the heart to pump the transiently increased preload. Hepatic enlargement due to causes other than passive venous congestion of the liver does not produce hepatojugular reflux.

---

372   How is the hepatojugular reflux demonstrated?

☐ Hepatojugular reflux is demonstrated as follows: (1) patient must be in the recumbent position; (2) patient is advised to relax, to avoid straining, talking, holding his/her breath, or carrying out a Valsalva maneuver (these actions might distend the jugular veins independently of abnormal compression); and (3) the right upper quadrant of the abdomen should be compressed firmly, gradually, and continuously for about one minute while the jugular veins at the neck are observed. Hepatojugular reflux is present (positive sign) if neck veins distend while performing this maneuver, and absent (negative sign) if jugular veins fail to enlarge.

---

373   What are the physical examination findings of patients with congestive hepatomegaly?

☐ Pain in the right upper quadrant of the abdomen that is spontaneous or elicited on palpation and percussion might occur in patients with congestive hepatomegaly. Liver tenderness or pain is due to stretching of the organ capsule. It develops with rapid and recent hepatomegaly whereas it disappears with long-standing passive congestion (despite persistent liver enlargement). Inspection of the abdomen might reveal fullness/distention of the right upper quadrant and epigastric areas. Percussion of these areas elicits dullness because this enlarged solid organ (liver) displaces hollow organs (stomach). The enlarged and congested liver might also have pulsations recognized on palpation.

---

374   What hemodynamic parameters of patients with heart failure correlate with the development of hepatic dysfunction?

☐ The venous pressure of the systemic circulation and the cardiac index can be used to predict the presence of liver abnormalities in heart failure. Sustained high levels of venous pressure and low cardiac index that exceed 14 cm H_2O and fall short of 1.5 L/min/m^2, respectively, are generally associated with clinical and laboratory manifestations of hepatic dysfunction.

---

375   Can severe jaundice occur as a complication of heart failure in the absence of a primary liver disease?

☐ Yes. A syndrome that resembles acute viral hepatitis might be observed in patients with severe congestive heart failure. Serum AST (aspartate aminotransferase, 0 to 35 U/L) can be as high as ten times the normal levels and bilirubin can increase to 15 to 20 mg/dL in some patients. In contrast with viral hepatitis, the successful treatment of heart failure in these patients rapidly ameliorates the clinical and laboratory abnormalities of liver dysfunction.

---

376   What causes of pulsation of the liver might be detected in patients with congestive hepatomegaly?

☐ Expansion of the liver during ventricular systole producing a palpable pulsation might be recognized in patients with tricuspid regurgitation. A different hepatic pulsation that occurs in presystole and is due to a forceful right atrial contraction might be evident in patients with pulmonary hypertension, pulmonic stenosis, tricuspid stenosis, restrictive cardiomyopathy of the right ventricle, and constrictive pericarditis. The presystolic pulsation of the liver coincides with the "a" wave of the jugular venous pulse detected on examination of the patients's neck.

---

377   What liver diseases might be caused by heart failure?

☐ Congestive hepatomegaly and cardiac cirrhosis (i.e., liver cirrhosis due to passive congestion and reduced blood perfusion of this organ in patients with cardiac disease/failure) are responsible for most of the abnormal liver function studies observed in severe congestive heart failure. Centrilobular hepatic necrosis might also develop, possibly leading to hepatic coma. The latter might be the final outcome of cardiac cirrhosis.

378   What components of the physical examination provide clues to the presence of a high cardiac output state independent of its specific cause?

☐ Cardiovascular examination in states of high cardiac output frequently reveals abnormalities in the arterial pulses, systemic veins, and the precordial area that are common to all conditions responsible for a hyperdynamic circulation. We shall succinctly evaluate these abnormalities in the following questions.

379   What are the physical findings on examination of the systemic veins in high cardiac output states?

☐ A cervical venous hum is a continuous murmur with diastolic accentuation heard over the deep internal jugular veins (more often on the right side) in states of hyperdynamic circulation. Although cervical hums in the sitting position might be found in normal children, venous hums in adults (especially in the recumbent posture) are abnormal and indicate an accelerated circulation. Venous hums might occasionally be detected in the femoral area and have a similar pathogenesis.

380   What findings might be detected on physical examination of the precordial area in high cardiac output states?

☐ Increased intensity of the first cardiac sound and either a third sound (protodiastolic or ventricular gallop) or a fourth sound (presystolic or atrial gallop) are commonly encountered. A midsystolic murmur located in the second and third intercostal spaces in the absence of diastolic murmurs is also characteristic of high cardiac output states. Furthermore, aortic and mitral diastolic murmurs are occasionally detected in hyperkinetic states.

190Blackwell's Basics of Medicine Series

---

381 What changes in the arterial pulses might be recognized in high cardiac output states independent of the specific cause or etiology?

☐ Abnormalities in the heart rate and the morphology of the pulse might be evident on examination of systemic arteries (e.g., carotid, femoral, radial). Heart rate is increased at rest but is usually below 110 beats/min in the absence of both overt heart failure and a severe form of the underlying disease (e.g., acute blood loss, thyroid storm, complicating tachyarrhythmia). The pulse is bounding and has a quick upstroke. The increased left ventricular stroke volume is responsible for the wide pulse pressure that is in turn due to a combination of increased systolic blood pressure and decreased diastolic blood pressure. Auscultation of the carotid arteries might reveal a systolic bruit and that of femoral arteries might disclose pistol-shot sounds and flow murmurs (Duroziez's sign or murmur). Patients with aortic regurgitation might have signs on examination of the arterial pulse that are identical to those described above.

---

382 Might systemic and pulmonary congestion be evident in high cardiac output states?

☐ Yes. Hyperkinetic states might produce a syndrome of congestive heart failure (i.e., pulmonary congestion, systemic congestion, or both are present) despite an elevated cardiac output and little or no response to digitalis preparations. Thus, the presence of systemic and pulmonary venous congestion is not specific for low cardiac output heart failure because it might be observed in hypokinetic and hyperkinetic circulatory states.

---

383 Name important clinical conditions that might cause high output heart failure.

☐ Clinical conditions that might cause high output heart failure include anemia, thyrotoxicosis (hyperthyroidism), congenital and acquired arteriovenous fistulae, beriberi, Paget's disease of bones, and multiple myeloma.

384   Describe the major abnormalities in the cardiovascular examination of high output heart failure due to anemia.

☐ Such patients have bounding arterial pulses, subungual capillary pulsations (Quincke's pulse), and pistol-shot sounds that can be heard over the femoral arteries (Duroziez's sign). The heart sounds are accentuated and a midsystolic murmur of up to 3/6 in intensity (i.e., without a palpable thrill) due to high blood flow is commonly observed. In addition, cardiac auscultation reveals a left ventricular gallop. Hepatomegaly and peripheral edema might be present, but their pathogenesis might involve factors other than heart failure. Neck vein distention is generally absent. Cardiovascular examination of patients with severe anemia resembles that found in aortic regurgitation with respect to the peripheral circulation.

385   What are the most common findings on the chest x-ray, ECG, and echocardiogram of high output heart failure due to anemia?

☐ Common findings of high output heart failure due to anemia include: (1) mild to moderate cardiomegaly on chest-x-ray; (2) T wave inversions in the lateral precordial leads on ECG; and (3) symmetrical increase in the size of all cardiac chambers of moderate degree observed on echocardiogram.

386   What are the principal physical findings related to the cardiovascular system in high output heart failure due to thyrotoxicosis?

☐ The high output state of the circulation in these patients is manifested by tachycardia, brisk carotid pulsations (carotid, femoral, radial), a widened pulse pressure, a hyperkinetic heart apex, a loud first heart sound, and a midsystolic murmur along the left sternal border.

387   What are the most common findings on the chest x-ray, ECG, and echocardiogram, of high output heart failure due to thyrotoxicosis?

☐ Common findings of high output heart failure due to hyperthyroidism include: (1) a normal cardiac silouhette on chest x-ray; (2) nonspecific ST segment elevation, T wave inversion, shortening of the QT interval, and atrial fibrillation on the ECG; and (3) normal or increased ejection fraction and augmented left ventricular wall thickness and chamber dimension observed on echocardiogram.

---

388   Summarize the general characteristics common to all systemic arteriovenous fistulas that cause high output heart failure.

☐ Physical examination generally reveals mild tachycardia, brisk arterial pulses (e.g., carotid, femoral), and a widened pulse pressure. Manual compression of the fistula produces bradycardia (Branhan's sign) and increases arterial pressure. Other physical findings depend on the size and location of the shunt as well as the underlying disease. A continuous "machinery" murmur accompanied by a palpable thrill and warmer skin are present at the location of the fistula. Auscultation of the heart might reveal a midsystolic "flow" murmur, as well as ventricular and atrial gallops. Left ventricular hypertrophy is common and can be demonstrated by electrocardiography.

---

389   Name the most clinically relevant systemic arteriovenous fistulas.

☐ Congenital and acquired systemic arteriovenous fistulas might lead to high output heart failure. Congenital fistulas include a wide range of lesions and diseases. The fistulas might be localized to one body region as exemplified by a "strawberry mark" that is barely tangible. More evident fistulas include the large hemangiomas that comprise cyanotic areas rich in varicose veins that cover a swollen and deformed extremity. On the other hand, fistulas might be widespread as a generalized disease involving many body areas (e.g., hereditary hemorrhagic telangiectasia or Osler-Weber-Rendu disease). Patients with congenital fistulas manifested as cutaneous hemangiomas might have additional vascular deformations involving internal organs (e.g., hemangioendothelioma of the liver). Acquired fistulas might result from trauma (e.g., stab or gunshot wounds), surgery (e.g., vascular access for long-term hemodialysis), tumors (e.g., Wilms's tumor of the kidney in children), and other diseases (e.g., spontaneous rupture of aortic aneurysm into the inferior vena cava).

390 What diagnostic procedures are of special value in the evaluation of patients suspected to have congenital and acquired fistulas?

    ☐ Angiography and Doppler studies can establish the anatomy and functional characteristics of congenital and acquired fistulas. These techniques also guide therapy and allow follow-up of patients with these diseases.

391 What are the clinical manifestations of beriberi heart disease leading to high output heart failure?

    ☐ Severe thiamine or B_1 vitamin deficiency produces biventricular heart failure, wide pulse pressure, and an apical systolic "flow" murmur with a ventricular gallop on cardiac auscultation. Important additional findings include abnormalities in the: (1) ECG, such as low voltage of the QRS complex, prolongation of the QT interval, and low voltage or inversion of T waves; (2) chest x-ray, such as biventricular enlargement, pulmonary congestion, and hydrothorax; (3) cardiovascular laboratory showing diminished left ventricular ejection fraction; and (4) biochemical laboratory, such as increased serum levels of pyruvate and lactate, a low transketolase level in red blood cells, and diminished thiamine concentration in body fluids. An almost immediate correction of several cardiovascular abnormalities occurs after administration of thiamine.

392 What noncardiovascular clinical manifestations are commonly present in beriberi?

    ☐ Multiple vitamin deficiency (several members of the B complex of vitamins) and generalized malnutrition are frequently present in beriberi. Consequently, peripheral neuropathy manifested by paresthesias, sensory and motor deficits, depressed or absent knee and ankle reflexes, skin hyperkeratosis, painful glossitis, and anemia are commonly observed.

393 What are "dry" and "wet" beriberi and which are the conditions leading to these diseases?

☐ "Dry beriberi" refers to thiamine deficiency manifested by isolated peripheral neuropathy, whereas "wet beriberi" has signs and symptoms of high output heart failure and generalized edema. The conditions leading to a deficiency of vitamin B_1 include excessive alcohol intake, ingestion of faddist diets (rich in carbohydrate content), and low nutrient intake. Although the first two causes are most frequently observed in the Western world, the latter condition is more prevalent in Asia and Africa.

394 How might Paget's disease of bones (osteitis deformans) cause high output heart failure?

☐ Increased blood flow to areas of the skeleton with abnormally rapid bone formation and reabsorption might produce a symptomatic high output state especially in patients with an associated heart disease (e.g., coronary artery disease). Additional findings in Paget's disease include sclerosis and metastatic calcifications. The latter condition might involve several body regions including the heart where abnormalities of atrioventricular or interventricular conduction might develop.

395 Name other causes of high output heart failure.

☐ Conditions that might cause high output heart failure other than those previously considered include pregnancy, obesity, cor pulmonale, polycythemia vera, glomerulonephritis, carcinoid syndrome, multiple myeloma, and fibrous dysplasia (Albright's syndrome).

396 What abnormalities in blood and urine chemistries might be present in heart failure?

☐ Abnormal results of laboratory studies indicative of renal or hepatic dysfunction are commonly observed in patients with severe heart failure, but not with mild cardiac impairment.

Reduction of renal blood flow or glomerular filtration rate plays a role in the urinary (e.g., decreased urine output, high urine specific gravity, low urinary [Na$^+$], increased urinary protein excretion) and blood abnormalities (e.g., hyponatremia, prerenal azotemia leading to high levels of blood urea nitrogen and creatinine). Reduced blood flow and congestion of the liver produce high serum levels of several liver enzymes including aspartate aminotransferase (AST), alanine aminotransferase (ALT), lactic dehydrogenase (LDH), and alkaline phosphatase. In addition, liver dysfunction might be evident by prolongation of the prothrombin time, hyperbilirubinemia, hypoalbuminemia, and occasionally hypoglycemia.

---

397   What main abnormalities in the serum electrolytes might be observed in heart failure?

☐ Low serum [Na$^+$] with reduced serum osmolality (i.e., hypotonic hyponatremia) and abnormally low or high serum K$^+$ levels might be observed in patients with severe heart failure. This hypotonic hyponatremia might be due to the combined effects of excessive dietary Na$^+$ restriction, intensive diuretic therapy, a relatively high water intake, and inappropriately low water excretion. Hypokalemia and hyperkalemia might be due to diuretic usage and abnormally low renal excretion of K$^+$, respectively. Serum electrolyte levels are usually normal in patients with mild to moderate heart failure before initiating therapy for this condition.

---

398   What is the significance of hyponatremia (abnormally low serum [Na$^+$]) in patients with congestive heart failure?

☐ Hyponatremia is an important laboratory finding in patients with congestive heart failure. Except for patients with heart failure whose hyponatremia is induced by overaggressive diuretic treatment and salt restriction (wherein discontinuation of such practice will allow correction of the hyponatremia) or excessive water intake, a diminished serum [Na$^+$] indicates significant activation of the neurohormonal system (e.g. vasopressin) as well as poor prognosis with respect to long-term survival. Serum [Na$^+$] correlates inversely with plasma renin activity, aldosterone, and PGE$_2$ (vasodilator prostaglandin).

Consequently, activation of the intrinsic vasoconstrictor system (renin-angiotensin-aldosterone, catecholamines, vasopressin) as well as the vasodilator system (vasodilator prostaglandins, atrial natriuretic factor, kinins) occurs in patients with severe heart failure and hyponatremia. A diminished serum [Na^+] predicts a brisk response to ACE inhibitors (greater likelihood of developing hypotension and renal insufficiency with these drugs) as well as warns of likely development of nephrotoxicity due to NSAIDs which depress intrinsic vasodilator mechanisms, promoting acute ischemic renal damage.

---

399   What is the role of exercise testing in the diagnosis of heart failure?

☐ Exercise testing by means of the stairmaster, bicycle ergometer, or treadmill might be helpful in the diagnosis of heart failure. Patients might develop dyspnea at low levels of exercise, a finding consistent with the diagnosis of heart failure. The maximal level of exercise that the patient can reach helps to diagnose heart failure as well as to determine its severity because it correlates with oxygen delivery by the circulatory system and tissue oxygen uptake. Exercise testing might precipitate symptomatic heart failure, cardiac arrhythmias, and even sudden death. Consequently, close supervision of patients undergoing exercise testing is mandatory.

---

400   Is an abnormal performance during exercise testing a specific indicator of heart failure?

☐ No. Many conditions including malingering, extreme sedentary life-style, obesity, peripheral vascular disease, anemia, and pulmonary diseases can limit performance during exercise testing. Measurement of other parameters during exercise testing (e.g., respiratory quotient, lactate production) helps to establish whether heart failure is responsible for the decreased performance.

401 What is the role of echocardiography in the evaluation of patients with heart failure?

☐ Echocardiography helps to establish whether a valvular disease (which is potentially correctable) is present, if wall motion abnormalities exist, and whether they are regional or diffuse. Although diffuse or global left ventricular dysfunction suggests a cardiomyopathy, regional wall motion abnormalities are more consistent with coronary artery disease. Doppler echocardiography permits measurements of blood flow. However, suboptimal sound penetration prevents optimal evaluation in some elderly patients, as well as others having chronic obstructive pulmonary disease or obesity.

402 What is the role of radionuclide ventriculography, coronary angiography, and cardiac catheterization in the evaluation and management of patients with heart failure?

☐ Radionuclide ventriculography is a noninvasive technique that can assess ventricular function at rest and during exercise. Coronary angiography allows recognition of coronary artery disease and it guides subsequent treatment with angioplasty or coronary artery bypass surgery. Cardiac catheterization is of special value in assessing the effect of drugs (e.g., vasodilators, inotropic agents) in patients with heart failure refractory to standard medical therapy. In addition, cardiac catheterization might help to establish the cause of heart failure.

403 Compare the information obtained with radionuclide ventriculography, echocardiography, and Doppler studies in the evaluation of patients with heart failure.

☐ Radionuclide ventriculography can measure ejection fraction of left and right ventricles, thereby helping to establish what cardiac chamber is primarily or more severely affected. The echocardiogram and Doppler studies can assess cardiac function and identify valvular and congenital defects. Regional wall motion abnormalities due to myocardial infarction can be recognized with all three techniques.

404   What is compensated congestive heart failure?

□ Compensated congestive heart failure is an expression commonly used by physicians to describe patients with heart failure in whom excessive fluid retention and pulmonary/systemic congestion have greatly improved or have completely resolved so that the patient's signs and symptoms of cardiac disease are ameliorated. Thus, the clinician's use of the term compensated congestive heart failure does not refer to the previously discussed compensatory mechanisms of heart failure.

405   What is intractable heart failure?

□ Intractable heart failure refers to a condition in which all conventional medical and surgical therapies pertinent to the management of the patient's cardiac disease fail to relieve signs and symptoms present at rest or with minimal activity. Patients with intractable heart failure might have a ventricular ejection fraction less than 20%, stroke volume 40 mL or less, serious ventricular arrhythmias, or other important signs and symptoms despite optimal treatment of their disease. Circulatory support with mechanical hearts or heart transplantation should be considered in these patients.

406   What is the overall prognosis in heart failure?

□ Heart failure is a disease with high morbidity and mortality, the latter being dependent on the severity of the disease. Patients with class IV heart failure have a one-year survival rate of only about 40%, whereas the survival rate for all classes combined is 55% for women and 40% for men at 5 years. Sudden death occurs in 33% to 47% of patients with severe heart failure, and ventricular arrhythmias play a major role in this outcome. The prognosis of heart failure and the survival of patients with this disease appear to improve with the use of afterload-reducing agents (vasodilator drugs), especially ACE inhibitors.

407 How might the prognosis in heart failure be determined?

☐ The prognosis in heart failure might be established according to clinical (e.g., NYHA class I through IV), hemodynamic (e.g., ventricular ejection fraction), biochemical (e.g., presence or absence of hyponatremia), and ECG (e.g, presence of ventricular arrhythmias) criteria. Integration of the elements obtained with these four categories of prognostic indicators allows the clinician to determine the expected morbidity and mortality for a given patient.

408 How do signs and symptoms help to estimate prognosis (e.g., survival) in heart failure? Does the cause of heart failure have any role on survival?

☐ The NYHA classification of the patient's clinical status is a major clinical indicator of prognosis. Patients belonging to class IV (symptomatic at rest and unable to carry on any physical activity without discomfort) have a 60% mortality per year, whereas those in class III (asymptomatic at rest but with marked limitation of physical activity) have a 20% mortality rate per year. A high resting heart rate detected on physical examination (e.g., above 120/min), a ventricular gallop, low systolic blood pressure, and low pulse pressure are also important indicators of severe disease and poor prognosis. The etiology of heart failure is also an important element of prognosis because mortality is higher when cardiac dysfunction is due to coronary artery disease.

409 What hemodynamic criteria help to determine prognosis (e.g., survival) in heart failure?

☐ Major hemodynamic criteria indicative of a poor prognosis are low levels of both ventricular ejection fraction (left or right chamber) and cardiac index. Patients with left ventricular ejection fraction of 20% or less have a mortality of about 30% per year, whereas those with ejection fraction of 31% to 40% have a mortality rate of 10% per year. Important additional hemodynamic criteria that are indicators of a bad prognosis are severely elevated ventricular filling pressures (left or right chamber) and increased systemic vascular resistance.

---

410   What biochemical criteria predict survival in heart failure?

☐ High plasma levels of norepinephrine, renin, vasopressin, and atrial natriuretic peptide (all indicative of neurohormonal activation) predict short survival in patients with heart failure. The high concentration of these substances, largely due to severe heart failure, might adversely affect cardiac function by augmenting ventricular afterload, increasing myocardial oxygen consumption, and inducing ventricular tachyarrhythmias. Hyponatremia is associated with high mortality, possibly reflecting a very low cardiac output, activation of the renin-angiotensin-aldosterone system, the use of an intense diuretic regimen, and presence of K^+ depletion.

---

411   What ECG findings might indicate a poor prognosis in heart failure?

☐ Sinus tachycardia (i.e., especially when resting heart rate is higher than 120 beats/min), ventricular extrasystoles, ventricular tachyarrhythmias, left intraventricular conduction defects, atrial fibrillation, and atrial flutter predict poor prognosis and short survival in heart failure. ECG evidence of myocardial ischemia worsens the prognosis of heart failure (see main factors that determine survival). Because death in patients with heart failure occurs suddenly or unexpectedly in about one half of them and it is presumed to occur because of an arrhythmia, the ECG findings are considered among the most important indicators of prognosis (survival).

---

412   Summarize the determinants of survival in heart failure.

☐ The main determinants of survival in congestive heart failure are: (1) etiology of heart disease (e.g., coronary artery disease entails a poor prognosis); (2) degree of left ventricular dysfunction (e.g., assessed by left ventricular ejection fraction); (3) symptomatic status, evaluated by exercise tolerance and NYHA class (e.g., low exercise tolerance or class IV have poor prognosis); (4) degree of neurohormonal activation, evaluated by serum [Na⁺], plasma renin activity, and plasma norepinephrine level (e.g., a higher level of neurohormonal activation has worse prognosis); and (5) ventricular arrhythmias (e.g., complex ventricular arrhythmias are commonly observed in heart failure and predict higher mortality and sudden death).

413   What are the causes of death in patients with heart failure?

□ Cardiac arrhythmias and pump failure account for about 80% of patients dying of heart failure (each of these causes is responsible for one half of the deaths). Cardiac arrhythmias are presumed to account for most, if not all sudden deaths in this population. The remaining 20% of deaths are secondary to pneumonia, pulmonary embolism, and other causes.

414   What is the prevalence and mortality of heart failure?

□ About 1% of the American population has congestive heart failure and for those over 75 years old, the prevalence of this syndrome is about 10%. The incidence and prevalence of heart failure increases at advanced age and this disease represents the most common hospital discharge diagnosis of patients over 65 years old. The mortality from congestive heart failure depends on the functional class of the disease, having the highest level (about 60% at one year) in patients with symptoms at rest (NYHA class IV). The overall combined mortality for all functional classes is 45% in women and 60% for men at 5 years (men afflicted with this disease have a more serious prognosis).

415   What abnormalities might be detected on macroscopic and microscopic examination of the liver in patients with heart failure?

□ Pathologic findings in the liver are characteristically present with right-sided heart failure, whereas lung abnormalities typically occur with left-sided heart failure. When right heart failure is severe but short lasting, the liver is enlarged, firm, and filled with fluid. The central hepatic veins and sinusoids are congested on microscopic examination. Long-standing heart failure reduces the size of the liver, which is no longer enlarged and might even significantly shrink in the advanced stage of the disease producing liver cirrhosis (i.e., cardiac cirrhosis). The dark red areas due to congestion of the central vein of the hepatic lobules surrounded by the lighter fatty area in the periphery of these lobules produces the "nutmeg" appearance detected on pathologic examination. Extensive fibrosis in association with central lobular necrosis, overall liver atrophy, and sclerosis of the hepatic veins are observed in cardiac cirrhosis.

416 What is the main determinant for the development of cardiac cirrhosis and what specific cardiac diseases most commonly lead to this hepatic illness?

☐ The severity of the elevated hepatic venous pressure and the duration of such abnormality are the main determinants for the development of cardiac cirrhosis. The specific heart diseases that most commonly produce cardiac cirrhosis are chronic constrictive pericarditis and organic tricuspid disease (including tricuspid atresia successfully corrected with surgery).

417 What pathologic findings might be disclosed in biopsy specimens of patients with severe hepatic damage due to advanced heart failure?

☐ Hepatocyte necrosis and red blood cell extravasation due to damaged endothelial cells are characteristic pathologic findings in these patients. The hepatic abnormalities might be transient if hemodynamic recovery occurs.

418 What abnormalities might be detected in the spleen, pancreas, and gastrointestinal tract of patients with heart failure?

☐ Congestive splenomegaly (enlargement of the spleen) due to portal hypertension might be present. Microscopic examination reveals widening of spleen sinusoids with fibrosis. The pancreas and the gastrointestinal tract also show venous congestion, which is occasionally associated with an ischemic noninfectious enterocolitis with areas of hemorrhagic necrosis.

Patients with heart failure and long-standing atrial fibrillation might also exhibit small infarcts in the spleen as well as in the kidneys.

MANAGEMENT OF HEART FAILURE

419   Outline the overall management of symptomatic or decompensated heart failure.

☐ The management of symptomatic or decompensated heart failure mandates that the clinician consider a three-pronged strategy aimed at: (1) removing the precipitating factors or causes of heart failure (e.g., arrhythmia, pulmonary embolism, sepsis); (2) controlling of signs and symptoms of heart failure (i.e., correction of fluid excess, decrease the cardiac work load, increase myocardial contractility); and (3) treating the underlying cardiac disease (e.g., hypertension, congenital malformation, acquired valvular lesions). Although the specific therapeutic measures vary widely among patients, these three elements must always be considered when the management strategy of patients with symptomatic or decompensated heart failure is reviewed.

420   What general measures might be required to control the signs and symptoms of heart failure?

☐ Control of the clinical manifestations of heart failure might require: (1) correction of fluid excess, which is the principal cause of most signs and symptoms (e.g., edema, dyspnea) in these patients; (2) reduction of the heart's work load by two mechanisms: a decrease in the blood flow demands of peripheral tissues and a decrease in the perfusion pressure that must be generated by the heart to supply the tissues with blood; and (3) enhancement of pumping action of the heart by means of drugs (e.g., digitalis glycosides) or electrical stimulation (e.g., pacemaker). These three groups of measures might be implemented on recognition of symptomatic heart failure.

421   Describe the treatment of localized and generalized edema.

☐ The treatment of localized and generalized edema must be directed, if possible, at the primary cause of fluid accumulation. Effective treatment of the primary cause leads to resolution of edema. Thus, in localized edema due to thrombophlebitis or lymphangitis, administration of antibiotics or anti-inflammatory agents corrects the primary process and helps in the resolution of edema. Patients with generalized edema due to severe nutritional deficiency leading to profound hypoalbuminemia must be treated with protein supplementation and other measures aimed at correcting this basic defect. Therapy of the primary process in congestive heart failure frequently involves the use of positive inotropic agents ("cardiotonics") or afterload-reducing agents. Likewise, therapy of the primary process in cirrhosis of the liver includes correction of nutritional deficits (vitamins, including B complex and K^+), avoidance of hepatotoxic agents (e.g., ethanol), and prevention of hepatic encephalopathy (e.g., low-protein diet, oral lactulose, nonabsorbable antibiotics in the digestive tract). In nephrosis, therapy of this condition with corticosteroids and cytotoxic drugs might favorably modify the glomerular disease. Patients with generalized edema most frequently require treatment of the fluid overload in addition to that directed at the primary disease. Correction of fluid overload involves restriction of dietary NaCl and, if this is unsuccessful, diuretic therapy.

---

422   What other measures are important in the treatment of edema?

☐ All forms of edema, localized and generalized, inflammatory and noninflammatory, are ameliorated by bed rest and elevation of the edematous body area (e.g., placement of swollen body region above the heart level such as the head in facial phlegmon following dental surgery, and the lower extremity in thrombophlebitis of the calf). The benefits derived from bed rest and elevation of edematous body region derive from: (1) facilitation of fluid exit from the edematous region due to the salutary effect on Starling forces (caused by reduction in arterial and increment in venous blood flow) accompanied by decreased metabolic demands of resting tissues, as well as to the hydrostatic effects of elevating the edematous region; (2) bed rest diminishes venous blood pooling, increasing venous return to the heart that augments atrial natriuretic factor, leading to renal vasodilation and increased NaCl excretion; and (3) bed rest suppresses the renin-angiotensin-aldosterone system and α-adrenergic-mediated vasoconstrictor influences, and these effects increase renal excretion of NaCl. Bed rest, extended for several days, or intermittent (a few hours of daytime rest in addition to nocturnal sleep), helps mobilization of dependent edema.

---

423 Describe the dietary management of generalized edema.

☐ Reduced dietary salt intake (in this book, the term "salt" is used interchangeably with sodium chloride or NaCl) is indicated in states of generalized edema. Mild NaCl restriction is accomplished by avoiding both the ingestion of salty foods and the addition of salt at the table. Moderate NaCl restriction requires measures outlined for mild restriction plus avoiding NaCl addition during meal preparation (cooking). Severe NaCl restriction mandates the exclusive ingestion of foods with very low NaCl content. The daily NaCl intake with these regimens is as follows: (1) normal diet contains 10 to 15 g NaCl (4 to 6 g or 174 to 261 mEq Na^+); (2) mild NaCl restriction provides 8 to 10 g NaCl (3.2 to 4 g or 139 to 174 mEq Na^+); (3) moderate NaCl restriction provides 4 to 6 g NaCl (1.6 to 2.4 g or 70 to 104 mEq Na^+); and (4) severe NaCl restriction provides 1 to 2 g NaCl (0.4 to 0.8 g or 17 to 35 mEq of Na^+).

---

424 Is water restriction routinely prescribed for the treatment of generalized edema?

☐ No. Water restriction is usually unnecessary in the management of edematous patients. Excessive water intake, however, should be always discouraged in patients on low-NaCl intake or receiving diuretics. If a very low NaCl intake is prescribed, water restriction must be enforced to prevent the development of hypotonic hyponatremia. The high ADH levels in patients on severe salt restriction or high doses of diuretics further increase the risk of hyponatremia

---

425 Name the best foods, very low in NaCl, recommended for patients with generalized edema.

☐ Very low-NaCl foods include: (1) grain products such as rice, corn, and pastas; (2) potatoes, cucumbers, Swiss chards, asparagus, sweet peas, lentils, mushrooms; (3) salt-free butter; (4) fresh fruits; and (5) tea, beer, and wines. The Na^+ content of these products is less than 25 mg (about 1 mEq) per cup.

---

426   Name the low-NaCl foods indicated for patients at risk of salt retention or experiencing mild edema.

☐ Low-NaCl foods include: (1) freshwater fish; (2) low-salt bread; (3) milk, cream, egg yolk; and (4) carrots, spinach, artichokes, cabbage. The Na^+ content of these products is less than 125 mg (about 5 mEq) per cup.

---

427   Name the NaCl-rich foods, the intake of which should be limited in patients predisposed to salt retention and encouraged in those predisposed to salt depletion.

☐ Sodium chloride-rich foods include: (1) meats such as pork, beef, lamb, and poultry; (2) egg whites; (3) "low-Na^+" cheese; (4) celery stems, paprika, nutmeg; and (5) chocolate, cocoa, instant coffee. These foods have up to 250 mg (about 11 mEq) Na^+ per cup.

---

428   Name the foods very rich in NaCl that are strictly forbidden to patients with generalized edema and specially valuable to those experiencing salt depletion.

☐ Very rich-NaCl foods include: (1) regular bread; (2) seafood; (3) canned meats and vegetables; (4) all cheeses other than those of "low-Na^+" content; (5) regular butter; and (6) salt-cured meats. The Na^+ content of these foods is between 500 and 7500 mg (22 to 326 mEq) per cup in canned goods, seafood and salt-cured meats. The last two have the highest salt content.

---

429   Outline the main steps for dietary salt (NaCl and other Na^+ salts) restriction that might be prescribed in accordance with the severity of heart failure.

☐ Discontinued use of a salt shaker at the table and avoidance of salt-rich foods represent the first step aimed at prevention of fluid retention or management of mild forms of congestive heart failure. The second step is the elimination of salt added, both during meal cooking and at the table, as well as avoiding salt-rich foods. Patients with heart failure ranging from mild to severe require implementation of the second step of salt restriction. The third step of salt restriction allows consumption of only low-Na^+ foods plus the limitation of salt intake described for step two. In general, only patients with the most severe forms of congestive heart failure require application of measures outlined in step three for the long-term management of their disease. The simultaneous prescription of diuretics permits a more liberal dietary salt intake that improves patient satisfaction and compliance.

430 How important is dietary salt restriction in the management of heart failure?

☐ Salt restriction is a critical therapeutic measure in patients with heart failure. Discontinuation of salt shaker use at the table and avoidance of salty foods (e.g., smoked and salt-cured meats and fish, potato chips, pretzels, salted nuts, pickles, olives) are standard measures required for most patients. Because adequate nutrition usually requires the ingestion of tasty foods, it might be advisable to continue using a modest amount of salt while cooking meals. Addition of spices and herbs to food during preparation enhances its flavor. The moderate salt restriction achieved with these measures might be complemented with diuretic drugs to secure optimal salt balance. If generalized edema refractory to moderate salt restriction and diuretics is present, severe salt restriction (e.g., Kempner's diet of rice and fruits) must be prescribed, at least temporarily.

431 Should restriction of water intake be generally enforced in the management of heart failure?

☐ No. Restriction of dietary salt is usually followed by a parallel salutary reduction in the spontaneous intake of water by the patient. Thus, the decrease in salt content of body fluids observed with correction of fluid overload (with low salt intake or diuretics) is not accompanied by hyponatremia (reduction in serum sodium concentration). By contrast, in advanced heart failure, especially when dietary salt is greatly reduced and the diuretic regimen is intensive, hyponatremia might develop if water intake is not restricted. Severe heart failure increases plasma ADH concentration and impairs urine dilution by multiple mechanisms. Thus, patients with severe heart failure are predisposed to hypotonic hyponatremia. Under these conditions, severe dietary salt restriction combined with generous water intake can lead to hypotonic hyponatremia.

432   What are so-called salt substitutes?

☐ Salt substitutes are K^+ salts (usually KCl) that mimic the taste of NaCl. Whenever a patient is told to reduce the NaCl (salt) intake, these salt substitutes are often recommended. Because these products are available over the counter, patients frequently use them whether they are endorsed by physicians or not. A low-NaCl intake reduces the ability to maximally excrete K^+ by the kidney. The simultaneous ingestion of salt substitutes (K^+ salts) can lead to hyperkalemia because the increased K^+ intake is accompanied by reduced renal K^+ excretion.

433   When should diuretics be used in volume expansion?

☐ The physician should consider the use of diuretics when dietary NaCl restriction and bed rest fail to correct salt and water retention. Diuretics promote natriuresis (increased urine Na^+ excretion) and diuresis (increased urine volume) by their actions on the renal tubules. Major indications for the use of diuretics include deterioration of cardiac function due to fluid overload, respiratory dysfunction due to pulmonary congestion, peripheral edema, or the mechanical effects of massive ascites.

434   Name the major classes or types of diuretics available for the management of volume expansion.

☐ Thiazides, loop diuretics, K^+-sparing diuretics, and acetazolamide are diuretics that might be recommended in the treatment of volume expansion. Thiazides and loop diuretics are commonly prescribed agents that can be used in most patients with generalized edema independently of its cause. By contrast, K^+-sparing diuretics and acetazolamide are indicated in specific conditions discussed in subsequent answers.

---

435 Describe how diuretic agents or drugs (or simply diuretics) increase natriuresis.

☐ All diuretic agents enhance natriuresis by diminishing NaCl reabsorption in the renal tubules. The potency of these agents and their effect on K^+ excretion are greatly dependent on the site of action on the renal tubule (e.g., proximal tubule, loop of Henle, distal tubule). Diuretics that inhibit salt reabsorption only in the proximal tubule, such as acetazolamide and mannitol, are not potent diuretics when used as single agents, because the increased salt and water that leave the proximal nephron promote increased salt and water reabsorption at more distal sites (loop of Henle and distal nephron). The so-called loop diuretics (furosemide, ethacrynic acid, bumetanide) exert their action on the medullary and cortical thick ascending limb of the loop of Henle and can promote excretion of up to 40% of the filtered load of NaCl. Loop diuretics are the most potent diuretics and are also characterized by their effectiveness in patients with either acidosis or alkalosis (as opposed to acetazolamide that is ineffective in patients with metabolic acidosis). Thiazides inhibit salt reabsorption in the cortical ascending limb of Henle's loop and in the early distal tubule; these drugs have less diuretic potency compared to loop diuretics. Diuretic agents whose action is mediated by inhibition of salt reabsorption in the collecting duct include the K^+-sparing diuretics (spironolactone, amiloride, and triamterene). The K^+-sparing diuretics are characterized by their moderate potency and reduced effectiveness in patients with metabolic alkalosis. All diuretic agents except for those acting in the collecting duct (K^+-sparing diuretics) enhance both natriuresis and kaliuresis.

436   Compare the potency of diuretic agents in terms of the fractional urinary excretion of sodium (FE_{Na^+}).

□   The K^+-sparing diuretics including spironolactone, triamterene, and amiloride are the least potent diuretics with a FE_{Na^+} 2% to 3%. Acetazolamide is also a very mild diuretic with a FE_{Na^+} between 3% and 5%. The most widely used agents are the thiazides or metolazone, with a FE_{Na^+} of 5% to 8%, and the "loop" diuretics (furosemide, ethacrynic acid, bumetanide) with a FE_{Na^+} of 20% to 25%. When massive doses of "loop" agents are used, FE_{Na^+} values as high as 40% can be attained.

437   Explain further fractional excretion of Na^+ (FE_{Na^+}).

□   The percent of filtered Na^+ being excreted defines the fractional excretion of Na^+. Its calculation requires urinary Na^+ excretion (urinary $[Na^+] \times$ urine flow) and filtered load of Na^+ (glomerular filtration rate $\times [Na^+]_p$). Glomerular filtration rate (GFR) is estimated as the ratio of urinary creatinine excretion (urinary creatinine concentration $\times$ urine flow) to plasma creatinine concentration. Thus,

$$FE_{Na^+} = \frac{U_{Na^+} \times V}{\dfrac{U_{cr} \times V}{P_{cr}} \times P_{Na^+}} \times 100$$

where U_{Na^+} is urinary $[Na^+]$; V is urinary flow; U_{cr} is urinary creatinine concentration; P_{cr} is plasma creatinine concentration; P_{Na^+} is $[Na^+]_p$; one hundred (100) is used to express the FE_{Na^+} as a percent value.

Because V is present in both numerator and denominator of the equation, its value is canceled; thus,

$$FE_{Na^+} = \frac{U_{Na^+} \times P_{cr}}{U_{cr} \times P_{Na^+}} \times 100$$

which is the formula most frequently used to calculate FE_{Na^+}.

---

438 What are the loop diuretics (also known as high-ceiling diuretics)?

☐ The loop diuretics are drugs that promote increased renal excretion of salt and water by inhibiting NaCl reabsorption in the thick ascending limb of Henle's loop. The term "high-ceiling" diuretics relates to the high intensity of their effects, which might trigger mechanisms that oppose the fluid loss. The loop diuretics include furosemide (sulfonamide derivative of anthranilic acid, brand name Lasix), bumetanide (Bumex), ethacrynic acid (a phenoxyacetic acid derivative, brand name Edecrin), piretanide (Arelix, Diumax, Taulig), and other compounds that are likely to be approved for general usage (muzolimine and torasemide that have a long-acting effect and a sustained antihypertensive action, respectively).

---

439 What are the most salient properties of loop diuretics?

☐ Loop diuretics, the most potent among all diuretic drugs, include furosemide (Lasix), ethacrynic acid (Edecrin), and bumetanide (Bumex). These agents inhibit NaCl reabsorption in the thick ascending limb of Henle's loop. This action takes place on the luminal membrane after the diuretic reaches Henle's loop by secretion into the proximal tubule and by glomerular filtration. The diuresis and natriuresis promoted by loop diuretics might additionally be due to increased renal blood flow partly mediated by increased secretion of vasodilatory prostaglandins. Administration of NSAIDs, drugs known to diminish renal prostaglandin synthesis, can decrease the diuretic action of loop diuretics. The onset of action occurs within minutes with peak effects occurring within two hours, and duration of action is up to six hours. Daily dosages are: (1) furosemide, 20 to 80 mg, maximal dose is 1000 mg/d; (2) ethacrynic acid, 50 to 100 mg but it can be given up to 400 mg/d; and (3) bumetanide, 0.5 to 2.0 mg, maximal dose is 10 mg/d. The most salient adverse effects are K^+ depletion with hypokalemia, metabolic alkalosis, hyponatremia, and muscle cramps. Furosemide can also cause glucose intolerance, deafness, and thrombocytopenia. Loop diuretics have synergistic effects with thiazides so that their combination can be useful in the management of edematous patients who fail to respond to a single agent.

---

440 What is the specific pharmacologic effect of loop diuretics on the thick ascending limb of Henle's loop?

☐ Loop diuretics inhibit a cotransport system located in the apical membrane of the medullary and cortical thick ascending limb of Henle's loop. This system promotes the simultaneous reabsorption of $Na^+/K^+/2$ Cl^- by an electrically silent process that moves these ions from the tubule lumen to the cell interior. Most K^+ reabsorbed by this mechanism leaks back into the tubule lumen due to the high membrane permeability to this ion and thereby causes a lumen-positive potential in this nephron segment. The inhibition of the $Na^+/K^+/2$ Cl^- cotransport system by loop diuretics has several consequences. (1) It delivers large amounts of Na^+, Cl^-, and water to the distal nephron greatly exceeding the reabsorptive capacity of this segment, leading to enhanced diuresis and natriuresis. (2) It increases K^+ secretion and urinary acidification by the distal nephron because of the large Na^+ load delivered to this segment. (3) It reduces electrolyte-free water reabsorption by the collecting duct (ADH-sensitive epithelium) because of a diminished osmotic gradient between the renal medulla and tubule lumen that promotes water transport; the diminished tonicity of medullary interstitium occurs because loop diuretics inhibit salt reabsorption from the water-impermeable thick ascending limb of Henle's loop, reducing the gradient for water movement from the collecting duct in the presence of ADH.

---

441 Do loop diuretics have extrarenal hemodynamic effects other than those secondary to natriuresis-induced ECF volume depletion?

☐ Yes. Loop diuretics increase capacitance of the venous system and thereby augment the fraction of total blood volume held in this compartment, with a secondary reduction in cardiac filling pressure during diastole. These hemodynamic effects of loop diuretics are potentially salutary in patients with both cardiogenic and noncardiogenic pulmonary edema.

The drug-induced venodilation is most evident after short-term administration of furosemide is blunted by inhibitors of prostaglandin synthesis (e.g., NSAIDs), and is absent in anephric patients. Short-term administration of furosemide might also have hemodynamic effects due to increased left ventricular afterload secondary to a rise in systemic vascular resistance. The arteriolar constriction induced by IV furosemide administration, which is due to stimulation of renin release (and a secondary rise in angiotensin level), might be harmful to patients with acute myocardial ischemia.

442   Describe further the effects of diuretics (e.g., furosemide) on systemic vascular resistance and on pulmonary function in congestive heart failure.

☐ Although the dominant vascular effect of furosemide administration occurs in the systemic venous system (producing venodilation that increases peripheral venous capacitance) and thereby reduces venous return to the heart, chronic therapy with this agent (and other diuretics) most frequently decreases systemic vascular resistance in congestive heart failure. Such salutary reduction in left ventricular outflow resistance might be due to decreased arteriolar stiffness caused by a reduced vessel wall Na^+ and water content. Diuretic therapy in congestive heart failure can decrease lung water, airway resistance, pulmonary compliance, and respiratory work, reversing at least in part the abnormalities in pulmonary function observed in patients with heart failure.

443   Compare the dose-response relationship for the hemodynamic and natriuretic effects of furosemide.

☐ Changes in both venous capacitance and systemic vascular resistance are nearly maximal after an IV dosage of only 20 mg furosemide. This dose-response relationship differs from the natriuretic effect of furosemide, which increases linearly with dosage. The hemodynamic effects of bumetanide are of less intensity in comparison with those of furosemide.

444   What are the similarities and differences among loop diuretics (furosemide, ethacrynic acid, bumetanide, and piretanide)?

☐ The therapeutic efficacy of all loop diuretics is similar. Nevertheless, the potency of bumetanide and piretanide is greater than that of furosemide per mg of drug (40:1 and 6:1, respectively compared to furosemide). These two drugs also have higher bioavailability and slightly less ototoxicity compared to furosemide. Considering that ethacrynic acid has considerable ototoxicity, other loop diuretics should be prescribed to patients for whom this class of diuretics is indicated. Exceptions to this rule include patients with a previous history of allergy or interstitial nephritis secondary to loop diuretics other than ethacrynic acid or to sulfonamides.

445   What features distinguish loop diuretics from other diuretic drugs?

☐ Loop diuretics are the most potent diuretic drugs. They can transiently increase renal blood flow without changing the GFR, and augment urinary Na^+ excretion up to 40% of its filtered load. These drugs enter the lumen of the target nephron segment mostly by proximal tubule secretion (organic acid secretory pathway) to produce their effects. Only a small fraction of the loop diuretic enters the lumen by glomerular filtration. Consequently, these drugs remain effective in states of diminished GFR but their action might be delayed/diminished when proximal tubule secretion of loop diuretics decreases (e.g., competitive inhibition of the organic acid secretory pathway by indomethacin, probenecid, and by the metabolic byproducts of uremia). Unlike thiazides and other diuretics agents that decrease GFR by activating the tubuloglomerular feedback mechanism (i.e., an increased delivery of NaCl to the macula densa of the distal tubule activates the renin-angiotensin system leading to increased renin release as well as other mechanisms that generally reduce the rate of filtration by the glomerulus), loop diuretics do not decrease GFR because these drugs appear to inhibit NaCl reabsorption in macula densa cells. Blood flow to the renal medulla is decreased by loop diuretics and this effect can be prevented by administration of angiotensin II antagonists.

446   What is the preferred route for administration of loop diuretics?

☐ The oral route should be used whenever possible except in clinical situations that demand a very prompt response. The oral route cannot be used effectively in patients experiencing vomiting, diarrhea, or paralytic or mechanical ileus. A prompt therapeutic response is needed in patients with acute pulmonary edema for whom IV or IM (if IV is not possible) administration of the diuretic is the preferred route.

447   Describe the absorption, distribution, and duration of effects of loop diuretics.

☐ Loop diuretics are usually absorbed rapidly after oral administration but to a variable degree. The bioavailability (absorption) of furosemide is about 60% and is markedly reduced if it is taken with meals, whereas that of bumetanide is nearly 100% and not altered by meal ingestion. Although their bioavailability is not significantly reduced in congestive heart failure, the onset of the natriuresis and its intensity after oral administration of loop diuretics is diminished in this condition. These drugs are extensively bound to plasma proteins and enter the lumen of renal tubules mostly by the organic acid transport system of the proximal tubule. The half-lives of furosemide, bumetanide, and ethacrynic acid are only 1 to 2 hours and the duration of action is 3 to 6 hours.

448   How is the dose-response relationship of the natriuresis caused by loop diuretics modified by the presence of acid-base disorders?

☐ Respiratory acidosis (primary retention of carbon dioxide) combined with hypoxemia (e.g., this association commonly occurs in patients with chronic obstructive pulmonary disease) decrease the renal clearance and the natriuretic effects of loop diuretics. Metabolic alkalosis, a relatively common complication of therapy with loop diuretics, does not significantly reduce the potency of these drugs as long as depression of ventilation and the consequent respiratory acidosis does not develop.

449   How do NSAIDs modify the action of loop diuretics?

☐ The inhibitory effects of NSAIDs on the production of renal prostaglandins reduce the natriuresis and diuresis induced by loop diuretics. These hormones increase renal blood flow and urinary salt excretion and loop diuretics commonly augment their levels. Prostaglandins are important to sustain the natriuresis induced by the loop-acting drugs. Inhibition of prostaglandin synthesis decreases the response to high-ceiling diuretics. The degree and clinical importance of this interaction differs among NSAIDs, being maximal with indomethacin, mild with sulindac, and absent with a low-dosage aspirin regimen of less than 1.0 mg / kg / d (the latter is prescribed to inhibit platelet aggregation).

450   What are the mechanisms responsible for the adverse effects of NSAIDs on renal function and electrolyte balance?

☐ Suppression of renal prostaglandin synthesis can produce acute renal failure in disease states in which vasodilator prostaglandins counterbalance the norepinephrine or angiotensin II-induced renal vasoconstriction. NSAIDs can also cause hyperkalemia because they inhibit prostaglandin-induced stimulation of the renin-aldosterone system. Sodium retention might complicate therapy with NSAIDs because suppression of prostaglandin synthesis diminishes the natriuresis mediated by the diuretic-induced stimulation of renal prostaglandins. Water retention and hyponatremia can also develop with these drugs due to inhibition of renal prostaglandins, because these humoral agents promote water diuresis by antagonizing ADH effects on the collecting tubules.

451   Compare the effects of loop diuretics and thiazides on serum $[Ca^{++}]$.

☐ Loop diuretics increase urinary excretion of Ca^{++} and, as a consequence, decrease serum $[Ca^{++}]$. Thiazides, on the other hand, decrease urinary Ca^{++} excretion and might produce hypercalcemia (rare). The effects of diuretics on Ca^{++} homeostasis are independent of parathyroid hormone and 1,25-dihydroxyvitamin D_3 levels.

452   Describe the thiazide diuretics and related compounds.

☐ The thiazide diuretics and related drugs have in common a benzothiadiazine nucleus. These agents act directly on the kidney to inhibit NaCl reabsorption in the cortical ascending limb of Henle's loop and the early distal tubule, promoting increased urinary excretion of Na^+, Cl^-, K^+, and water. Because about 90% of filtered NaCl is reabsorbed before the site of action of thiazide(s), the diuretic effect of these drugs is relatively mild. Their specific action is inhibition of electroneutral $Na^+ - Cl^-$ cotransport. Although all thiazides also inhibit the enzyme carbonic anhydrase (located predominantly in the proximal tubule), the diuretic action for most compounds of this class of drugs is unrelated to those effects. By contrast, metolazone (Zaroxolyn) is a thiazide with relatively potent carbonic anhydrase inhibitory effect that resembles that of acetazolamide (a nonthiazide proximal tubule diuretic). Consequently, metolazone combined with loop agents is a powerful diuretic regimen useful in the treatment of refractory edema.

453   What are the most salient properties and adverse effects of thiazide diuretics?

☐ Thiazides have an intermediate potency between loop diuretics, which have the highest potency, and K^+-sparing diuretics/acetazolamide that have the lowest potency. Thiazides inhibit NaCl reabsorption in the renal tubule acting on its luminal side. The onset of action is 1 to 2 hours, peak effect 2 to 6 hours, and duration of action varies with the preparation (chlorothiazide and hydrochlorothiazide, 6 to 18 hours; chlorthalidone, 24 hours; and metolazone 24 to 48 hours). Thiazides increase K^+ excretion (kaliuresis) and decrease water diuresis (impairment of maximal urine dilution). The oral dosages in mg/d are as follows: (1) chlorothiazide, 500 to 1000; (2) hydrochlorothiazide, 50 to 100; (3) chlorthalidone, 25 to 100; and (4) metolazone, 2.5 to 10. The most salient adverse effects are K^+ depletion with hypokalemia, metabolic alkalosis, hyponatremia, hypercalcemia, hyperuricemia, carbohydrate intolerance, pancreatitis, hepatic encephalopathy, thrombocytopenia, and agranulocytosis.

---

454   Provide the pharmacologic and the corresponding registered or trade names, as well as daily dosages of commonly prescribed thiazide diuretics.

☐ Available thiazide diuretics are chlorothiazide (Diuril, 500 to 1000 mg IV or PO), hydrochlorothiazide (Hydrodiuril 50 to 100 mg/d PO), chlorthalidone (Hygroton, 25 to 100 mg/d PO), metolazone (Zaroxolyn, 2.5 to 10 mg/d PO), indapamide (Lozol, 2.5 to 5 mg/d PO), trichlormethiazide (Metahydrin, 1 to 4 mg/d PO), cyclothiazide (Anhydron, 1 to 6 mg/d PO), hydroflumethiazide (Diucardin, 25 to 200 mg/d PO), polythiazide (Renese, 1 to 4 mg/d PO), quinethazone (Hydromox, 50 to 100 mg/d PO), methyclothiazide (Enduron, Aquatensen, 2.5 to 10 mg/d PO), and bendromethiazide (Naturetin, 2.5 to 30 mg/d PO).

---

455   What distinct features do metolazone and indapamide have as compared to other thiazides?

☐ Metolazone is among the most potent thiazides because it also inhibits salt reabsorption in the proximal nephron in addition to its distal tubule effects. In addition, metolazone might cause a smaller reduction in glomerular filtration rate compared to other thiazides. Indapamide is a most useful thiazide for the treatment of hypertension because it has significant vasodilatory effects in addition to its diuretic action. Thus, low dosage of indapamide might reduce peripheral vascular resistance in both hypertension and heart failure, and the relatively low daily dosage causes fewer side effects compared to other thiazides (e.g., less K^+ and Mg^{++} losses, minimal or absent increase of plasma cholesterol and triglycerides). It must be recognized that all thiazide diuretics are more effective antihypertensive agents than the loop diuretics in patients with normal renal function. This differential effect is likely due to the longer duration of action of the former group of drugs.

456 Describe the K$^+$-sparing diuretics.

☐ The K$^+$-sparing diuretics are drugs that promote increased urinary NaCl excretion not accompanied by increased urinary K$^+$ excretion. This group of drugs act on the distal tubule and collecting duct and includes the aldosterone antagonists (e.g., spironolactone, which operates indirectly on the tubules by preventing aldosterone effects due to competition for cellular receptors) and agents that directly inhibit Na$^+$ reabsorption in the renal tubule (i.e., amiloride, triamterene). The most serious side effect of all K$^+$-sparing diuretics is clinically significant hyperkalemia.

457 What are the most salient properties and adverse effects of K$^+$-sparing diuretics?

☐ The K$^+$-sparing diuretics are triamterene, amiloride, and spironolactone. These drugs have a mild natriuretic effect accompanied by renal conservation of K$^+$. The indications for their use include: (1) the induction of mild natriuresis without kaliuresis that is of special value in the treatment of ascites due to liver cirrhosis; and (2) the treatment of congestive heart failure and other forms of generalized edema in combination with diuretics having K$^+$-losing effects. Triamterene and amiloride inhibit Na$^+$ reabsorption in the distal tubule and collecting duct, and indirectly decrease K$^+$ and H$^+$ excretion (the latter two effects depend in part on distal Na$^+$ delivery and reabsorption). Spironolactone competitively inhibits the effect of aldosterone in the collecting duct. The onset of action of triamterene and amiloride is within two hours, whereas that of spironolactone takes 1 to 2 days; the peak effects of the first two drugs are at 6 to 10 hours and that of spironolactone occurs after a few days. The duration of action of triamterene and amiloride is 12 to 24 hours and that of spironolactone is 2 to 3 days. The daily dosages of amiloride, triamterene, and spironolactone are 5 to 10 mg, 25 to 300 mg, and 25 to 400 mg, respectively. The K$^+$-sparing diuretics are contraindicated in patients with hyperkalemia and those at risk for its development. Because the most serious side effect of these drugs is hyperkalemia, K$^+$-sparing diuretics should not be used in patients with acute or chronic renal insufficiency. Additional side effects are impotence and gynecomastia for spironolactone and renal calculi for triamterene.

---

458   Elaborate further on the action of aldosterone antagonists.

☐ Spironolactone and canrenone belong to the group of aldosterone antagonists, agents that competitively bind to a receptor protein located in the cytoplasm of aldosterone-responsive cells of the collecting duct. As a consequence, these drugs interrupt the biochemical events that normally lead to the synthesis of physiologically active transport proteins (e.g., Na^+, K^+-ATPase). The mechanism of action explains two major characteristics of these drugs, namely: (1) diuretic action occurs only in the presence of endogenous or exogenous aldosterone; and (2) the effects of aldosterone-antagonists might be overcome by high concentrations of aldosterone. These drugs are weak natriuretics when used as single agents, but they are generally prescribed in combination with loop diuretics or thiazides. The urinary $Na^+:K^+$ ratio, which is an indirect index of aldosterone activity, is significantly increased by spironolactone. This agent also increases urinary Ca^{++} excretion. Spironolactone (Aldactone) is available in 25-, 50-, and 100-mg oral tablets. Initial daily dosage is 100 mg (single or divided doses) with a dosage range of 25 to 400 mg/d. A fixed-dose combination of spironolactone and hydrochlorothiazide (Aldactazide, containing either 25 or 50 mg of each drug) is available.

---

459   Describe additional properties of amiloride and triamterene.

☐ Amiloride and triamterene are weak diuretic agents with a mode of action that is independent of aldosterone and mineralocorticoids. These drugs inhibit electrogenic Na^+ reabsorption in the renal collecting duct and therefore reduce or prevent the development of a lumen-negative electric potential that normally facilitates K^+ secretion into the urine. Administration of amiloride or triamterene as single agents induces a modest increase in Na^+ and Cl^- excretion with either no change or a slight increase in the urinary excretion of K^+. However, these drugs greatly blunt the urinary K^+ excretion induced by kaliuretic diuretics (e.g., loop agents, thiazides), mineralocorticoid excess, or high K^+ intake. Amiloride (Midamor) is available as 5-mg tablets and daily dosage is 5 to 10 mg. A combination of amiloride and hydrochlorothiazide (Moduretic, having 5 mg and 50 mg, respectively) is also available. Triamterene (Dyrenium) is prescribed by the oral route at dosages of 50 to 300 mg/d. A combination of triamterene and hydrochlorothiazide (Dyazide, containing 50 mg and 25 mg, respectively) is also available.

---

460 What are the most salient characteristics of acetazolamide (Diamox)?

□ Acetazolamide is a carbonic anhydrase inhibitor that diminishes $NaHCO_3$ reabsorption in the renal proximal tubules. This diuretic has relatively low potency that is comparable to that of K^+-sparing diuretics. Because the increased natriuresis is accompanied by urine HCO_3^- excretion, acetazolamide is useful in metabolic alkalosis due to loop diuretics, thiazides, and other causes. Acetazolamide is generally prescribed for oral administration at a dosage of 250 mg three times a day for 2 to 4 days. The onset of action, peak effects, and duration of action are 1 hour, 2 to 4 hours, and 6 to 8 hours, respectively. The most significant adverse effects include metabolic acidosis and renal calculi.

---

461 Describe the effects of acetazolamide on urinary electrolytes, acid-base balance, and extrarenal tissues.

□ Acetazolamide increases urinary excretion of Na^+, K^+, and bicarbonate (HCO_3^-). The main effect of this drug on acid-base balance is the induction of metabolic acidosis. This acid-base disorder blunts the pharmacologic action of acetazolamide on the proximal nephron, ameliorating the severity of the acid-base disturbance. The systemic acid-base effect of this drug accounts for its use in the treatment of metabolic alkalosis caused by other diuretics. The extrarenal effects of acetazolamide include stimulation of ventilatory drive (useful in respiratory depression, cor pulmonale with hypercapnia, acute mountain sickness), and depression of intraocular pressure (useful in the treatment of glaucoma).

462   What are the main properties and principal site of action of mannitol?

☐ Mannitol (Osmitrol) is the most widely used osmotic diuretic (other compounds include urea, glycerin, isosorbide). All of these agents are: (1) freely filtered at the glomerulus; (2) relatively inert pharmacologically; and (3) minimally reabsorbed in the renal tubules. The site of diuretic action is primarily the proximal tubule wherein the progressively higher concentration of the non-reabsorbable solute (due to fluid removal leaving mannitol behind) prevents the normal reabsorption of water leading to a decreased $[Na^+]$ in the lumen of the proximal tubule. The mannitol-induced natriuresis occurs because of: (1) decreased Na^+ reabsorption due to abnormally low luminal $[Na^+]$; (2) increased back-flux of Na^+ from peritubular fluid to lumen due to the favorable $[Na^+]$ gradient; and (3) increased renal medullary blood flow mediated by stimulation of renal prostaglandins; these hormones promote a partial washout of medullary hypertonicity, leading to diminished Na^+ reabsorption in Henle's loop.

463   Describe the effects of mannitol on urinary electrolytes and extrarenal tissues, as well as its daily dosage.

☐ Mannitol (Osmitrol) increases the urinary excretion of Na^+, Cl^-, and water acting as an osmotic diuretic. The most important extrarenal actions of this compound include a transient expansion of ECF volume, and decreases in both intracranial (e.g., treatment of cerebral edema) and intraocular pressures. The usual dosage of mannitol is 1 to 1.5 g/kg and 50 to 200 g/d administered intravenously.

464   What is the specific treatment of fluid excess in heart failure?

☐ The specific treatment of fluid excess in heart failure depends on many factors including: (1) severity of fluid retention; (2) response to prior treatment; (3) intensity of cardiorespiratory failure (e.g., extreme hypoxemia due to pulmonary edema); and (4) associated diseases (e.g., advanced renal failure wherein diuretic usage is ineffective and ultrafiltration with or without dialysis might be necessary).

Consequently, specific measures might include options that range from simple (e.g., salt restriction) to complex ones (e.g., continuous arteriovenous ultrafiltration). The specific treatment measures might include: (1) low Na^+ diet, especially NaCl; (2) diuretics; (3) evacuation of fluid from body cavities with a needle or catheter (e.g., thoracentesis, paracentesis); and (4) ultrafiltration techniques (e.g., intermittent or continuous arteriovenous or venovenous ultrafiltration with or without dialysis). The specific indications for these measures are explained in the answers to subsequent questions.

---

465   What are the main indications of diuretics in heart failure?

☐ Patients with symptomatic or decompensated congestive heart failure with obvious fluid retention (e.g., peripheral edema, fluid accumulation in body cavities) should be prescribed diuretic agents if not already in use, and should receive a more intense diuretic regimen if they are currently taking these medications. Afterload-reducing agents used in the treatment of heart failure might promote salt and water retention by the kidney and this side effect might either diminish or abolish the therapeutic efficacy of these drugs. Consequently, salt and water retention of only mild degree manifested by increasing body weight (absence of obvious fluid retention including peripheral edema and fluid accumulation in body cavities) due to afterload-reducing agents is an indication for initiation of diuretic drugs. On the other hand, symptomatic heart failure not associated with significant fluid retention can be generally managed with dietary salt restriction (without diuretics) and other measures including afterload-reducing agents and inotropic drugs.

---

466   How important are diuretics in the treatment of heart failure?

☐ Diuretics, a term that refers to drugs that promote increased urinary salt and water excretion, are among the most important pharmacologic agents available in the treatment of heart failure. The diuretic-induced negative fluid balance might effectively control signs and symptoms of congestion as well as slow down progressive dilation of heart chambers by reducing preload (i.e., diminished end-diastolic volume and pressure), and afterload because of antihypertensive effects of these drugs. Nevertheless, diuretics may not favorably influence natural history of the primary disease responsible for the cardiac dysfunction (e.g., ischemic myocardium).

---

467   What other drugs used in heart failure have diuretic effects despite not being true diuretics?

☐ Digitalis preparations and dopamine (when given at 1 to 3 μg/kg/min) might increase renal excretion of salt and water in heart failure predominantly due to their effects on the renal circulation rather than on the renal tubules (site of action of true diuretic agents). Digitalis and dopamine enhance renal plasma flow and glomerular filtration rate (RPF and GFR, respectively) thereby increasing the amount of salt and water reaching the kidney (RPF) and the amount delivered to the renal tubules (largely determined by the GFR). The combination of increased RPF and filtered load of NaCl and water, and decreased reabsorption of these substances by the renal tubules (this effect occurs mostly in the proximal nephron and is the dominant mechanism responsible for the natriuresis), accounts for their diuretic effects. Digitalis and dopamine at low dosage (1 to 3 μg/kg/min) also decrease the renal filtration fraction (ratio of GFR to RPF, which is normally about 20% and rises in heart failure) because these drugs induce larger increases in RPF than in GFR. A high filtration fraction generally causes salt and water retention whereas a low one promotes natriuresis and diuresis. Digitalis and dopamine prescribed to patients with decompensated congestive heart failure increase cardiac output and reduce renal sympathetic tone as well as angiotensin II production, thereby attenuating, at least partially, the decreased renal perfusion characteristic of this disease. In addition, dopamine induces renal vasodilation by stimulation of renal vascular dopaminergic receptors and directly inhibits salt and water reabsorption in the renal tubules.

468 How does the dose-response relationship for the loop diuretics-induced natriuresis compare in normal individuals and patients with heart failure?

☐ The dose-response relationship to loop diuretics is shifted to the right (i.e., a higher dose is required to obtain a specific level of urinary Na^+ excretion) in patients with heart failure in comparison to that of normal individuals. The diminished response in heart failure is mostly due to increased salt reabsorption in the proximal tubule, which decreases NaCl delivery to the loop of Henle and distal nephron where loop diuretics and thiazides, respectively, exert their action. The shift to the right of the dose-response relationship is not due to impaired gastrointestinal absorption of loop diuretics in heart failure because this rightward shift is also observed after IV administration of these agents. Increasing the dose of the loop diuretic or adding a different drug that exerts effects at another nephron site (e.g., thiazides or K^+-sparing agents acting on the distal tubule and the collecting duct, respectively) might increase natriuresis. Very high doses of furosemide (250 to 4000 mg/d) have been recommended for the treatment of refractory edema in patients with heart failure, but clinical toxicity becomes significant when single IV doses are higher than 500 mg. The usual dosage of furosemide given PO or IV is 20 to 1000 mg/d. Its IV administration should be performed over several minutes as opposed to bolus injection to diminish the risks of toxicity (e.g., hypoacusia). The usual dosage of bumetanide is 0.5 to 2.0 mg/d PO and that of piretanide is 6 to 20 mg/d PO. Ethacrynic acid is now used less commonly and its dosage is 50 to 200 mg/d PO.

469 Outline the indications for each type of diuretic in the treatment of heart failure.

☐ A diuretic of moderate potency such as a classic thiazide or metolazone is commonly chosen at the initiation of diuretic therapy in heart failure (first step). If the response to these drugs is inadequate, a more powerful agent of the group of loop diuretics (furosemide, bumetanide, ethacrynic acid) should be prescribed (second step). Persistent fluid retention after a trial with loop diuretics or K^+ depletion secondary to these agents prompts the clinician to combine a loop diuretic and a distal tubule (K^+-sparing) diuretic (third step). Finally, the combined use of the three types of diuretics including a thiazide, loop agent, and K^+-sparing drug (fourth step) might be necessary in cases refractory to the previous therapeutic strategies.

---

470 What is the rationale for the combined use of loop diuretics and thiazides in the management of edema secondary to congestive heart failure?

☐ Patients with edema refractory to a single diuretic drug might experience a salutary synergistic effect on salt and water excretion using a combination of a thiazide and a loop diuretic. The larger diuretic response observed with this combined regimen of drugs might be due to: (1) "unmasking" the inhibitory effects of thiazides (e.g., metolazone) on proximal tubule reabsorption (which would otherwise lead to increased salt reabsorption in the loop of Henle, blunting the diuretic response) by the concomitant inhibitory effects of high ceiling drugs on salt reabsorption of Henle's loop; and (2) the thiazide-induced inhibition of salt reabsorption in the distal tubule prevents the otherwise expected increased salt reabsorption in this segment when a loop diuretic is administered. Loop diuretics combined with thiazides might be used effectively at low dosages of both drugs, thereby decreasing the risk of toxicity. Combined diuretic use might also cause serious adverse effects including profound intravascular volume depletion, prerenal azotemia, hyponatremia, hypokalemia, and increased risk of toxicity due to cardiac glycosides.

---

471 Describe common causes of diuretic resistance, also known as the "breaking phenomenon."

☐ Decreased responsiveness to chronic diuretic administration in congestive heart failure, a common problem, prevents marked intravascular volume depletion and its adverse consequences in these patients. Consequently, the "breaking phenomenon" might represent a salutary homeostatic response to preserve ECF volume. Common causes of diuretic resistance include: (1) insufficient delivery of the drug to the tubular lumen (required for all diuretics to be effective except for "distal" diuretics) because of low GFR or competition with the organic acid transport pathway for proximal secretion (e.g., probenecid); (2) severe reduction of fluid delivery to the site of diuretic action because of diminished GFR (e.g., severe heart failure, volume depletion, renal failure secondary to any cause); (3) marked activation of both the renin-angiotensin and the adrenergic systems causing renal vasoconstriction and decreased renal blood flow; (4) severe electrolyte imbalance including hyponatremia (the associated high ADH levels promote excessive water retention), as well as hypokalemia and hypomagnesemia (that might depress myocardial performance and secondarily, renal perfusion); (5) concomitant use of NSAIDs that block the synthesis of prostaglandins and blunt the response to diuretic drugs; and (6) ACE inhibitors and other vasodilators that might produce excessive hypotension, thereby reducing the action of diuretics. Thus, multiple mechanisms acting either independently or more commonly in combination are responsible for diuretic resistance in patients with heart failure.

---

472 Should diuretics of the same class be prescribed simultaneously to achieve more pronounced urinary salt and water loss in patients who require immediate effects (i.e., pulmonary edema) or who have had an inadequate pharmacologic response (i.e., those with refractory edema)?

☐ No. Diuretic agents of the same class should not be simultaneously prescribed in any clinical situation because their identical site of action (e.g., loop of Henle for high-ceiling diuretics) prevents summation of effects while increasing the risk of clinical toxicity. Consequently, there is no scientific basis for concomitant administration of two loop diuretics, two thiazides, two K^+-sparing agents, etc. It is apparent that a more pronounced urinary loss of salt and water can be achieved if needed by the simultaneous use of one drug from each class (e.g., furosemide plus amiloride, hydrochlorothiazide and bumetanide, metolazone plus spironolactone).

473   Does the use of K^+-sparing agents in combination with thiazides or loop-acting drugs have any significant role in the treatment of congestive heart failure?

☐ Yes. Prevention of diuretic-induced K^+ depletion is steadily gaining importance among clinicians in the management of congestive heart failure. Consequently, K^+-sparing agents are commonly prescribed as a second drug because these compounds are useful when combined with loop diuretics or thiazides (K^+-sparing agents decrease the kaliuresis induced by the other two groups of diuretics), are relatively safe, and they are of moderate cost. In addition, all the K^+-sparing diuretics diminish Mg^{++} and K^+ loss (e.g., K^+-sparing agents can produce hyperchloremic metabolic acidosis, whereas loop agents and thiazides are more likely to cause hypochloremic metabolic alkalosis) induced by loop agents, thiazides, and other diuretics acting proximally to the collecting duct.

474   What are the indications of carbonic anhydrase inhibitors (e.g., acetazolamide) in the management of congestive heart failure?

☐ Acetazolamide (Diamox) is a weak diuretic that promotes bicarbonaturia because of inhibition of carbonic anhydrase activity in the proximal nephron, an enzyme that allows the normal reabsorption of filtered bicarbonate in this nephron segment. The main indications of carbonic anhydrase inhibitors in heart failure are: (1) metabolic alkalosis associated with volume expansion or hyperkalemia, conditions wherein NaCl and/or KCl infusions (alternative treatment of metabolic alkalosis) are contraindicated; (2) cor pulmonale with hypercapnia and metabolic alkalosis (this acid-base disturbance depresses ventilation further and the consequent respiratory acidosis induces diuretic resistance); (3) prevention of non-cardiogenic pulmonary edema and cerebral edema in patients at risk of developing acute mountain sickness; and (4) urine alkalinization to transiently increase the renal excretion of certain drugs or facilitate dissolution of uric acid crystals.

475   What are the indications of osmotic diuretics such as mannitol in the management of fluid overload in congestive heart failure?

☐ Osmotic diuretics such as mannitol (Osmitrol) are contraindicated in patients with decompensated congestive heart failure because they promote a transient increase in ECF volume that might precipitate or worsen acute pulmonary edema. On the other hand, mannitol may be used in patients with compensated heart failure to transiently enhance the effectiveness of loop diuretics by increasing fluid delivery to the Henle's loop when glomerular filtration is low and resistance to diuretics is present.

476   What is the major indication for fluid removal by thoracentesis or abdominal paracentesis in patients with heart failure?

☐ Patients with acute respiratory distress due to large pleural effusion(s) or ascites who fail to respond to diuretic therapy might benefit from direct fluid removal by thoracentesis or abdominal paracentesis, respectively. These procedures, if uncomplicated, can promptly improve dyspnea. By contrast, pneumothorax, hemothorax, or hemopneumothorax (immediate complications), as well as pleural infection (delayed complication), might occur and worsen the patient's clinical status and increase the risk of death. Abdominal paracentesis that is either large (i.e., in excess of 1500 mL of fluid) or too fast (i.e., more than 200 mL/h) might also have serious consequences including circulatory collapse and even death.

477   How does the presence of renal insufficiency alter the natriuresis induced by thiazides and loop diuretics?

☐ Renal insufficiency blunts the response to all diuretic agents. Thiazides as single agents are not effective diuretic drugs when the GFR is less than 30 mL/min (about one third of normal level), whereas loop diuretics used at high dosage might still produce natriuresis. A combination of loop diuretics and thiazides might have synergistic effects on salt and water excretion in patients with an abnormally low GFR. Diuretic drugs are contraindicated in patients with anuria (lack of urine output).

478   Explain further the effects of renal insufficiency on the response to diuretics.

    ☐ Renal insufficiency decreases the response to diuretics and increases their clinical toxicity. Yet, diuretics are valuable therapeutic agents in patients with heart failure and renal insufficiency except for those with end-stage renal failure (state in which diuretics are contraindicated because of absence of meaningful effects and high risks of toxicity). Thiazides are generally of no value when the GFR is less than 30 mL/min and might further decrease overall renal function. Loop agents, on the other hand, have diuretic effects in patients with low GFR, yet higher dosage is generally required. Ethacrynic acid is not recommended for the treatment of heart failure associated with renal insufficiency because of the increased risk of ototoxicity. Potassium-sparing diuretics generally are contraindicated in patients with renal insufficiency because of the risk of hyperkalemia. Renal insufficiency is a common associated condition in patients with heart failure. It has multiple causes including a reduced blood flow to this organ due to heart disease, a concomitant vascular illness (e.g., atherosclerosis, hypertensive glomerulosclerosis), associated metabolic or other diseases (e.g., diabetic nephropathy), and as a complication of diuretic therapy.

479   How does the clinician monitor the response to diuretic therapy (insufficient, adequate, or excessive) and assess for evidence of toxicity?

    ☐ Monitoring the clinical response to diuretic therapy is accomplished through the history and physical examination obtained in follow-up visits, and by measurement of body weight in the physician's office as well as at home by the patient on a daily basis. Monitoring of the biochemical response to diuretics is accomplished by measurement of serum electrolytes (e.g., hypokalemia or hyperkalemia, hyponatremia), uric acid levels, blood glucose, and digoxin levels (if applicable).

480   What are the causes and management of refractory edema?

    ☐ Refractory edema, or resistance of generalized edema to conventional diuretic therapy (e.g., lack of response to more than 200 mg/d furosemide) can be due to: (1) high NaCl intake, detected by measuring urine Na^+ excretion; (2) decreased intestinal absorption of diuretics, due to bowel wall edema, which is overcome with IV administration of these agents; (3) decreased drug availability at the lumen of renal tubules that can occur in severe heart failure and renal failure and is managed with massive doses of loop diuretics, combination of diuretics, hemofiltration, or dialysis; in hepatic cirrhosis the use of albumin, loop diuretics, and spironolactone can help; and (4) enhanced renal reabsorption of salt and water with low GFR; these defects might respond to acetazolamide, thiazides, K^+-sparing diuretics, combination of diuretics, aminophylline, IV dopamine infusion, and rarely, to glucocorticosteroids.

481   What is the role of high-dosage furosemide or ultrafiltration in the management of heart failure with severe and refractory fluid overload?

    ☐ High-dosage furosemide (250 to 4000 mg/d) in combination with vasodilators or inotropic drugs might be useful in patients with refractory heart failure. A combination of two to four diuretics acting on different segments of the renal tubule (e.g., loop agent, thiazide, acetazolamide, K^+-sparing drug) simultaneously administered, might produce a substantial natriuresis in patients who failed to respond to a high-dosage furosemide regimen. Ultrafiltration is an effective therapeutic option for fluid removal in patients who fail to respond to diuretics or those with severe renal insufficiency (the response to diuretic agents is poor or absent in this condition). The ultrafiltration technique (e.g., arteriovenous or venovenous access to the circulation) is relatively simple, cost effective, and might achieve sustained symptomatic improvement in selected patients.

482   Outline the major features of extracorporeal ultrafiltration (intermittent or continuous) and its use in the management of heart failure.

□ Extracorporeal ultrafiltration or hemofiltration is a therapeutic modality that allows fluid removal from the circulation (with the use of a filtering-membrane device interposed between an arterial and a venous access or a venovenous access) in patients with severe fluid overload unresponsive to diuretics. Fluid can be removed at rates of up to 500 mL/h for a 2 to 6 hour treatment (intermittent modality), or at relatively low rates (e.g., 100 mL/h) for prolonged periods (continuous modality for 24 to 72 hours or longer duration). Ultrafiltration is an effective temporary method for the control of fluid overload that requires close monitoring because of its potential for inducing serious hemodynamic instability and major fluid and electrolyte losses. Patients with congestive heart failure and intractable fluid overload with significant renal insufficiency should receive ultrafiltration (intermittent or continuous) plus dialysis. Extracorporeal ultrafiltration (or simply 'ultrafiltration') promotes fluid loss due to a hydrostatic pressure gradient across the semipermeable membrane that separates the blood compartment from the collecting receptacle. In contrast with ultrafiltration, hemodialysis promotes solute removal from the blood compartment to a dialysate fluid that circulates on the other side of the semipermeable membrane, driven by a concentration (chemical) gradient.

483   Describe the alterations in K^+ homeostasis that might be observed in heart failure as complications of therapy.

□ Low dietary intake due to anorexia and increased urinary losses secondary to thiazides and loop agents (drugs most commonly responsible) can lead to K^+ depletion in patients with heart failure. Serum K^+ tends to be diminished (hypokalemia) in those conditions, especially if other complications of diuretic drugs that include metabolic alkalosis and severe secondary hyperaldosteronism are also present. Hyperkalemia (elevated serum K^+) might be also observed if K^+-sparing diuretics or ACE inhibitors are used, dietary intakes of this electrolyte and supplements are high, or renal ciency develops. Both hypokalemia and hyperkalemia might have serious consequences including cardiac arrhythmias and even circulatory arrest (cardiac standstill or ventricular fibrillation). The risk of digitalis toxicity is significantly increased in patients with hypokalemia (see therapy with cardiac glycosides).

---

484 Which patients are at greatest risk of hypokalemia and significant K^+ depletion due to prolonged use of diuretics?

☐ Diuretics used in the treatment of edematous states (e.g., congestive heart failure, cirrhosis of the liver, and nephrotic syndrome) produce substantial urine K^+ loss. Conversely, diuretics cause only limited kaliuresis when used in nonedematous states (e.g., hypertension). Consequently, a formal plan for K^+ supplementation must be instituted when diuretics are used for long periods in the treatment of the former group of patients.

---

485 What mechanisms might account for increased cardiovascular morbidity and mortality in states of K^+ depletion?

☐ Potassium depletion might increase cardiovascular morbidity and mortality through several mechanisms including: (1) direct effects on vascular smooth muscle producing arteriolar constriction (e.g., cerebral, coronary, renal vessels); (2) sympathetic activation, which in turn might lead to cardiac stimulation as well as arteriolar constriction (most vascular beds); and (3) Na^+ retention with secondary increase in ECF and plasma volume, and high cellular levels of Na^+. All the previously mentioned effects increase arterial pressure. Consequently, K^+ depletion might increase the risk of cardiovascular disease including hypertension, strokes, coronary artery disease, heart failure, cardiac arrhythmias, and renal failure.

---

486 Describe the overall strategy for the prevention and management of hypokalemia due to K^+ depletion.

☐ Prevention and management of K^+ depletion can be accomplished by either increasing K^+ intake or by decreasing K^+

loss. Potassium supplementation by the oral route, whenever possible, should be used to increase K^+ intake. Excessive K^+ loss, by renal and extrarenal mechanisms, can be controlled by specific therapeutic interventions. ACE inhibitors and K^+-sparing diuretics help to diminish kaliuresis. A variety of antidiarrheal agents can help to diminish excessive K^+ excretion in the stools or through intestinal fistulas.

487   What is the role of K^+-rich foods in the prevention and management of K^+ depletion?

□ It is always advisable to prescribe a diet that includes K^+-rich foods as the initial step in the management of K^+ depletion before considering the use of oral K^+ pharmaceutical preparations. Among the K^+-rich foods are fruit and fruit juices (1 cup of orange juice and a medium-size banana have identical K^+ content, about 15 mEq each), which have a K^+ content equivalent to two tablets/capsules of K^+ salts for each portion of fruit/fruit juice.

488   What are the indications for K^+ replacement with oral K^+ supplementation, K^+-sparing diuretics, and ACE inhibitors in patients with heart failure?

□ Prescription of K^+ replacement with oral K^+ supplements, K^+-sparing diuretics, or ACE inhibitors is generally recommended for patients with heart failure, adequate renal function, $[K^+]_p$ less than 3.5 mEq / L and: (1) chronic use of diuretics, which predispose to K^+ depletion; (2) excessive extrarenal K^+ losses (e.g., diarrhea); (3) therapy with cardiac glycosides, because their toxicity increases with hypokalemia; (4) a history of atrial or ventricular arrhythmias; (5) significant cardiac enlargement; (6) ischemic heart disease, which predisposes to malignant ventricular arrhythmias; and (7) hepatic dysfunction due to advanced right heart failure or other causes because correction of K^+ depletion decreases hepatic and renal ammonia production and might protect from hepatic encephalopathy.

489   Provide examples of very K^+-rich foods, whose intake should be recommended for patients with K^+ depletion and prohibited in patients predisposed to hyperkalemia.

☐ Examples of very K^+-rich foods include: (1) dried fruits (i.e., raisins, apricots, prunes); (2) dried legumes (i.e., peanuts, pecans, dates, almonds, walnuts); and (3) spinach and cocoa powder. These foods have more than 30 mEq K^+ per cup.

490   Provide examples of K^+-rich foods, whose intake should be encouraged in patients predisposed to K^+ depletion and limited in patients predisposed to hyperkalemia.

☐ Examples of K^+-rich foods include: (1) red and white meat as well as fish; (2) most legumes (i.e., corn, beans, peas, avocados, artichokes); (3) most fruits and their juices (i.e., bananas, oranges, cantaloupes, grapes, nectarines, pineapples, watermelons, tomatoes, papayas, prunes, cherries, lemons, peaches, plums, strawberries); (4) potatoes (regular and sweet), mushrooms, carrots, cabbage; and (5) chocolate. These foods have 10 to 30 mEq K^+ per cup.

491   Provide examples of low-K^+ foods that are of special value in patients predisposed to hyperkalemia.

☐ Examples of low-K^+ foods include: (1) grain products such as bread, rice, and pastas; (2) eggs and milk products (milk, cheese); (3) certain fruits (apples, pears, and tangerines); and (4) certain legumes such as lettuce and onions. These foods have less than 10 mEq K^+ per cup.

492   How is oral K^+ supplementation usually prescribed?

☐ The usual dosage of K^+ supplementation is 40 to 120 mEq/d and should be taken with or after meals to diminish gastrointestinal side effects.

493 Describe commonly used preparations for oral K⁺ supplementation.

☐ Several K⁺ salts such as KCl, K⁺ phosphate, and KHCO₃ (or HCO₃⁻ precursors such as citrate, acetate, or gluconate) are available for oral administration (liquid, powder, tablet, capsule). The strength of these preparations is as follows: each tablet/capsule (Slow-K, Micro-K) has 8 to 10 mEq; each packet of powder (K-lor, Kay Ciel, Klyte/Cl) has 15 to 25 mEq; the liquid forms (KCl, Kay Ciel, Kaon) have 1 to 3 mEq/mL.

494 What criteria help the clinician to decide whether K⁺ should be administered parenterally?

☐ The parenteral administration of K⁺ should be considered when the oral route for K⁺ replacement is either not possible or when immediate action is mandatory to correct a life-threatening condition that is likely to respond to K⁺ therapy. Examples for the mandatory use of IV K⁺ salts include hypokalemic patients with digitalis-induced arrhythmias or severe skeletal muscle paresis or paralysis. It must be recognized that even when immediate effects of the administered K⁺ salt are desired, an oral preparation, if available, can be used, and its effects might become evident by the time the K⁺ salt for IV administration is ready for infusion. Whether the full dose of IV K⁺ salt initially considered for administration is given or not will depend on the results of a close follow-up of the clinical and laboratory data.

495 Describe the prevention and management of K⁺ depletion by measures other than K⁺ supplementation.

☐ Effective prevention and management of K⁺ depletion can be accomplished with the use of K⁺-sparing diuretics (spironolactone, amiloride, triamterene), as well as with ACE inhibitors. Because the major risk in the prevention and management of K⁺ depletion is hyperkalemia, it is unwise to superimpose two or more modes of therapy for K⁺ depletion.

Thus, the physician must choose the best strategy to be used in a particular patient among the various alternatives in the prevention and management of K^+ depletion.

---

496 Compare the risks of K^+ administration by oral and parenteral routes.

☐ Although 50 mEq of K^+ can be safely given as a single bolus dose by the oral route, a similar dose administered IV requires a constant infusion of several hours' duration. The oral route obligates administered K^+ to go through the splanchnic circulation in which uptake by the hepatocytes and other cells prevents a large rapid entry of K^+ to the systemic circulation. Furthermore, oral K^+ triggers insulin release and activates the sympathetic nervous system, thereby increasing internal disposal of the K^+ load. Oral K^+ administration promotes a smoother repletion of K^+ stores. The mechanisms that protect against iatrogenic hyperkalemia during K^+ supplementation described above for the oral route are not available with IV administration of K^+. Consequently, IV administration of K^+ should generally not exceed 10 mEq/h. If the rate of IV K^+ administration exceeds 10 mEq/h (given, for example because of life-threatening digitalis intoxication), continuous ECG monitoring is mandatory. An exception to this rule is the K^+ replacement therapy given to patients undergoing recovery from diabetic ketoacidosis.

---

497 Compare the therapeutic options for immediate and long-term management of K^+ depletion.

☐ When immediate correction (acute management/ therapy) of hypokalemia is desired, the exclusive option is K^+ supplementation. Neither the administration of K^+-sparing diuretics or ACE inhibitors have an immediate effect on $[K^+]_n$. By contrast, long-term correction (chronic management/therapy) of hypokalemia can be achieved effectively and safely with the use of one of the three following options: (1) K^+ supplementation (oral, parenteral); (2) K^+-sparing diuretics (spironolactone, triamterene, amiloride); and (3) ACE inhibitors (captopril, enalapril, lisinopril).

498   Describe the relative potency/efficacy of the various options for the prevention or long-term management of K⁺ depletion.

☐   The potency/efficacy of the three options, namely K⁺ supplementation, K⁺-sparing diuretics, and ACE inhibitors, for the prevention or management of K⁺ depletion is of comparable value. The selection of a particular form of K⁺ replacement is based on multiple factors including the patient's tolerance to any of these options (e.g., gastrointestinal intolerance to oral K⁺ intake), adverse effects of medication (e.g., K⁺-sparing diuretics are unsafe in diabetics, especially elderly patients), the patient's hemodynamic condition (e.g., ACE inhibitors are not indicated in patients with normal or low blood pressure), and the physician's previous experience/expertise.

499   Is there any condition wherein the simultaneous use of two treatment modalities for hypokalemia is justified?

☐   Yes. Patients with persistent and clinically significant hypokalemia that fails to respond to any one of the three treatment modalities used as monotherapy require a combination of two treatment modalities for K⁺ repletion. It should be recognized that this particular situation is the exception and K⁺ depletion in most patients is effectively managed with a single modality of K⁺ repletion.

500   Describe a standard prescription for IV K⁺ supplementation.

☐   Because available ampules of K⁺ salts contain 2 mEq K⁺/mL, IV K⁺ supplementation requires dilution of this concentrated K⁺ salt solution. In most conditions 20 to 40 mEq K⁺ (2 to 4 ampules) are added to each liter of saline or dextrose-containing solution.   Because   dextrose   solutions stimulate insulin secretion, a given dose of K⁺ salt will produce a smaller rise in $[K^+]_p$ when this cation is infused in a glucose-containing solution instead of a saline infusion. If the aim of therapy is to restore the depressed $[K^+]_p$ very promptly, it is advisable to dilute the K⁺ ampules in   NaCl-containing solutions. On the other hand, when correction of the overall K⁺ deficit is the main goal of therapy, K⁺ salts diluted in glucose-containing solutions are the first choice.

501 What is the importance of the overall level of renal function (GFR) in patients who are being considered for K^+ replacement (K^+ supplementation and drugs that diminish K^+ excretion)?

 ☐ It is of critical importance that adequate mechanisms for K^+ excretion are present in patients considered for K^+ replacement. Adequate renal function will generally protect the patient from extreme hyperkalemia that can result from K^+ supplementation. Patients with significant renal insufficiency (GFR as low as 20 to 30 mL/min), especially of chronic nature, can have substantial kaliuresis that provides some protection from iatrogenic hyperkalemia. Patients with acute renal insufficiency who are already in the nonoliguric phase are also somewhat protected from iatrogenic hyperkalemia.

502 What is the importance of daily urine output (diuresis or urine volume) in patients considered for K^+ supplementation?

 ☐ Patients receiving K^+ supplementation should have a daily urine output of at least one liter to provide a basic level of renal protection against iatrogenic hyperkalemia, independently of the associated GFR. This applies because urine $[K^+]$ is usually severalfold the $[K^+]_p$ unless the patient is concomitantly receiving a K^+-sparing diuretic.

503 What is the best overall indicator of renal K^+ excretory capacity in patients about to receive K^+ replacement?

 ☐ Daily urine volume is the best indicator of renal K^+ excretory capacity. Neither blood urea nitrogen (BUN) nor plasma creatinine values provide comparable information. Lack of diuresis results in zero kaliuresis, whether blood chemistries that indicate overall renal function (BUN and creatinine) are normal or not. Furthermore, the levels of BUN and creatinine might misrepresent the current renal function in patients who are seriously ill, because these patients' chemistries are not stable (a steady-state condition has not been reached). A dramatic example is that of a patient in the immediate postsurgical period following bilateral nephrectomy (e.g., due to trauma or tumor) in whom BUN and plasma creatinine levels are normal, yet urine output and renal K^+ excretion are zero.

---

504 How common and serious are the risks of K^+ replacement therapy?

☐ At least one in 20 patients receiving K^+ supplementation will develop adverse effects including significant hyperkalemia. Occasionally, life-threatening hyperkalemia is observed in patients receiving measures aimed at preventing K^+ depletion.

---

505 What patients are at greatest risk for the development of hyperkalemia as a result of K^+ replacement therapy?

☐ Patients with limited renal K^+ excretion are at great risk for developing hyperkalemia with K^+ supplementation. Included in this category are patients with renal insufficiency, those receiving ACE inhibitors (captopril, enalapril, etc.), or K^+-sparing diuretics (amiloride, triamterene, spironolactone), and elderly individuals (especially diabetics). Elderly patients have diminished GFR and a less effective renin-angiotensin-aldosterone axis for their defense against hyperkalemia during K^+ supplementation.

---

506 List drugs that impair external K^+ balance and therefore can cause hyperkalemia.

☐ Drugs that diminish renal K^+ excretion include the K^+-sparing diuretics (spironolactone, amiloride, and triamterene), angiotensin II-converting enzyme inhibitors (captopril, enalapril, lisinopril, etc.), NSAIDs (indomethacin, ibuprofen, etc.), heparin, and cyclosporine. In addition, any drug that causes renal failure can lead to hyperkalemia.

507 What is the clinical relevance of diuretic-induced magnesium (Mg^{++}) deficiency in patients with heart failure?

□ Urinary Mg^{++} wasting might occur during long-term diuretic therapy with loop agents and thiazides (less severe) but not with K^+-sparing diuretics. Clinically significant Mg^{++} deficiency might occur in response to diuretics in patients ingesting a low Mg^{++} diet or who have additional mechanisms of urinary Mg^{++} wasting (e.g., excessive alcohol intake, aminoglycoside antibiotics such as gentamicin and tobramycin, amphotericin B, cisplatin, digitalis preparations). The cardiac effects of hypomagnesemia might include: (1) coronary artery constriction leading to arterial spasms, extension of myocardial infarction, and sudden death in ischemic heart disease; (2) cardiac arrhythmias including ventricular premature contractions, ventricular tachyarrhythmias, supraventricular tachycardia, atrial fibrillation, augmented chance of ventricular fibrillation, increased risk of digitalis toxicity, torsade de pointes (a form of ventricular tachycardia characterized by polymorphic QRS complexes that change in amplitude and cycle length, that might be caused by Mg^{++} deficiency or K^+ deficiency); and (3) ECG abnormalities including T wave flattening as well as prolonged PR and QT intervals. Because the severity of Mg^{++} depletion does not closely correlate with the serum Mg^{++} level, evaluation of the changes in body stores of this element requires serial measurements of serum Mg^{++} levels (normal range is 1.6 to 2.1 mEq / L).

508 What are the routes of administration and dosage for Mg^{++} replacement?

□ Oral supplementation of Mg^{++} should be considered in patients with heart failure and hypomagnesemia who have predisposing factors for the development of significant Mg^{++} deficiency (see answer to previous question). Daily oral dosage 10 to 30 mEq (120 to 360 mg) of elemental Mg^{++} administered for 2 to 4 weeks generally corrects Mg^{++} deficiency. IV administration of Mg^{++} might be considered in patients with atrial or ventricular arrhythmias presumably due to Mg^{++} deficiency. In those instances 1 g of Mg^{++} might be administered over 20 minutes (e.g., treatment of torsade de-pointes) but dosages of up to 12 g of Mg^{++} administered over 6 hours under careful blood pressure and ECG monitoring might be necessary for the treatment of other cardiac arrhythmias (e.g., multifocal atrial tachycardia).

---

509 What are the risks of Mg^{++} supplementation in patients with heart failure?

☐ Magnesium replacement by oral or parenteral routes as well as therapy with Mg^{++}-containing antacids might lead to hypermagnesemia in patients with renal insufficiency. The most common manifestations of Mg^{++} toxicity include sedation, hypotension, nausea, and muscle weakness. Severely symptomatic patients with serum Mg^{++} levels higher than 5 mEq/L might temporarily improve with IV Ca^{++} administration until a more effective treatment that includes hemodialysis or peritoneal dialysis is provided.

---

510 What are the most salient complications of diuretic therapy with loop agents and thiazides?

☐ The most salient complications of diuretic therapy are alterations in the volume and composition of body fluids. Malaise, asthenia, and symptoms of volume depletion commonly occur after rapid mobilization of edema, even in patients with an expanded ECF volume. Intense therapy with diuretics might also cause ECF volume depletion with or without hyponatremia that responds to discontinuation of the diuretic agent and increased dietary salt intake. A commonly observed complication is hypotonic hyponatremia (abnormally low $[Na^+]_p$ accompanied by decreased serum osmolality) in patients with expanded ECF volume and persistent edema. The hypotonic hyponatremia is due to the combined effects of diuretic therapy, the underlying disease (i.e., congestive heart failure decreases the ability for maximal urine dilution and water diuresis), and overzealous dietary salt restriction combined with relatively high water intake. The most effective therapy of hypotonic hyponatremia is water restriction. Potassium depletion and metabolic alkalosis are other salient complications of therapy with loop agents and thiazides. Diuretic agents might also produce adverse metabolic effects that are described in the answer to another question.

---

511   What is the management of hyponatremia in patients with heart failure?

☐ Because hyponatremia in patients with heart failure is commonly a complication of diuretic therapy, its management includes temporary discontinuation of these drugs, a more liberal salt intake, and limitation of water intake. Hyponatremia in patients with heart failure is generally mild (e.g., 120 to 135 mEq/L), well tolerated, and responds favorably to the above-mentioned therapy. Patients with severe, symptomatic hyponatremia (e.g., under 120 mEq/L), on the other hand, might require IV 0.9% NaCl or rarely 3% NaCl in combination with loop diuretics to prevent excessive ECF volume expansion secondary to these NaCl-rich infusions.

---

512   What are the most salient metabolic complications of diuretic therapy?

☐ Hyperuricemia, carbohydrate intolerance, and hyperlipidemia are the most important metabolic complications of diuretic therapy. The increment in plasma uric acid levels is a relatively common adverse effect of loop agents, thiazides, and K^+-sparing diuretics, which might occasionally produce acute gouty arthritis (secondary gout) or uric acid nephropathy (including stones). Carbohydrate intolerance that might precipitate or aggravate type II diabetes mellitus (noninsulin-dependent diabetes) is partially due to K^+ depletion and possibly to other mechanisms (thiazides are the drugs most frequently implicated). Hyperglycemic hyperosmolar nonketotic state might also develop due to diuretic-induced volume depletion in type II diabetic patients. Hyperlipidemia, manifested by increases in plasma triglycerides, total cholesterol, and low-density lipoprotein cholesterol might occur with prolonged use of thiazides. A diet low in saturated fat and cholesterol might minimize or prevent the hyperlipidemia caused by thiazides.

513   How commonly are adverse effects of diuretics observed?

☐ Adverse effects are frequently observed with this widely prescribed medication. Major complications of diuretics include prerenal azotemia with orthostatic hypotension and disturbances arising from volume depletion. Abnormalities in body fluid composition with respect to Na^+ (hyponatremia, hypernatremia), and H^+ (metabolic alkalosis and acidosis) are also commonly encountered. In addition, carbohydrate intolerance (hyperglycemia or worsening of diabetes mellitus), hyperuricemia (secondary gout), and disorders of Ca^{++} homeostasis (hypercalcemia, hypocalcemia) can develop in the course of diuretic treatment. The nature of the adverse effect (e.g., glucose, $[Na^+]_p$, etc.), and the direction of the alteration (e.g., hyponatremia, hypernatremia) depends on multiple factors including the specific diuretic prescribed, the patient's underlying disease and associated conditions, and the oral/parenteral intake of water, electrolytes, and other nutrients.

514   Do loop diuretics have any unique toxic effects?

☐ Yes. Ototoxicity due to sensorineuronal damage is a rare but important untoward effect, unique to loop diuretics. Ethacrynic acid might cause transient or permanent deafness, whereas furosemide appears to induce only transient ototoxicity. Consequently, it is advisable to avoid loop diuretics in patients receiving another potentially ototoxic drug (e.g., aminoglycoside antibiotic such as gentamicin or tobramycin). In addition, loop diuretics decrease the renal elimination of lithium (possibly leading to exceedingly high plasma levels) and increase the nephrotoxic effects of cephaloridine. A rare adverse effect of furosemide is exocrine pancreatitis, which might be due to increased levels of secretin that stimulate pancreatic secretion.

515   What other manifestations of clinical toxicity might be caused by loop diuretics?

☐ Allergic reactions to furosemide are occasionally observed due to cross sensitivity with other sulfonamides (e.g., for the therapy of infections). Other manifestations of toxicity include gastrointestinal symptoms, skin rashes, paresthesias, depression of formed elements in the blood, hypoglycemia, hepatic dysfunction, and renal abnormalities. Carbohydrate intolerance due to loop diuretics is of lesser severity than that observed with thiazides. Acute allergic interstitial nephritis leading to reversible renal failure is an important but unusual side effect of both loop diuretics and thiazides.

---

516 What are the major manifestations of clinical toxicity of aldosterone antagonists and other K⁺-sparing diuretics?

☐ The most serious toxic manifestations of aldosterone antagonists and other K⁺-sparing diuretics (amiloride, triamterene) is hyperkalemia, which derives from the major action of these drugs. Hyperkalemia is likely to develop in patients with significant renal insufficiency or with high K⁺ intake. Spironolactone might also cause gynecomastia in men, androgen-like side effects (e.g., hirsutism in women), and minor gastrointestinal symptoms. All these manifestations of clinical toxicity reverse on discontinuation of the drug. Amiloride might produce headache and gastrointestinal symptoms, whereas triamterene might cause nephrolithiasis, megaloblastic anemia, and gastrointestinal manifestations.

---

517 What are the potential problems arising from the use of diuretics in geriatric patients with heart failure?

☐ The potency of all diuretic drugs decreases in the elderly and such reduction of effects is due, at least in part, to the age-induced decrement in GFR. However, geriatric patients are also at greater risk of diuretic-induced toxicity (e.g., hyponatremia, volume contraction) because of decreased baroreceptor responsiveness, poor tolerance to electrolyte depletion, and lower blood flows (e.g., cerebral, coronary, splanchnic, renal) as compared to young adults. In addition, loop diuretics might induce Ca⁺⁺ depletion in the elderly. Thus, Ca⁺⁺ supplementation might be needed in geriatric patients.

518   What diuretics are preferentially used in infants and children with heart failure, and what untoward effects of these drugs might be relevant in this patient population?

☐   Furosemide, bumetanide, metolazone, and K^+-sparing agents are widely used diuretics in children and infants, and their bioavailability after oral administration as well as effects are generally similar to those observed in adults. Displacement of bilirubin from albumin-binding sites might cause kernicterus with hyperbilirubinemia in premature infants receiving large doses of furosemide. In addition, this loop diuretic might cause significant hypercalciuria in infants, leading to secondary hyperparathyroidism and pathologic fractures, as well as contribute to the development of nephrocalcinosis and Ca^{++} nephrolithiasis. Thiazides (e.g., metolazone), on the other hand, reduce urinary Ca^{++} excretion and might prevent the hypercalciuria due to loop agents if the two drugs are used in combination. Treatment of congestive heart failure in children involves the use of a single drug or combination of diuretic agents in a fashion similar to that previously described for adult patients. The usual pediatric dosage of furosemide is 1 mg/kg, which might be increased to a maximum of 6 mg/kg.

519   What general measures, other than those specifically directed toward management of the cardiac disease, should be prescribed for patients with asymptomatic heart failure?

☐   Measures aimed at reducing risk factors for heart failure should be enforced in asymptomatic (as well as symptomatic) patients including: (1) cessation of smoking; (2) correction of obesity; (3) dietary or drug management of hyperlipidemia; and (4) adequate control of hypertension. It must be recognized that treatment of the underlying cardiac disease in a given patient might not be indicated or feasible (e.g., valvular disease at early stage) and only measures aimed at reducing risk factors might be applied in asymptomatic heart failure. The role of ACE inhibitor drugs in the management of asymptomatic heart failure is discussed elsewhere.

520 What restrictions of physical activity are necessary in the management of symptomatic heart failure?

☐ Restricting the physical activity of patients with heart failure of mild to moderate severity might be limited to discontinuation of heavy labor and exhausting sports. More advanced heart failure that includes patients with moderate to severe incapacitation requires the introduction of rest periods during the daily activities and discontinuation of full-time work or equivalent physical demand. Patients with the most advanced forms of heart failure require confinement to their house and in cases of extreme severity, they must be confined to a chair or bed. The degree to which physical activity is restricted depends not only on the disease severity but also on a compromise reached between the treating physician and the patient based on advice of the former and needs plus physical capacity of the latter.

521 How important is restriction of physical activity in the management of heart failure?

☐ Careful restriction of physical activity to levels dependent on the patient's symptoms and functional stage (e.g., class I to IV of NYHA) is of critical importance in the management of chronic heart failure. All activities or sports that demand intense physical exercise, especially those of competitive nature, should be discontinued in all patients with heart failure (including those with asymptomatic stages of the disease). In addition, physical activities that elicit symptoms related to the cardiac disease (e.g., persistent dyspnea and palpitations) should be avoided. Not infrequently, patients develop symptoms of heart failure with activities that appear to be less demanding but are capable of performing more strenous activities without symptoms. In such cases, those specific activities that elicit symptoms should be discontinued. Physical exercise that involves the upper extremities is generally not tolerated as well as those activities that are mostly restricted to the lower extremities (e.g., walking). Nevertheless, excessive restriction of physical activity is counterproductive in the management of heart failure. Patients should generally be advised to remain active short of becoming symptomatic. A reduction in the pace of an activity or recreational endeavor ("slow-down") commonly allows patients to successfully complete a chosen task over a longer time period.

---

522   Should physical activity be restricted to a similar degree in acute and chronic heart failure?

☐ No. Physical activity must be maximally restricted and emotional stress avoided in patients with acute heart failure. These criteria are of great importance and are at variance to those recommended for patients with chronic heart failure. Complete physical rest is generally attained by either temporarily confining the patient to a sofa or bed according to preference. Patients are usually more comfortable in the sitting as compared to the supine position. Preference for the sitting position is likely due to the decreased venous return and thereby reduced cardiac preload attained in the upright posture. Use of the bathroom instead of a bedpan can usually be allowed. Additionally, emotional and mental rest is of great importance as is securing adequate sleep. The duration of severe restriction of activities depends primarily on the patient's overall response to treatment and on the specific cause of acute heart failure (e.g., 2 to 4 weeks in patients with acute myocardial infarction).

---

523   What specific measures might be used in the management of emotional and mental stress of patients with acute heart failure?

☐ The physician's role as a friendly listener who comforts the patient and offers a hopeful and realistic outlook of the clinical condition is of utmost importance. Hospitalization might help to provide the emotional, mental, and physical rest that the patient needs. Restrictions on visitation and telephone calls must be enforced. Medication to control anxiety (e.g., diazepam 2 to 5 mg twice a day) and to help securing sleep at night (e.g., furazepam 15 to 30 mg, triazolam 0.125 to 0.25 mg) might be beneficial.

524 How important is the patient's nutrition in the management of heart failure?

☐ A weight-reduction program for obese patients with heart failure is as important in the prevention and treatment of this condition as prophylaxis and therapy of cardiac cachexia in patients having these extremes of abnormal caloric balance. The latter group of patients might require continuous feeding by means of a nasogastric tube or percutaneous endoscopic gastrostomy (PEG).

525 What measures might be used to facilitate adequate bowel movements in patients with heart failure?

☐ Excessive strain during bowel movements must be avoided in patients with heart failure by using various measures to facilitate intestinal transit. Stool softeners such as dioctyl sodium sulfosuccinate, 50 to 200 mg daily, might be prescribed to patients prone to constipation, especially when physical activity has been significantly restricted. A mild laxative might also be required to control severe constipation and to avoid fecal impaction. In addition, increased dietary fiber content might help to prevent constipation.

526 What clinical and laboratory evaluations are routinely performed in the follow-up of patients with heart failure?

☐ The routine follow-up evaluation of patients with heart failure requires a complete cardiovascular examination including body weight and laboratory determinations comprising BUN, creatinine and serum electrolytes. In addition, a more thorough evaluation might be done periodically consisting of measurement of plasma cardiac glycoside levels and noninvasive cardiac procedures to assess ventricular ejection fraction.

527   What measures might decrease the risk of phlebothrombosis and pulmonary embolism in patients with heart failure whose activities have been maximally restricted (e.g., prolonged bed rest or confinement to chair or sofa)?

☐ Patients with heart failure confined to the bed, chair, or sofa might be routinely advised to perform deep-breathing and leg exercises as well as to wear elastic stockings. In addition, enteric-coated aspirin 325 mg daily or anticoagulation with minidoses of heparin (i.e., 1000 to 5000 U subcutaneously every 8 to 12 hours) or coumadin might be recommended. Patients with advanced heart failure including those with ejection fraction under 20% might be prescribed long-term anticoagulation with coumadin or related compounds because of the exceedingly high risk of systemic and pulmonary embolism.

528   How might cardiac work load be reduced?

☐ Reduction of the cardiac work load might be accomplished by: (1) decreasing the blood flow demands of peripheral tissues with physical and emotional rest, and a weight-reduction program in obese patients; (2) ameliorating or correcting specific conditions that produce an abnormally higher preload or afterload (e.g., congenital heart diseases, valvular abnormalities, arteriovenous fistulas) with appropriate interventions including surgery; and (3) reducing the resistance to blood flow along the circulation, thereby facilitating ventricular ejection of blood through the arterial vascular bed as well as diminishing venous return or preload. Consequently, arterial pressure in the systemic (aorta) and pulmonary circulations might be reduced by means of either vasodilator therapy (afterload-reducing agents) or assisted circulatory devices (e.g., intraaortic balloon, left ventricular assist device, artificial heart). In addition, venodilators (e.g., nitrates) might help to reduce venous return and cardiac preload. Measures aimed at decreasing the blood flow demands of peripheral tissues should always be prescribed and might be the only measures necessary to relieve symptoms. Yet, symptomatic heart failure might require utilization of multiple measures designed to reduce cardiac work load.

529 How might vasodilators relieve the signs and symptoms of heart failure?

☐ Vasodilators diminish the metabolic cost of cardiac work during systole (by reducing ventricular preload and afterload) allowing the heart to better meet the metabolic demands of the tissues (by increasing regional blood flows). Consequently, vasodilators (as single agents or combined with digitalis or diuretics) might ameliorate or completely correct signs and symptoms of heart failure. Vasodilators might exert their actions on arteries, veins, both arteries and veins, or have additional properties on the circulatory system due to inhibition of the renin-angiotensin system.

530 Classify and name the commonly used vasodilators in heart failure.

☐ Commonly used vasodilators for the management of heart failure are conveniently classified as follows: (1) venodilators (e.g., nitrates including nitroglycerin and isosorbide dinitrate) that relax smooth muscle of systemic veins, distending these vessels and thereby increasing the capacity of the systemic venous bed (also referred to as the capacitance bed); consequently, venodilators redistribute blood from the pulmonary to the systemic circuit, decreasing pulmonary venous congestion and left ventricular preload; (2) arteriolar vasodilators (e.g., Ca^{++} entry blockers, hydralazine, minoxidil) that relax smooth muscle of systemic arterioles, reducing the systemic vascular resistance, thereby acting as afterload-reducing agents (diminish left ventricular afterload); consequently, arteriolar vasodilators reduce wall stress of the left ventricle, increasing cardiac output per beat (i.e., larger stroke volume) due to augmented myocardial fiber shortening; (3) combined arteriolar and venous dilators (e.g., nitroprusside, trimethaphan, and α blockers such as prazosin) that relax smooth muscle of arterioles and veins of the systemic circulation, thereby reducing left ventricular preload and afterload; and (4) combined arteriolar and venous dilators with additional effects on the circulatory system due to inhibition of the angiotensin-aldosterone system (e.g., ACE inhibitors including captopril, enalapril, lisinopril); this group of agents has properties comparable to those of the previous group plus those properties related to ACE inhibition (depression of angiotensin II and aldosterone levels).

531   Are the salutary actions of the various types of vasodilators due to effects on specific abnormalities present in congestive heart failure?

☐ Yes. Patients with congestive heart failure frequently have an inappropriately high level of constriction of the arterial and venous beds of the systemic circulation, as well as activation of the renin-angiotensin-aldosterone system. Consequently, all classes of vasodilators might theoretically have desirable effects in this disease. The choice of vasodilator is generally based on the relative importance of abnormalities of preload, afterload, or activation of the renin-angiotensin-aldosterone system in the patient's signs and symptoms, as described below.

532   What determines the inappropriately high level of constriction of arterioles and veins in patients with heart failure?

☐ The maintenance of perfusion of vital organs such as the brain and heart in states of low cardiac output (including heart failure and hypovolemic shock) occurs at the expense of the skin, gut, and kidney that are vascular beds not immediately essential for survival. Stimulation of sympathetic activity and of the renin-angiotensin-aldosterone system, acting as compensatory mechanisms, triggers arterial and venous constriction, and promotes salt and water retention. Cardiac preload and afterload increase allowing maintenance of systemic blood pressure. Yet, the increased systemic vascular resistance augments impedance to left ventricular ejection, thereby depressing left ventricular function (which in turn decreases cardiac output). This vicious cycle leads to a new steady state characterized by a lower cardiac output and higher systemic vascular resistance that worsens the patient's signs and symptoms of heart failure. The mechanisms involved in the vasoconstriction observed in heart failure are: (1) sympathetic activation of constrictor tone mediated by vascular nerve endings; (2) high concentration of circulating catecholamines; (3) increased renin secretion leading to augmented production of angiotensin II, a potent vasoconstrictor; (4) high levels of circulating arginine vasopressin (AVP); and (5) thickening of arteriolar walls, presumably due to fluid accumulation.

---

533 Describe the hemodynamic effects of venodilator drugs.

☐ The acute hemodynamic effect of a venodilator agent (e.g., nitrates) in normal individuals consists of a decrease in left ventricular end-diastolic pressure and a secondary reduction in cardiac output (frequently leading to postural hypotension). In contrast, administration of venodilators to patients with congestive heart failure and high ventricular filling pressure can relieve symptoms of pulmonary congestion due to a reduction in the elevated filling diastolic pressure without depressing cardiac output. These drugs (e.g., nitrates) might also decrease cardiac output in patients with heart failure without venous congestion (normal diastolic filling pressure). Venodilator drugs are generally well tolerated in patients with heart failure. The hemodynamic effects of venodilators partially resemble the venodilator action of diuretics (e.g., loop agents). In addition, depletion of intravascular volume observed with all types of diuretics occurs predominantly in the capacitance beds and produces hemodynamic effects that are additive to those previously described for venodilator agents (e.g., nitrates). Consequently, the simultaneous use of diuretics and venodilator drugs imposes a risk of hypotension and forward circulatory failure.

---

534 How are nitrates used and what effects does each formulation have in heart failure?

☐ Nitrates including nitroglycerin and the long-acting preparations (isosorbide dinitrate, erythrityl tetranitrate, and pentaerythritol tetranitrate) dilate systemic veins as their principal action, as well as the pulmonary arterial bed and the systemic arterioles to a lesser degree. A continuous IV infusion of nitroglycerin (initial dosage of 10 μg/min that may be increased every 5 minutes by steps of 10 μg/min to a maximum of 100 μg/min) might be used in acute heart failure and pulmonary edema, when venodilation is the desired effect. Nitroglycerin administered sublingually in a dose of 0.4 to 1.2 mg might help in the management of acute congestive heart failure associated with normal blood pressure; the effects persist for 15 to 30 minutes and left ventricular filling pressure might decrease from about 20 mmHg to 10 mmHg. Effects that last at least 3 hours are obtained with topical nitroglycerin when a 0.5- to 4-inch strip of ointment is applied on the chest skin. Alternatively, nitroglycerin patches or discs might be used, and they allow showering and provide steady absorption. The long-acting nitrate, isosorbide dinitrate (Isordil), can be prescribed as a sublingual (e.g., 2.5 to 10 mg every 2 hours) or oral (e.g., 20 to 60 mg every 4 hours) formulation. The side effects of all nitrates include headache, postural hypotension, and methemoglobinemia (rare).

---

535   Describe the main properties of nitrates that are relevant for the treatment of heart failure.

☐   The commonly used nitrates include nitroglycerin and isosorbide dinitrate (Isordil), drugs having similar pharmacologic action (i.e., a strong [+ + +] venous dilating effect and a mild [+] arteriolar dilating action). These drugs exert direct influences on the vascular wall. Nitroglycerin can be used by multiple routes including sublingual (SL) 0.4 mg tablets, patch (5 to 10 mg/24 h), cutaneous ointment (1/2 to 1 inch every 6 hours or 5 to 60 mg as daily transdermal dosage), IV (initial dosage of 5 to 10 μg/min and maximal dosage of 100 μg/min). Tolerance to nitrates might develop with continuous usage. Nitrates in combination with hydralazine can increase survival of patients with heart failure.

---

536   How can nitrate tolerance (loss of hemodynamic efficacy over time at sustained constant dosage) be overcome in long-term therapy of heart failure?

☐   Tolerance to nitrate therapy can be significantly attenuated with a drug regimen that secures medication-free intervals of several hours' duration on a daily basis. The medication-free interval selected for a given patient is tailored according to the least symptomatic time frame over 24-hour periods. For example, patients with paroxysmal nocturnal dyspnea (PND) should receive nitrates before and during night rest with medication-free interval during the day.

537 How effective are nitrates in the long-term treatment of heart failure?

☐ Nitrates increase exercise tolerance, reduce symptoms, and prolong survival (if used in combination with other vasodilators) in patients with heart failure. Consequently, nitrates are effective drugs in the long-term management of this condition.

538 What patients with heart failure are likely to respond favorably or unfavorably to venodilator agents?

☐ Patients with heart failure whose principal manifestations are secondary to pulmonary congestion are likely to respond favorably to venodilator agents because of the reduction in intrathoracic blood volume elicited by these drugs. Venodilators are also useful in combination with arteriolar dilators in patients having signs and symptoms of heart failure secondary to both pulmonary congestion and reduced systemic perfusion. On the contrary, venodilators would be most likely counterproductive in heart failure with normal diastolic pressure (e.g., due to concomitant diuretic therapy).

539 Describe the hemodynamic effects of arteriolar vasodilators.

☐ The reduction in systemic vascular resistance observed with arteriolar vasodilators in both normal individuals and patients with heart failure produces different overall hemodynamic effects in these two groups. A greater increase in stroke volume is observed in the failing heart than in the normal heart at any given reduction of afterload (decreased systemic vascular resistance). Consequently, administration of arteriolar vasodilators to normotensive individuals without heart failure might produce reflex tachycardia and postural (orthostatic) hypotension (due to a reduction in systemic vascular resistance), because cardiac output fails to significantly increase. Administration of arteriolar vasodilators to patients with heart failure reduces systemic vascular resistance but increases cardiac output so that blood pressure remains unchanged or declines only slightly. It should be recognized that in patients with heart failure without elevated diastolic filling pressure, the administration of arteriolar vasodilators might produce only a small increase in cardiac output accompanied by a decreased arterial pressure.

---

540   What patients with heart failure are likely to respond favorably or unfavorably to arteriolar vasodilators?

☐ Arteriolar vasodilators are most useful in patients with forward failure due to low cardiac output and progressive reduction in perfusion of vital organs as a result of intense vasoconstriction. In addition, a favorable response to arteriolar vasodilators might be observed in patients with heart failure due to mitral or aortic regurgitation, because these drugs decrease regurgitation (backflow) and augment forward stroke volume by reducing afterload. On the other hand, arteriolar vasodilators might produce unfavorable effects in patients with ischemic heart disease. The reflex tachycardia might significantly increase myocardial oxygen consumption, and the excessive hypotension might further reduce coronary blood flow.

---

541   Describe the main properties of hydralazine (Apresoline) that are relevant for its use in heart failure.

☐ Hydralazine is a potent (+ + +) arteriolar vasodilator that has a direct action on the vascular wall. The usual oral dosage is 10 mg every 6 hours or every 8 hours (q.i.d. and t.i.d., respectively) with maximal dosage of 200 to 300 mg/d. Because sustained benefit is not observed in heart failure when hydralazine is used as the sole vasodilator, this drug is frequently combined with other agents (e.g., ACE inhibitors, nitrates) to obtain long-term benefits. Complications of therapy include headache, nausea and vomiting, fluid retention, drug fever, skin rash, positive antinuclear antibodies, and systemic lupus erythematosus-like syndrome; the latter side effect occurs in 10% to 20% of patients receiving a daily dosage higher than 400 mg.

542 Describe the main properties of prazosin (Minipress) that are relevant for its use in heart failure.

☐ Prazosin (α_1-adrenergic blocker) is a mixed vasodilator with a potent (+++) arteriolar action and a moderate (++) venous effect. Its vascular action is indirectly mediated because of its property as a selective α-adrenoceptor blocker. The usual dosage is 1 mg every 8 hours and maximal dosage is 24 mg/d. Because initial dosage might produce severe hypotension, the first dose of this drug is often given at bedtime (patient is recumbent so that postural hypotension will not develop) to reduce the symptoms due to this potential side effect. Complications of therapy include postural hypotension, fluid retention, and polyarthralgia.

543 Is there any relationship between the toxic effects of hydralazine (e.g., lupus syndrome) and the rate of metabolism of this drug?

☐ Yes. The risk of toxicity from hydralazine, including the development of a lupus syndrome, is significantly higher in patients who metabolize (degradation and elimination of this drug occurs by acetylation) this compound slowly, known as slow acetylators. This group represents about 50% of patients receiving hydralazine, and the rest of the population, labelled as rapid acetylators, might require a higher dosage of this medication to obtain comparable pharmacologic effects or develop toxic effects secondary to this agent.

544 What is the role of hydralazine (Apresoline) in the long-term management of heart failure?

☐ Long-term treatment with hydralazine is most beneficial in patients with severe cardiomegaly and markedly elevated systemic vascular resistance as well as in patients with moderate to severe aortic regurgitation. Other vasodilators such as ACE inhibitors have more favorable long-term results than hydralazine in the management of most patients with heart failure. Hydralazine might be added to supplement the effects of ACE inhibitors in the treatment of patients who can benefit from this drug. Nitrates might be effectively used in combination with hydralazine in the long-term management of heart failure.

---

545 What is the role of prazosin (Minipress) in the long-term management of heart failure?

☐ Although prazosin has favorable acute hemodynamic effects in heart failure, the development of drug tolerance (loss of hemodynamic efficacy over time at sustained constant dosage) and the high frequency of side effects makes this agent a poor choice for use as a single vasodilator in the long-treatment of heart failure. ACE inhibitors produce better long-term results than prazosin in most patients with heart failure. Nevertheless, prazosin, which is a potent α-adrenoreceptor blocking agent with effective antihypertensive properties, might be added to a regimen of vasodilators to supplement the effects of ACE inhibitors.

---

546 Describe the main properties of minoxidil (Loniten) that are relevant for its use in heart failure.

☐ Minoxidil is a potent (+ + +) arteriolar vasodilator that acts directly on the vascular wall activating ATP-dependent K^+ channels (blockade of ATP-dependent K^+ channels with oral sulfonylureas such as glyburide produce vasoconstriction, the opposite effect). The usual oral dosage is 2.5 mg once or twice a day, and maximal dosage is 40 mg/d. Side effects of minoxidil include hirsutism, Na^+ retention, and pericardial effusion.

---

547 Describe the main properties of nitroprusside (drug that releases nitric oxide, a potent vasodilator) and trimethaphan (nondepolarizing ganglionic blocking agent) that are relevant for the treatment of heart failure.

☐ Nitroprusside and trimethaphan are mixed vasodilators for IV administration. These drugs are potent (+ + +) dilators of both veins and arterioles. Nitroprusside is used at an initial dosage of 10 to 25 μg/min and maximal dosage of up to 300 μg/min. Because nitroprusside is a light-sensitive compound, the drug container must be covered with foil paper during administration. Medical complications of therapy include thiocyanate toxicity and methemoglobinemia. Trimethaphan dosage is 1 to 15 mg/min and complications of therapy include postural hypotension (blockade of sympathetic ganglia interrupts adrenergic tone on arterioles), bowel and bladder atony, and respiratory depression.

---

548 What is the role of nitroprusside, how is it prescribed, and which are the major complications of its use in heart failure?

☐ Nitroprusside is among the most commonly used vasodilators in the treatment of acute congestive heart failure. It must be administered as a continuous IV infusion because of its very short-lasting effects (when the nitroprusside molecule comes in contact with red blood cells, it decomposes, releasing nitric oxide that has a half-life of 2 to 30 seconds). Nitroprusside is most useful in severe heart failure associated with uncontrolled hypertension, acute myocardial infarction, mitral or aortic regurgitation, in acute exacerbations of chronic heart failure, and acute heart failure following cardiac surgery. The initial dosage in adults in 10 μg/min, which can be increased by 5 to 10 μg/min every 5 minutes if necessary. In addition, positive inotropic agents such as dobutamine might be infused in combination with nitroprusside. The most important complication of therapy is drug-induced hypotension, which reverses within 10 minutes of discontinuation of the nitroprusside (if necessary, phenylephrine or norepinephrine might be administered to correct severe or persistent hypotension). Cyanide poisoning (due to the release of hydrocyanic acid from the nitroprusside) is most unusual because hydrocyanic acid is converted to thiocyanate and excreted by the kidney. Consequently, if renal failure is present, thiocyanate toxicity might develop, which is characterized by dizziness, muscle twitching, abdominal pain, psychosis, and convulsions. Additional complications include hypoxemia due to increased blood flow of poorly ventilated alveoli, methemoglobinemia, and vitamin B_{12} deficiency.

549   What are the hemodynamic effects of "balanced" or "mixed" vasodilators?

☐ Balanced or mixed vasodilators are terms used to describe drugs that relax the vascular smooth muscle of both arterial and venous vessels (e.g., α_1-blockers such as prazosin, ACE inhibitors). The same terms also describe the combined use of a venodilator (e.g., isosorbide dinitrate) and an arteriolar vasodilator (e.g., hydralazine). The balanced vasodilators combine the hemodynamic effects of pure venous and pure arterial dilators acting simultaneously. Thus, balanced vasodilators in normal subjects and in patients with heart failure but without congestion (i.e., normal ventricular filling pressure) usually decrease preload, cardiac output, and arterial pressure. Balanced vasodilators in patients with heart failure and pulmonary congestion can reduce left ventricular filling pressure and relieve pulmonary congestion as well as decrease systemic vascular resistance and increase cardiac output. Because most patients with heart failure have symptoms of both low cardiac output and pulmonary congestion, they have a salutary response to "mixed" vasodilators (e.g., ACE inhibitors) or the simultaneous use of a venodilator and an arterial dilator (e.g., isosorbide dinitrate and hydralazine). Mixed vasodilators are generally preferred to the combination of two drugs with pure venous and arteriolar dilator actions. Although mixed vasodilators are unlikely to produce immediate beneficial effects in patients with heart disease without manifestations of overt failure (e.g., elevated filling pressure, depressed cardiac output, elevated systemic vascular resistance), long-term salutary effects might occur (e.g., diminished incidence of overt heart failure and cardiac dilation, as well as increased survival).

550   Do venous and arteriolar dilators act exclusively by reducing preload and afterload, respectively, or does each type of dilator reduce both preload and afterload?

☐ Venodilators and arteriolar dilators decrease both preload and afterload but the main action of each type of drug is on one of these determinants of cardiac output. Because afterload is a function of intraventricular pressure and volume, reduction of ventricular volume by a pure venodilator decreases afterload (in addition to the characteristic preload-reducing effects). In a comparable manner, arterial dilators decrease systemic vascular resistance, thereby augmenting stroke volume and producing a more complete ventricular emptying; consequently, ventricular diastolic volume decreases so that cardiac preload is reduced. It should be apparent that the classic view of venodilators as exclusively preload-reducing drugs and that of arteriolar dilators as exclusively afterload-reducing drugs is somewhat arbitrary.

---

551 What effect does systemic hypertension have on the selection of vasodilators (as opposed to diuretics and digitalis) for the treatment of heart failure?

☐ Hypertension (also called systemic hypertension) in patients with heart failure constitutes a major reason to select vasodilators (e.g., mixed or arterial) as first-line agents for the therapy of this condition (as opposed to diuretics and digitalis). Patients with heart failure and a history of long-standing hypertension might significantly improve their heart function with a vasodilator-induced reduction in blood pressure, even if this parameter is within normal limits. Those patients usually have concentric hypertrophy with normal or small left ventricular cavity (absence of ventricular dilation) and reduced ventricular diastolic compliance. Calcium entry blockers, drugs with properties of mixed vasodilators, effectively reduce systemic vascular resistance as well as improve diastolic relaxation in these patients; yet, these drugs might depress myocardial contractility (i.e., systolic function). In addition, ACE inhibitors appear to be beneficial in patients with heart failure and hypertension (of mild, moderate, and severe degree) and they might improve survival.

---

552 What effect does the presence of severe vasoconstriction in the renal, splanchnic, and cutaneous circulations have on whether vasodilators should be selected (as opposed to diuretics and digitalis) for the treatment of heart failure?

☐ The presence of severe vasoconstriction of cutaneous and abdominal circulations (e.g., renal, hepatic, gastrointestinal tract) in patients with heart failure represents a major reason to select vasodilators (e.g., mixed or arteriolar) as first-line agents for the therapy of this condition (vasodilators alone or combined with diuretics or digitalis). ACE inhibitors and hydralazine might increase renal blood flow, improve overall renal function, and enhance the renal response to loop diuretics. GFR might remain unaltered, increased, or decreased with ACE inhibitors. These drugs might precipitate a reversible but severe reduction in GFR (even acute renal failure) in patients with volume depletion or those with a severe angiotensin-induced efferent arteriolar constriction of the renal circulation. Prazosin (α_1-adrenergic blocker) has no major effects on renal blood flow but might significantly improve splanchnic extrarenal hypoperfusion.

553   What are the clinical conditions wherein vasodilator-induced reflex tachycardia might be particularly harmful?

☐ Vasodilator therapy in patients with acute heart failure (of any cause) and those with ischemic heart disease (acute and chronic) might increase myocardial oxygen consumption due to reflex tachycardia, the latter having detrimental effects on the patient's condition. Yet, vasodilator agents can be used with caution in these patients and might have salutary actions. In fact, ACE inhibitors (e.g., captopril, enalapril) might improve exercise tolerance in patients with coronary artery disease. Because the myocardial norepinephrine stores are depleted and the baroreceptor reflex is blunted in patients with chronic heart failure, the vasodilator-induced reflex tachycardia might not be a significant problem in this patient population (except for ischemic cardiomyopathy described above).

554   How important is attenuation of the response to vasodilators (known as drug tolerance or tachyphylaxis) in the therapy of heart failure, and what are its underlying mechanisms?

☐ Drug tolerance to vasodilators represents a significant problem in the therapy of heart failure. The underlying mechanisms for the attenuated response to these agents might include: (1) progression of the primary myocardial disease;

(2) activation of neurohormonal mechanisms (primary or secondary); (3) alterations in drug responsiveness or available tissue receptors; and (4) differences among the various vasodilators with respect to tolerance (large with nitrates and unimportant with ACE inhibitors).

555 Describe the main properties of ACE inhibitors (e.g., captopril, enalapril, lisinopril) that are relevant for their use in heart failure.

☐ The ACE inhibitors are mixed vasodilators with moderate (++) effects on both arterioles and veins. The oral route is generally used for the administration of ACE inhibitors in heart failure. The action of these drugs on the vessels is indirectly mediated by their properties as ACE inhibitors, preventing the transformation of angiotensin I to angiotensin II, the latter being a powerful constrictor of vascular smooth muscle. The usual and maximal dosages of captopril (Capoten) are 6.25 to 25 mg every 8 hours and 450 mg/d, respectively; the corresponding dosages for enalapril (Vasotec) are 2.5 to 10 mg daily or every 12 hours and 30 mg/d, respectively; the corresponding dosages for lisinopril (Prinivil, Zestril) are 10 to 20 mg daily and 80 mg/d. Captopril has the shortest duration of action (requiring daily dosing of 2 to 4 times), enalapril has intermediate duration (once or twice daily dosing), and lisinopril has the longest duration (once daily dosing). Intravenous enalapril (solution contains 1.25 mg/mL) produces effects that are apparent in 15 minutes. The most relevant complications of all ACE inhibitors in the treatment of heart failure are hypotension, renal failure, hyperkalemia, angioedema and laryngeal edema, and agranulocytosis. In addition, nonproductive cough, skin rash, proteinuria, and taste disturbances are observed with the use of some ACE inhibitors.

556 What renal effects of angiotensin II are ameliorated by ACE inhibitors?

☐ Angiotensin II constricts both afferent and efferent arterioles, but the effects on the latter are dominant. The overall influences of angiotensin II comprise increases in renal vascular resistance with decreases in renal blood flow, glomerular filtration, urinary flow, and Na^+ excretory rates. The filtration fraction increases because the reduction in renal blood flow generally is larger than that of GFR in response to angiotensin II. Although ACE inhibitors reverse the effects of angiotensin II on the kidney, the response to these drugs is not uniform among patients. Although renal blood flow generally increases with these agents, the GFR response is variable (most commonly unchanged but it might increase or decrease) if salt intake is normal. By contrast, in states of ECF volume depletion or severe reduction of effective arterial blood volume (e.g., congestive heart failure), the GFR tends to decrease.

557   What are the benefits, if any, of ACE inhibition in the management of asymptomatic heart failure due to hypertension or myocardial ischemia?

☐   ACE inhibition (e.g., with captopril, enalapril) delays symptomatic heart failure in patients with left ventricular dysfunction due to hypertension and coronary artery disease. These drugs might be beneficial for both systolic and diastolic dysfunction of the left ventricle. In addition, ACE inhibitors might decrease left ventricular mass, a parameter known to correlate inversely with survival (i.e., a large left ventricular mass is associated with shorter survival or life span).

558   What are the effects of ACE inhibitors (e.g., captopril, enalapril) on the sympathetic and parasympathetic systems, function of arterial baroreceptors, and on the levels of arginine vasopressin and atrial natriuretic peptide (ANP)?

☐   ACE inhibition has profound effects on several regulatory mechanisms that play a role in the clinical manifestations and complications of heart failure. This group of drugs has effects on: (1) the sympathetic nervous system that include down-regulation of β receptors, as well as a decrease in both peripheral sympathetic activity and catecholamine concentrations at rest and during exercise; (2) the parasympathetic system that normalizes heart rate variability and augments parasympathetic tone; and (3) the diminished sensitivity of baroreceptor function in patients with heart failure is restored. These drugs might correct the diminished responsiveness of the circulatory system to ANP and normalize plasma ANP levels (increased in congestive heart failure). In addition, ACE inhibitors depress the high ADH levels observed in heart failure.

---

559 What are the most common problems and side effects of ACE inhibitors in heart failure?

□ ACE inhibitors commonly cause hypotension in patients with heart failure, particularly with the first dose. Subsequent doses are usually better tolerated. Hypotension is not actually a side effect but derives from the predicted action of these agents. To decrease the incidence and severity of the first dose-induced hypotension, treatment with ACE inhibitors might be initiated with a low dosage that can be increased gradually. In addition, the initial dose might be taken in the evening immediately preceding the nightly resting period to avoid hypotension-related symptoms. Systolic blood pressure levels of about 80 mm Hg are well tolerated by many patients with heart failure without symptoms of postural hypotension. The risk of ACE-induced hypotension (e.g., postural type or syncope after exercise) is higher in patients with superimposed volume depletion (e.g., due to diuretics) and in those who are taking other vasoactive medication (e.g., prazosin, nitrates). Side effects of ACE inhibition include renal insufficiency, hyperkalemia, coughing, taste disturbances, skin rash, impotence, and neutropenia.

---

560 What are the risk factors for and how common is the development of renal insufficiency during treatment of congestive heart failure with ACE inhibitors?

□ The main risk factors for the development of renal insufficiency (increment of serum creatinine greater than 1 mg/dl or reduction of GFR greater than 20% with respect to pretreatment level) with ACE inhibitors in patients with congestive heart failure include: (1) hyponatremia, because this electrolyte abnormality is associated with marked activation of the renin-angiotensin-aldosterone axis; (2) diabetes mellitus, a condition in which the autoregulation of GFR is impaired and the efferent arterioles are excessively constricted; and (3) the use of long-acting ACE inhibitors (e.g., enalapril, lisinopril). Prolonged dilation of the renal efferent arterioles with lisinopril (about 36 hours) as compared to captopril (only about 6 hours) might explain the greater risk of renal insufficiency with the former drug due to the sustained decrease in renal filtration pressure leading to a diminished GFR. The frequency of developing renal insufficiency with ACE inhibitors in congestive heart failure is about 10%, 40%, 80%, and 100%, if risk factors are absent or an increasing number of factors from one to three are present, respectively.

---

561   Summarize the various mechanisms responsible for an acute/subacute decline in renal function with ACE inhibitors.

☐ The mechanisms responsible for the ACE inhibitors-induced acute/subacute renal insufficiency are either of hemodynamic nature (common) or due to parenchymal injury (rare). The hemodynamic mechanisms that lead to renal insufficiency are commonly precipitated by Na^+ depletion (e.g., diuretic therapy, extrarenal fluid losses, low-salt diet) or a reduction in renal perfusion pressure. Conditions in which the hemodynamic mechanisms are responsible for ACE-induced renal failure include congestive heart failure, volume depletion, diabetes mellitus, hypertensive nephrosclerosis, chronic renal disease, polycystic renal disease, hepatic cirrhosis, and nephrotic syndrome. Alternatively, parenchymal injury (rare) might account for the renal insufficiency observed with ACE inhibitors. Lesions that might be observed include acute interstitial nephritis, membranous nephropathy, and acute tubular necrosis.

---

562   What is the role of ACE inhibitors in the treatment of hyponatremia in patients with congestive heart failure?

☐ ACE inhibitors (e.g., captopril) used as single agents or in combination with a loop diuretic might promote reversal of the hyponatremia observed in heart failure. The use of ACE inhibitors might correct, at least in part, the neurohormonal activation and improve survival, in addition to reversing the hyponatremia. This action of ACE inhibitors on serum $[Na^+]$ most likely represents a class effect common to all compounds of the group, but does not occur with other classes of vasodi-lators (e.g., hydralazine, prazosin). It should be recognized that ACE inhibitors might occasionally worsen or induce hy-ponatremia because of a greater urinary excretion of salt as compared to water.

---

563 Describe the main properties of nifedipine that are relevant for its use as vasodilator in heart failure.

□ Nifedipine (Procardia, Adalat) is a Ca^{++} entry blocker (also known as a Ca^{++} channel blocker) with properties of a mixed vasodilator (i.e., moderate [++] arteriolar dilation and mild [+] venodilation). The usual oral or sublingual dosage is 10 mg every 6 hours and maximal dosage is 160 mg/d. Side effects include headache and a negative inotropic action that might be evident in patients with severe congestive heart failu-re.

---

564 What is the role of Ca^{++} antagonists (Ca^{++} entry blockers or Ca^{++} channel blockers) in the long-term management of heart fai-lure?

□ Calcium antagonists are relatively potent vasodilators that can decrease preload and afterload, thereby improving left ventricular function in heart failure. Nevertheless, negative inotropic effects of clinical significance might be observed with any Ca^{++} antagonist, especially the nonselective agents (e.g., diltiazem, verapamil, nifedipine). Consequently, they must be used with caution in patients with heart failure. Short-term improvement of left ventricular function might oc-cur in selected patients receiving Ca^{++} antagonists, especially if hypertension or coronary artery disease is present. It must be recognized that Ca^{++} antagonists activate endogenous neurohormonal mechanisms including the sympathetic and renin-angiotensin-aldosterone systems, and that these effects might counterbalance the salutary action of these drugs. In fact, it appears that Ca^{++} antagonists do not have significant favorable effects in the long-term management of chronic con-gestive heart failure.

565   Compare the effects of nonselective (e.g., diltiazem [Cardizem], verapamil [Calan, Isoptin], nifedipine [Procardia, Adalat]) and vasoselective (e.g., felodipine [Plendil], amlodipine [Norvasc], isradipine [DynaCirc], nitrendipine) Ca^{++} antagonists in the management of congestive heart failure.

□ The vasoselective Ca^{++} antagonists are more effective drugs for the management of congestive heart failure than the nonselective type of Ca^{++} channel blockers because the former agents: (1) lack clinically significant negative inotropic effects on the myocardium; and (2) have high selectivity for precapillary resistance vessels (arteriolar dilatation). The vasoselective Ca^{++} antagonists are a second or third generation of dihydropyridines that, in contrast to first-generation Ca^{++} antagonists such as verapamil (Calan, Isoptin), diltiazem (Cardizem), and nifedipine (Procardia, Adalat), have negligible myocardial depressant effects and have not been associated with any clinical or hemodynamic deterioration in short-term studies of patients with heart failure. The preferential dilation of precapillary resistance vessels might decrease cardiac afterload and increase regional blood flows. The short-term effects of vasoselective Ca^{++} antagonists in congestive heart failure are excellent, but the consequences of long-term treatment are unknown.

566   Outline the use of each group of vasodilator drugs in the management of heart failure.

□ Two possible regimens that include either an ACE inhibitor or a combination of hydralazine and isosorbide dinitrate (or other nitrate agent) might be considered as initial therapy (first step). If the response to the initial regimen is inadequate, all three oral vasodilators might be combined and the daily dosages of each drug increased to the maximum tolerable level (second step). Failure of the oral vasodilator regimen might lead the clinician to decide prescribing IV vasodilators (e.g., nitroprusside) (third step). The use of vasodilator agents must be integrated with all other therapeutic measures to achieve optimal results in the management of heart failure.

567 How important is the effect of a vasodilator drug on the neuro-hormonal activation of heart failure with respect to its therapeutic benefits?

☐ Because neurohormonal activation might have short-term and long-term detrimental effects in patients with heart failure (including signs, symptoms, and survival), neurohormonal effects should be considered when choosing a vasodilator. ACE inhibitors (e.g., captopril, enalapril) have unique properties among all vasodilators because they produce effective blockade of neurohormonal activation (these drugs ameliorate sympathetic and angiotensin-mediated mechanisms). β-adrenergic antagonists and digitalis preparations (in addition to ACE inhibitors) can also oppose the neurohormonal activation and therefore these three groups of drugs might have long-term beneficial effects in the treatment of heart failure. Although all vasodilators appear to have salutary hemodynamic effects (especially after acute administration) in the therapy of heart failure, those agents that blunt the neurohormonal activation might have better long-term effects in these patients (e.g., ACE inhibitors).

568 What properties have made ACE inhibitors the most widely used vasodilators for the treatment of heart failure?

☐ ACE inhibitors have distinct properties and effects in heart failure including: (1) a "mixed" or "balanced" vasodilator action because these agents dilate both arterioles and veins (thereby reducing afterload and preload, respectively); (2) ameliorate activation of both sympathetic and angiotensin-aldosterone systems; (3) good acceptance by patients in long-term treatment, without tachyphylaxis (drug tolerance); (4) effective in patients who failed to respond to digoxin or diuretics; (5) beneficial in mild, moderate, and severe heart failure; (6) multiple salutary actions such as improving heart failure symptoms and NYHA functional class, prolonging exercise tolerance time, decreasing the number of hospitalizations, reducing left ventricular mass, improving cardiac hemodynamics, correcting hyponatremia, and diminishing the incidence of ventricular arrhythmias; and (7) improved survival.

569   How do currently available vasodilator agents differ with respect to drug tolerance in the treatment of heart failure?

□ ACE inhibitors are unique among all vasodilators because they produce little or no drug tolerance in the therapy of heart failure. In addition, ACE inhibitors decrease arterial blood pressure without (or with minimal) reflex tachycardia, blunt the baroreceptor reflex, and block neurohormonal mechanisms (e.g., prevent secondary rises in plasma catecholamines, decrease angiotensin and aldosterone levels) in patients with heart failure. On the contrary, drug tolerance is significant with nitrates (described elsewhere in this chapter), prazosin, hydralazine, and β-adrenergic receptor agonists (drugs that have positive inotropic effects on the heart and dilator action on blood vessels). Attenuation of the response to prazosin appears to be secondary to increases in the plasma levels of renin and norepinephrine. Drug tolerance to hydralazine might be due to alterations in its metabolism or receptor adaptation. Attenuation of the response to β-adrenergic receptor agonist (e.g., dobutamine and salbutamol, which reduce systemic vascular resistance in addition to increasing cardiac output) might be due to down-regulation of β-adrenergic receptors in the blood vessels and myocardium. Patients developing tolerance to one vasodilator might favorably respond to another vasodilator that has a different mechanism of action. Consequently, clinical tolerance is reduced by either alternating the use of several vasodilators or using two drugs combined.

570   What is the most commonly observed side effect with all vasodilator drugs in the treatment of heart failure?

□ A decrease in systemic blood pressure, occasionally severe, might be observed with all vasodilator drugs, particularly in patients with advanced heart failure. Such hypotensive effect is most notable with the initial use of these agents. Consequently, it is advisable to titrate the dosage of vasodilators starting with relatively low levels to test the patient's sensitivity to the hemodynamic effects of these drugs.

571 Should long-term therapy with oral vasodilators be prescribed to most patients with chronic heart failure due to left ventricular dysfunction?

☐ Yes. In the absence of contraindications including hypotension and renal failure, long-term therapy with oral vasodilators is recommended in patients with chronic heart failure due to left ventricular dysfunction. This therapy might include the use of ACE inhibitors alone or in combination with other vasodilators (e.g., isosorbide dinitrate, hydralazine) as well as combinations of vasodilators (e.g., hydralazine and isosorbide dinitrate) without ACE inhibitors. In addition, vasodilator therapy can be effectively used in combination with digitalis and diuretics in the treatment of heart failure.

572 How important is monitoring of arterial blood pressure and other hemodynamic parameters when vasodilators are used in the treatment of patients with significant ischemic heart disease?

☐ Close hemodynamic monitoring and great caution should be exercised when using vasodilator therapy in patients with severe obstructive disease of the coronary vessels. The risk of serious complications due to a further decrease in coronary blood flow as a result of vasodilator therapy (e.g., due to arterial hypotension or reduction of cardiac preload) is substantial in patients with acute ischemia or acute myocardial infarction. Because IV administration (as opposed to other routes) of vasodilators has more powerful effects and is prescribed to more seriously ill patients, monitoring for possible changes in arterial pressure (e.g., direct measurements through arterial catheters), ventricular filling pressure (e.g., determination of pulmonary artery pressure or pulmonary capillary wedge pressure), and cardiac output (e.g., serial measurements) might be required in acutely ill patients receiving parenteral treatment with these drugs. In the absence of ischemic heart disease, the follow-up of IV vasodilator therapy does not require invasive hemodynamic monitoring (although it might be desirable). Nevertheless, frequent measurements of blood pressure are mandatory in this condition as well as in patients receiving vasodilators administered by the oral, sublingual, and transdermal routes.

573   How do NSAIDs interact with vasodilator agents?

☐ NSAIDs diminish the effects of vasodilators in patients with heart failure. NSAIDs might increase systemic vascular resistance and reduce both renal blood flow and GFR due to inhibition of prostaglandins E_2 and I_2 production. In addition, NSAIDs might precipitate acute renal failure in patients with prerenal azotemia due to heart failure or other causes.

574   Name the vasodilator agents used in the treatment of acute pulmonary edema and those prescribed for chronic congestive heart failure (i.e., chronic pulmonary congestion/edema).

☐ Nitroglycerin (Nitro-Bid, Nitrostat, Tridil, Nitro-Dur) and sodium nitroprusside (Nipride) are the vasodilator drugs commonly used in patients with acute pulmonary edema. The management of chronic congestive heart failure might include isosorbide dinitrate or other nitrate agent, ACE inhibitors (e.g., captopril, enalapril), and hydralazine. Therefore, nitrates might be effective in both acute and chronic heart failure due to their predominant venodilator effect (at low dosage there is dilation of both arterioles and veins, but effects on veins are more intense), or dilation of both arterioles and veins (at high dosage both vessel types are dilated to a comparable degree). Thus, at high dosages, nitrates behave as combined vasodilators.

575   What medication might benefit patients with predominant right ventricular failure and significant pulmonary hypertension?

☐ Postcapillary (also known as venocapillary) pulmonary hypertension might respond to venodilators (e.g., nitroglycerin, isosorbide dinitrate) as well as to left ventricular afterload-reducing drugs such as the combined vasodilators (e.g., ACE inhibitors, prazosin). Precapillary pulmonary hypertension might be treated with Ca^{++} antagonists, hydralazine, and prostacycline. In addition, all forms of pulmonary hypertension might be ameliorated by diuretics due to a shift of blood from the thorax to the systemic venous circulation (e.g., venodilator effect of furosemide) and reduction of intravascular volume secondary to the negative salt and water balance. Furthermore, correction of the increased airway resistance that frequently accompanies congestive heart failure with bronchodilators (e.g., using aminophylline, terbutaline) might help to ameliorate all forms of pulmonary hypertension. Management of hypoxemia, if present, with oxygen-rich inspired mixtures might decrease pulmonary vascular resistance, thereby reducing pulmonary artery pressure. The salutary effects of oxygen administration on hemodynamic parameters of patients with cor pulmonale (e.g., patients with right ventricular failure secondary to chronic obstructive pulmonary disease) might be dramatic, producing brisk diuresis and prompt resolution of anasarca.

---

576 Restate the technique to prevent nitrate tolerance in long-term therapy of heart failure.

☐ Withholding therapy with nitrates for 8 to 12 hours daily might prevent tolerance (amelioration of the vasodilator effects) to these drugs. Because reduction of preload by nitrates has the largest beneficial effect when patients are recumbent (e.g., while sleeping at night), especially for those with paroxysmal nocturnal dyspnea or nocturnal angina pectoris, a daytime nitrate-free interval might be prescribed so that these drugs are exclusively administered (e.g., oral or transdermal route) at night. On the other hand, patients with exertional angina pectoris might benefit from taking the nitrates during the daytime and having a nocturnal nitrate-free interval.

---

577 What major measures might be used to increase cardiac output in patients with heart failure?

☐ The major measures aimed at increasing cardiac output might be: (1) correction of an abnormal heart rate (i.e., extreme tachycardia, symptomatic bradycardia) with or without altered myocardial contractility; abnormal heart rates might produce symptomatic heart failure secondary to decreased cardiac output due to reduced effective rate of cardiac contractions; (2) repairing ventricular dysfunction secondary to abnormalities in preload (i.e., diminished or excessive) and afterload (i.e., increased); and (3) augmenting contractility in states of myocardial depression with positive inotropic agents.

Patients with transient or sustained bradycardia might increase cardiac output in response to electrical stimulation with an implanted pacemaker. Positive inotropic agents such as digitalis glycosides, sympathomimetic drugs, and other pharmacologic substances might ameliorate the depressed myocardial contractility of heart failure. All patients with symptomatic or decompensated heart failure require treatment with one or more of the previously mentioned major measures to stimulate the heart's pumping action.

---

578 What inotropic agents might be used in the management of heart failure?

☐ Digitalis glycosides are the time-honored and most widely prescribed positive inotropic agents for the management of heart failure. Other inotropic agents of value in the therapy of this disease are dopamine, dobutamine, and amrinone. The specific indications of all inotropic agents are discussed in the answers to subsequent questions.

---

579 What are the digitalis glycosides?

☐ Digitalis glycosides or simply digitalis are terms that refer to steroid compounds derived from either the leaves of the foxglove plant, *Digitalis purpurea* (e.g., digitoxin) or *Digitalis lanata* (e.g., digoxin, lanatoside C), or from the seeds of *Strophanthus gratus* (e.g., ouabain). These compounds exert a clinically significant positive inotropic action on myocardial contractility and cause typical electrophysiologic effects. Digitalis glycosides have been used for more than 200 years and remain as a major tool in the management of congestive heart failure and certain cardiac arrhythmias (i.e., rapid ventricular rate in patients with atrial fibrillation or flutter). Digoxin and digitoxin are the two preparations most widely used. Digoxin is the drug of choice because of its more rapid onset of action, faster elimination, and easier control of toxic effects as compared to digitoxin.

580 What are the main characteristics of the inotropic effects of digitalis?

□ Main features that characterize the action of digitalis include: (1) an increase in the force and velocity of contraction of cardiac muscle but not of skeletal muscle; (2) the positive inotropic effects are observed in both normal and failing hearts; (3) a dose-response relationship characterized by a gradual increase in the positive inotropic effects as a function of higher daily dosage or plasma levels up to the development of arrhythmias due to digitalis toxicity; (4) the pharmacologic action is significantly modified according to the concentration in biologic fluids of several ions including K^+, Na^+, Ca^{++}, and Mg^{++}; (5) inotropic action persists after complete β-adrenergic blockade; (6) absence of a direct effect on contractile proteins and intermediate metabolism; and (7) increase in myocardial oxygen consumption acting on isolated cardiac muscle (similar to other positive inotropic agents), but a potential for reduction in myocardial oxygen consumption in patients with heart failure due to a diminished wall tension and heart size.

581 What are the major pharmacokinetic characteristics of digoxin? Compare the dosages, time of effect, and fate of digoxin and digitoxin.

□ Digoxin (Lanoxin), the most widely used digitalis compound in the United States, is well absorbed after oral intake (about 80% absorption), its excretion occurs predominantly by the kidney, and enterohepatic recycling is insignificant. The onset of action occurs in 15 to 30 minutes, peak effects are evident in 1.5 to 3 hours, the average half-life is 36 hours, and one third of digoxin body stores are lost daily when renal function is normal. Loading dosage of digoxin is generally administered over 24 hours in three or four equal amounts at 6- or 8-hour intervals for both oral (total dosage is 0.75 to 1.25 mg) and IV (total dosage is 0.5 to 1.0 mg) routes. The maintenance dosage in patients with normal renal function is 0.125 to 0.5 mg and 0.25 mg for oral and IV administration, respectively. Therapeutic digoxin levels can be also achieved in 5 to 7 days after starting with a maintenance dosage regimen in the absence of a loading dosage. The relatively short half-life (1.6 days) of digoxin has advantages with respect to toxicity because the effects of the drug disappear rapidly after discontinuation of administration. On the other hand, digitoxin has a long half-life (7 days), steady-state concentrations in plasma are attained slowly, and recovery from toxicity is protracted (thereby digoxin is the drug of choice). Digitoxin is administered orally, its loading dosage is 0.8 to 1.2 mg, and daily maintenance dosage is 0.05 to 0.3 mg. The onset of action and route of elimination of digitoxin are 3 to 6 hours and hepatic degradation/renal excretion of metabolites, respectively.

---

582 What are the loading and maintenance dosages of digoxin (Lanoxin) in infants and children?

□ The oral loading dosage of digoxin elixir is about 30 μg/kg lean body weight in infants and children (under 10 years of age) and about 15 μg/kg for children over age 10 years. The daily maintenance dosage is 25% of the oral loading dosage for patients with normal renal function and requires adjustments in the presence of renal insufficiency. IV loading and maintenance dosages are about 75% of the oral ones.

---

583 What is the purpose of measuring serum digoxin levels in the treatment of heart failure with this drug?

□ Determination of serum digoxin/digitoxin levels (e.g., radioimmunoassay) might help to adjust the daily dosage of the drug in patients with heart failure such that the risk/benefit ratio of toxicity versus therapeutic results is optimal. The therapeutic serum digoxin level is from 0.5 to 2 ng/mL (for digitoxin is 10 to 35 ng/mL), and adequate clinical response without toxicity is generally observed within this range. The higher therapeutic serum digitoxin level as compared to digoxin is due to higher binding to serum proteins (about 10 times) of the former drug. Because digoxin is the preparation of choice, we shall refer below to plasma levels of this drug. Evidence of clinical toxicity is usually associated with levels higher than 2 ng/ml. Yet, 10% of patients develop signs of digitalis toxicity at levels under 2 ng/mL, and 10% of patients are free of toxic signs at levels above 2 ng/mL. The serum digoxin level in adult patients receiving 0.25 mg/d is 1.25 ± 0.4 ng/mL.

---

584 What are the main indications for measuring serum digoxin/digitoxin levels in patients with heart failure?

□ The main indications for determination of serum digoxin/digitoxin levels are: (1) to establish the maintenance dosage that achieves serum levels within the therapeutic range and offers optimal risk/benefit ratio; (2) to monitor compliance with the prescribed regimen; (3) to adjust, if necessary, the maintenance dosage in patients with severe heart failure or in patients who fail to respond to digitalis therapy; (4) to evaluate whether absorption of the drug is adequate in patients with gastrointestinal disease or following abdominal surgery; (5) to investigate the possibility of digitalis toxicity in patients with clinical signs compatible with this entity but without overt ECG manifestations; and (6) to follow up treatment of patients who have demonstrated clinical signs of digitalis toxicity. Clinical evidence of toxicity due to digoxin or digitoxin generally develops at plasma levels that are two times higher than those measured in patients having adequate therapeutic response.

---

585 Describe succinctly how cardiac glycosides exert their pharmacologic effects.

□ Cardiac glycosides exert their effects by binding to the Na^+,K^+-ATPase in the myocardium (and other tissues), thereby leading to inactivation of this pump. Consequently, intracellular $[Na^+]$ rises, which in turn leads to an increase in the intracellular Ca^{++} pool due to several possible mechanisms: (1) a diminished Ca^{++} extrusion from cells via the Na^+/Ca^{++} exchanger (most important mechanism); (2) an increase in cellular entry of Ca^{++} via the same exchange mechanism; and (3) an increased Ca^{++} influx through sarcolemmal Ca^{++} channels, augmenting sarcoplasmic reticulum (SR) Ca^{++} content. The larger intracellular Ca^{++} pool is mostly stored within the SR via the SR-Ca^{++} ATPase and becomes available for release at the time of excitation-contraction coupling through a Ca^{++} channel. The release of a higher amount of Ca^{++} from the SR during depolarization might account for the pharmacologic effects of cardiac glycosides to increase myocardial contractility.

---

586   How do cardiac glycosides inhibit Na^+,K^+-ATPase (Na^+ pump)?

☐ The cell membrane Na^+,K^+-ATPase has its binding sites for cardiac glycosides facing the external surface of the cells. The binding site of the Na^+,K^+-ATPase is located in the α subunit (a 100-kd polypeptide), which, combined with the β subunit (50 kd) compose the whole enzyme. The Na^+,K^+-ATPase, also known as the Na^+ pump, represents an active transport protein for the monovalent cations Na^+ and K^+ that is intrinsic to the cell membrane. Glycoside binding is inhibited by extracellular K^+, and optimal interaction of digitalis and the pump requires Na^+, Mg^{++}, and ATP. Once digitalis binds to the Na^+,K^+-ATPase, complete inhibition of enzymatic and transport function of this protein occurs. The normal function of the cellular membrane Na^+ pump consists of the extrusion of three Na^+ and the concomitant uptake of two K^+ ions per cycle.

---

587   How does digitalis-induced inhibition of the Na^+ pump change the cytosolic $[Ca^{++}]$?

☐ Inhibition of Na^+,K^+-ATPase with cardiac glycosides increases cellular $[Na^+]$, decreasing the driving forces for cellular Na^+ entry. This leads to reduced activity of the Na^+/Ca^{++} exchange system in the cell membrane, which extrudes Ca^{++} from the cell in response to the downhill movement of Na^+ into the cell. The result is higher cytosolic $[Ca^{++}]$, which has a positive inotropic effect.

---

588   Do cardiac glycosides increase cytosolic free Ca^{++} concentration ($[Ca^{++}]_i$) in both systole and diastole?

☐ No. Cardiac glycosides increase the intracellular Ca^{++} content due to the previously explained effects on cell membrane Ca^{++} transport (i.e., facilitation of cellular Ca^{++} entry through the Na^+ / Ca^{++} exchanger represents the most important mechanism). The larger Ca^{++} pool is rapidly taken up into the SR, preventing a significant rise in intracellular $[Ca^{++}]$. Yet, the Ca^{++} buildup in the SR allows for a larger transient increase in $[Ca^{++}]_i$ during the cardiac action potential, thereby increasing myocardial contractility. Efficient retrieval of Ca^{++} from the cytosol to the SR secures normal relaxation of the heart during diastole. Thus, cardiac glycosides increase $[Ca^{++}]_i$ in systole but not in diastole.

---

589 What are the effects of cardiac glycosides on the ventricular function curves (e.g., relation between ventricular wall force and fiber length) of the intact heart in the normal state and in heart failure?

☐ Cardiac glycosides modify the ventricular function curves (e.g., Frank-Starling relationship) of normal and failing hearts causing a shift upward and to the left. Consequently, digitalis increases systolic function (e.g., stroke work) at any given level of diastolic filling pressure in normal individuals and in patients with heart failure. In addition, cardiac glycosides increase the velocity of myocardial shortening at any given load imposed. Nevertheless, the digitalis-induced augmentation of myocardial contractility does not lead to a higher cardiac output in normal subjects. The unaltered cardiac output in the normal condition is due to adjustments in the other determinants of cardiac output (e.g., preload, afterload, heart rate).

---

590 What is the relationship between dosage of digitalis (and the resulting plasma levels) and the therapeutic effects on myocardial contractility in patients with heart failure?

☐ The positive inotropic effects of cardiac glycosides increase progressively as a function of the dosage of those drugs, until arrhythmias due to clinical toxicity develop. Consequently, prescription of a low dosage of cardiac glycosides might improve myocardial contractility and therefore achieve desirable effects in patients with heart failure. This "low dosage" strategy might be used in patients at increased risk for serious side effects from digitalis. Thus, a digoxin dosage regimen that achieves lower plasma levels (e.g., 0.5 to

1 ng/mL) might still produce clinically significant salutary effects in patients with heart failure. The clinician should determine the appropriate dosage in a given patient that is likely to be free of toxic effects (margin of safety should be favorable). Patients with congestive heart failure and normal sinus rhythm receiving digoxin, the most commonly used preparation, obtain near-maximal positive inotropic effects with dosages leading to plasma levels not exceeding 1.5 to 2.0 ng/mL. Monitoring for evidence of clinical toxicity and periodic measurement of plasma levels is required, especially if daily dosages of cardiac glycosides are relatively elevated.

---

591   What are the major electrophysiologic effects of digitalis that account for its antiarrhythmic action?

□   Major electrophysiologic effects of digitalis include: (1) decreased conduction velocity through the AV node and Purkinje fibers; (2) increased effective refractory period of the AV node and Purkinje fibers; and (3) increased pacemaker automaticity of Purkinje fibers. The first two actions account for slowing the ventricular response to atrial fibrillation (and atrial flutter) and for prolonged PR interval in the presence of normal sinus rhythm. The third action explains the development of bigeminy (arterial pulse characterized by two beats close together with a pause following each pair due to intermittent premature ventricular beats) that might occur with digitalis toxicity.

---

592   What are the effects of cardiac glycosides on heart rate of patients with normal sinus rhythm and on ventricular rate of those with supraventricular tachyarrhythmias?

□   Although usual dosages of digitalis have no major direct effects on automaticity of the sinus node (normal heart rhythm), sinus tachycardia is often greatly ameliorated by these drugs in patients with heart failure. The underlying mechanisms of the digitalis-induced correction of sinus tachycardia include increased myocardial contractility that leads to a higher cardiac output and secondary amelioration of elevated sympathetic tone, vagal stimulation, as well as increase in baroreceptor sensitivity. In addition to this effect on the sinus node, cardiac glycosides characteristically reduce the ventricular response to supraventricular tachyarrhythmias (including atrial fibrillation and flutter), particularly in patients with mitral stenosis. Slowing the rapid ventricular rate in mitral stenosis is of critical importance to prolong the period of ventricular diastole, thereby partially ameliorating the hemodynamic consequences of stenosis of this AV valve (barrier to rapid ventricular filling).

---

593 Explain further the role of digitalis therapy in the improvement of cardiac function (increased cardiac output) independently of the inotropic action of these drugs.

□ The beneficial effect of slowing the ventricular rate with ouabain (used only intravenously because gastrointestinal absorption is unreliable, with total digitalis dosage of 0.3 to 0.5 mg) or digoxin in patients with mitral stenosis and atrial fibrillation/flutter fully accounts for the usefulness of digitalis in the management of these patients. Slowing the ventricular rate allows a more complete diastolic filling of the left ventricle and thereby increases cardiac output in mitral stenosis accompanied by atrial fibrillation. On the contrary, cardiac glycosides have no therapeutic effect in patients with mitral stenosis and normal sinus rhythm. The salutary action of digoxin or ouabain in the first group of patients (with high ventricular rate due to atrial fibrillation/flutter) is independent of digitalis-induced positive inotropic effects.

---

594 What are the effects of cardiac glycosides on Na^+ and water excretion by the kidney?

□ Administration of digitalis preparations to edematous patients with congestive heart failure increases renal Na^+ and water excretion due to salutary effects on renal hemodynamics (e.g., increases blood flow, reduces arteriolar resistance, augments GFR, and reduces salt and water reabsorption in the proximal tubule). The effect of digitalis on renal hemodynamics observed in patients with heart failure is largely due to indirect hemodynamic actions (e.g., increased cardiac output) that suppress the so-called compensatory mechanisms of heart failure including sympathetic activation and stimulation of the renin-angiotensin-aldosterone axis. The diuretic effects of digitalis are not observed in individuals with normal heart function. It must be recognized, however, that a very substantial natriuresis due to inhibition of salt reabsorption secondary to depression of the Na^+,K^+-ATPase within the kidney can be demonstrated by infusion of a large dose of ouabain into the renal artery of the experimental animal. Such an effect also occurs in humans beings but is unlikely to play any significant role in the diuresis observed with digitalis therapy in congestive heart failure.

---

595 How should the dosage of digoxin be modified in patients with renal insufficiency?

☐ The loading dosage of digoxin is unchanged in patients with renal insufficiency, but the maintenance dosage is reduced in proportion to the severity of renal dysfunction. Because the renal excretion of digoxin is proportional to the glomerular filtration rate, calculation of maintenance dosage is performed using the patient's serum creatinine level (marker of GFR), as follows:

$$\text{Daily maintenance dosage (mg)} = \% \text{ daily loss} \times$$
$$\text{Loading dosage (e.g., 0.75 mg)}$$

This formula indicates that when daily loss is zero, maintenance dosage is also zero because the latter is obtained as a product of percent daily loss and loading dosage. Estimation of percent daily loss as a function of serum creatinine is performed, as follows:

$$\% \text{ daily loss in men} = 11.6 + \frac{20}{\text{Serum creatinine}}$$

$$\% \text{ daily loss in women} = 12.6 + \frac{16}{\text{Serum creatinine}}$$

Thus, in anephric patients the maintenance dosage is 14% of loading dosage, whereas it is 37% if renal function is normal; it has a value intermediate between these extreme levels in patients with various degrees of renal insufficiency. The calculated maintenance dosage in patients with end-stage renal failure (anephric) is about 0.11 mg/d (14% × 0.75 mg) whereas that for normal renal function is 0.28 mg/d (37% × 0.75 mg).

---

596 What are the direct vascular effects of cardiac glycosides?

☐ Cardiac glycosides act directly on vascular smooth muscle to produce arteriolar and venous constriction. These effects are due to inhibition of Na^+,K^+-ATPase in vascular smooth muscle that are comparable to the action of these drugs on the heart. Consequently, generalized vasoconstriction due to the IV administration of digitalis (slow infusion over several minutes is preferred to rapid bolus injection) might be observed and have detrimental effects in patients with cardiogenic shock in whom the vasoconstrictor effects might outweigh any positive inotropic action. However, generalized vasodilation is commonly observed when digitalis is given to patients with heart failure (as opposed to generalized vasoconstriction observed in normal individuals and some patients with cardiogenic shock), presumably due to increased cardiac output mediated by positive inotropic effect of the drug, baroreflex-induced withdrawal of sympathetic vasoconstriction, and suppression of renin-angiotensin-aldosterone system. Thus, the increased sympathetic activity and other compensatory mechanisms that help to maintain cardiac output in patients with heart failure, and to produce systemic arteriolar and venous constriction that facilitate maintenance of blood pressure despite the low cardiac output, might be overcome when digitalis preparations are administered in this condition. Reduction in sympathetic discharge and improvement of baroreceptor sensitivity might explain, in part, the long-term salutary effects of these drugs in patients with heart failure.

---

597 Explain further the effects of digitalis on baroreceptors and on the autonomic nervous system.

☐ Heart failure is associated with significant desensitization of the normal baroreceptor reflexes and this abnormality contributes to the neurohormonal activation (e.g., stimulation of sympathetic outflow, increase in renin and vasopressin secretion) observed in this condition. Treatment of heart failure with digitalis reduces autonomic nervous system activation and increases baroreceptor sensitivity. The salutary effects of digitalis on these properties might be mediated, in part, by effects of these drugs on the sympathetic nervous system and on the baroreceptor cells possibly due to inhibition of the Na^+,K^+-ATPase in these tissues and to the overall improvement of the hemodynamic condition.

---

598 Name conditions wherein digitalis preparations are first-line drugs.

☐ Digitalis preparations are recommended as first-line drugs in patients with: (1) impaired systolic function and dilated hearts with evidence of cardiac failure (e.g., S_3 gallop); (2) advanced heart failure (class IV) with sinus rhythm, and low ventricular ejection fraction; (3) angina pectoris (that might improve) coexisting with cardiomegaly and congestive heart failure; (4) acute congestive heart failure with systolic dysfunction due to a precipitating process (e.g., sepsis, anemia, thyrotoxicosis), in which these drugs might be used temporarily; and (5) supraventricular arrhythmias including paroxysmal supraventricular tachycardia, atrial fibrillation, atrial flutter, and Wolff-Parkinson-White syndrome. The use of cardiac glycosides in patients with heart failure having any of these indications except the arrhythmias is generally prescribed in combination with other drugs (e.g., ACE inhibitors or diuretics).

---

599 How effective is the combination of cardiac glycosides and vasodilators in the therapy of chronic heart failure?

☐ The combination of ACE inhibitors and digoxin is very satisfactory, increasing exercise capacity and left ventricular ejection fraction, as well as prolonging survival. The effect of each drug is additive and side effects as well as toxicity of this combination are low. Vasodilators other than ACE inhibitors have been also successfully used in combination with digitalis in patients with symptomatic heart failure.

600 How is the dosage of digitalis selected according to the severity of congestive heart failure?

☐ Because the use of digitalis in the management of heart failure imposes risks of cardiac and noncardiac toxicity that are related to daily dosage (and plasma/tissue levels), the severity of heart failure mandates two possible dosage regimens of these drugs. Patients with heart failure of moderate to severe degree who are prescribed digitalis preparations should generally receive the usual recommended daily dosages, specifically avoiding high maintenance dosages (first step). Patients with refractory heart failure or those with disease of extreme severity might be prescribed maximum tolerable doses of digitalis (second step). The rationale for the use of high dosages of these drugs in the latter group of patients is based on the direct relationship between the plasma/tissue levels of digitalis and the intensity of positive inotropic effects.

601 What factors support the selection of a low-dosage regimen of digitalis for patients with heart failure chosen to receive this drug?

☐ Selection of the dosage of cardiac glycosides for the management of heart failure is based on the following factors: (1) positive inotropic effects that are clinically significant might be obtained with low dosages of digitalis; (2) other agents (e.g., diuretics, vasodilators) that are very effective for the treatment of heart failure are generally administered concomitantly with digitalis, thereby reducing the level of inotropic effect that must be achieved to improve cardiac function with cardiac glycosides; (3) toxic levels are close to those needed for maximal therapeutic effects so that the risk of clinical toxicity is high when attempts are made to achieve the greatest inotropic action; (4) digitalis toxicity might be life-threatening; and (5) factors known to increase the sensitivity and risk of toxicity to digitalis (e.g., hypokalemia, renal insufficiency, and many others described in a subsequent answer) are commonly present in patients with heart failure. Consequently, the dosage of digitalis to be prescribed in patients with heart failure should be, in most instances, in the low end of the range for therapeutic levels.

602   Should the criterion of "maximally tolerated dosage" be used routinely for the prescription of digitalis in patients with heart failure?

☐ No. Multiple reasons that have been presented in an answer to a previous question support the use of a low-dosage regimen of digitalis in most patients with heart failure receiving this medication. The criterion of "maximally tolerated dosage" for the prescription of digitalis has been used in the past when these drugs were the exclusive agents available for the treatment of heart failure. Consequently, attempts were made to achieve maximal inotropic effects with the use of digitalis. The current availability of other agents (e.g., ACE inhibitors, vasodilators) that are very effective in the management of heart failure is responsible, to a large extent, for the change in strategy from a "high-dosage" to a "low-dosage" regimen of digitalis in the therapy of this condition.

603   How important is a reduction of heart rate in assessing the adequacy of digitalis dosage?

☐ The importance of a reduction in heart rate in assessing the adequacy of digitalis dosage depends, among other factors, on the patient's cardiac rhythm. A reduction of heart rate to a normal value (e.g., 60 to 100 beats/min), assessed by the rate of ventricular contractions in patients with atrial flutter or fibrillation, represents an important therapeutic end point in gauging the adequacy of digitalis dosage. On the contrary, a reduction of heart rate in patients with sinus tachycardia (accompanied by the digitalis-induced ST segment and T wave changes) in the absence of salutary effects of signs and symptoms of heart failure has little importance in assessing the adequacy of digitalis dosage.

604   What are the most important drug interactions that might alter the efficacy or toxicity of digitalis preparations in patients with heart failure?

☐ Because patients with heart failure commonly receive multiple medications, the possibility of harmful drug interactions is high. Quinidine and verapamil increase serum digoxin level up to twofold due to a combination of reduced renal and non-renal elimination and decreased apparent volume of distribution; consequently, the dosage of digoxin must be accordingly reduced to half in patients receiving quinidine or verapamil. Neither procainamide nor nifedipine significantly changes digoxin levels. Diuretic agents might decrease GFR and renal excretion of digoxin, as well as induce hypokalemia, hypomagnesemia, and hypercalcemia (thiazides); therefore, the risk of digitalis toxicity is enhanced with this treatment modality. Sympathomimetic drugs and some agents used in anesthesia (e.g., cyclopropane, succinylcholine) also potentiate the arrhythmogenic action of digitalis. On the contrary, decreased serum levels of digoxin might occur in response to the concomitant intake of kaopectate, nonabsorbable antacids, cholestyramine, and neomycin due to decreased absorption of digoxin (oral administration).

---

605 What is the therapeutic value of digitalis in patients with cardiomegaly (concentric and eccentric hypertrophy) without cardiac failure?

□ Because digitalis preparations exert a positive inotropic action, and the systolic function of patients with cardiomegaly is frequently decreased (despite the normalcy of cardiac output) at any given end-diastolic pressure, these drugs might allow for a similar stroke work at lower ventricular filling pressure, thereby increasing inotropic reserve. Despite these theoretical advantages of digitalis therapy in patients with cardiomegaly and normal cardiac output (nonfailing heart), the value of these drugs in this setting is unknown.

---

606 What maneuver performed by the examiner might be useful for diagnosing impending digitalis toxicity?

□ ECG monitoring of cardiac conduction and rhythm during carotid sinus massage performed by the examiner can provide useful information indicative of impending digitalis toxicity. This maneuver might trigger abnormalities detectable in the ECG that were absent before the performance of the carotid massage. The most relevant defects that can be elicited include ventricular premature beats, bigeminy, second-degree AV block, and accelerated AV junctional rhythm.

---

607 What are the clinical manifestations of digitalis toxicity?

☐ Digitalis toxicity produces noncardiac and cardiac symptoms and signs that are characteristic of drug overdosage. Noncardiac manifestations include anorexia, nausea and vomiting, fatigue, agitation or drowsiness, restlessness, psychosis, and visual abnormalities including yellow halos, hazy vision, and scotomata. The most relevant cardiac manifestations include: (1) depression of cardiac conduction (e.g., second-degree AV block of Wenckebach type, third-degree AV block with junctional or ventricular escape, SA or AV junctional exit block); (2) increased automaticity of ectopic or subsidiary pacemakers (e.g., ventricular ectopic beats, ventricular bigeminy, ventricular tachycardia, ventricular fibrillation, nonparoxysmal AV junctional tachycardia); and (3) combined depression of conduction and increased automaticity of abnormal pacemakers (e.g., paroxysmal atrial tachycardia with AV block, simultaneous atrial and AV junctional tachycardia with AV dissociation).

---

608 What are the mechanisms responsible for the manifestations of digitalis toxicity?

☐ The commonly observed symptoms of anorexia, nausea and vomiting, are not due to local irritation of the gastrointestinal tract by the drug, but are secondary to stimulation of CNS mechanisms (i.e., activation of chemoreceptors located in the area postrema of the medulla). A combination of vagal stimulation and direct effects of digoxin on the sinus node contributes to sinus bradycardia and SA arrest. Sinus bradycardia predisposes to the emergence of escape rhythms that are junctional or ventricular. As with the sinus node, increased vagal activity and direct effect of digitalis on the AV node decrease conduction through this structure. The digitalis-induced appearance of new junctional or ventricular pacemakers is likely due to "oscillatory afterpotentials" or "transient depolarizations" that might develop in specialized cardiac conducting tissue. The differential effects of cardiac glycosides on ventricular and Purkinje fibers, as well as depression of conduction velocity in association with increased automaticity, might also lead to ventricular tachycardia and fibrillation.

609 How common is digitalis toxicity and what are its main predisposing conditions?

☐ Digitalis toxicity is observed in 8% to 25% of hospitalized patients who receive this drug. Conditions predisposing to digitalis toxicity include: (1) renal insufficiency; (2) electrolyte and acid-base abnormalities (e.g., hypokalemia hypomagnesemia, hypercalcemia, alkalemia); (3) acute myocardial infarction; (4) severe heart failure (NYHA class III or IV); (5) advanced age; (6) hypoxemia and acute or chronic pulmonary diseases; (7) thyroid diseases; (8) concomitant drug administration (e.g., sympathomimetic agents, verapamil, quinidine and other antiarrhythmic drugs, anesthetics); (9) cardiac conduction defects including SA and AV block; and (10) some cardiac conditions such as Wolff-Parkinson-White syndrome, hypertrophic obstructive cardiomyopathy, and amyloid heart disease.

610 Describe the manifestations of a massive digitalis overdose.

☐ Accidental or suicidal intake of a massive digitalis overdose can cause death due to ventricular standstill unresponsive to pacing or extreme hyperkalemia leading to circulatory or respiratory arrest (e.g., paralysis of respiratory muscles). Less severe forms might lead to sinus bradycardia, AV block, and ectopic rhythms that might respond to medications outlined in subsequent answers. The elevation of serum $[K^+]$ is due to inhibition of Na^+, K^+ ATPase throughout the body (especially in skeletal muscle), promoting the exit of cellular K^+ to the ECF following its electrochemical gradient. The high cellular $[K^+]$ as compared to that in the ECF (e.g., 150 mEq/L and 4 mEq/L in ICF and ECF, respectively) is due in part to the activity of Na^+, K^+ ATPase. Therefore, inhibition of this pump promotes the movement of K^+ and Na^+ in directions opposite to those generated by the normal operation of this transport process.

---

611 How and when might significant hyperkalemia develop in patients receiving digitalis preparations?

☐ Digitalis inhibits the Na^+,K^+-ATPase in all tissues including the heart and skeletal muscle. Consequently, cellular uptake of K^+ diminishes and $[K^+]_e$ tends to rise. Yet, significant hyperkalemia is found only with a large overdose of these drugs arising from accidental (e.g., children, demented adults) or intentional (e.g., suicidal attempt) intake. Extreme hyperkalemia leading to death can occur in these circumstances.

---

612 How is the diagnosis of digitalis toxicity made?

☐ Considering that digitalis inhibits the Na^+, K^+-pump, intracellular K^+ deficit might develop with digitalis intoxication, leading to disturbances in cardiac rhythm and conduction. The diagnosis of digitalis-induced hyperkalemia requires a high index of suspicion, ECG abnormalities suggestive of digitalis toxicity, and confirmation of toxic plasma levels of the digitalis preparation.

---

613 What is the overall treatment of digitalis intoxication?

☐ The treatment of digitalis intoxication differs according to the patient's clinical manifestations and total drug accumulation in body fluids. Patients with advanced life-threatening digitalis intoxication due to digoxin or digitoxin (including those who ingested very large doses accidentally or in a suicide attempt) might be treated with cardiac glycoside-binding resins, hemoperfusion, and glycoside-specific antibody Fab fragments. In addition, these patients might be treated with drugs that ameliorate or reverse the toxic effects on the heart (e.g., atropine, phenytoin, lidocaine, K^+, β-adrenergic blockers) or occasionally with DC countershock (this approach is considered only for patients unresponsive to pharmacologic therapy or whose arrhythmia is severe because it might induce ventricular fibrillation). Nevertheless, most patients with digitalis toxicity can be successfully treated with measures other than cardiac glycoside-binding resins, hemoperfusion, and infusion of specific antibodies. Additional information on the various modes of therapy of digitalis intoxication is presented in the answers to subsequent questions.

614 What are the indications for atropine, cardiac pacing, phenytoin, lidocaine, β-blockers, K$^+$, and DC countershock in the management of digitalis toxicity?

□ Sinus bradycardia, SA exit block, and AV block might be successfully treated with atropine. Sinus arrest and very slow ventricular rate due to second- or third-degree AV block might require temporary transvenous pacing. Phenytoin or lidocaine are effective drugs for the treatment of digitalis-induced ectopic arrhythmias including those of atrial, junctional, or ventricular origin. Phenytoin loading dosage is 100 mg infused IV slowly every 5 minutes until control of arrhythmia is achieved or drug toxicity develops, followed by a maintenance dosage of 400 to 600 mg/d. Because phenytoin also augments AV conduction, this agent has multiple beneficial effects in the treatment of digitalis intoxication. Lidocaine is administered as a 100-mg loading dosage followed by 1 to 3 mg/min of continuous intravenous infusion. Short-acting β-adrenergic blockers are potentially useful in the treatment of ectopic arrhythmias but might produce severe bradycardia or asystole. Potassium administration might revert ectopic tachyarrhythmias due to digitalis if hypokalemia is present, yet cardiac conduction abnormalities might worsen. DC countershock is reserved for patients with severe arrhythmias due to digitalis, who fail to respond to all other therapies because electrical therapy might lead to ventricular fibrillation.

615 What is the basis for the treatment of digitalis intoxication with cardiac glycoside-specific antibodies and their Fab fragments?

□ The IV infusion of purified cardiac glycoside-specific antibodies and Fab fragments allow effective binding of the drug within body fluids, rapidly reversing its toxic effects. The prompt renal excretion of Fab fragments decreases the immune response to the foreign protein. The efficacy and safety of this procedure is well documented and represents an important step in the therapy of advanced life-threatening digitalis toxicity.

---

616 What inotropic drugs other than digitalis preparations might be useful in the treatment of heart failure?

□ Positive inotropic drugs other than digitalis are commonly referred to as nonglycoside inotropic agents. This class of drugs includes the sympathomimetic amines (e.g., dopamine, dobutamine, levodopa, ibopamine, dopexamine, pirbuterol, terbutaline, salbutamol) and the phosphodiesterase inhibitors (e.g., amrinone, milrinone, enoximone, pimobendan). The sympathomimetic amines and the phosphodiesterase inhibitors can each be administered either IV or PO. A feature common to all nonglycoside inotropic agents is their efficacy in the short-term treatment of severe heart failure. On the contrary, nonglycoside inotropic agents have questionable or even harmful effects if used for long periods.

---

617 Recapitulate the mechanisms that control cytoplasmic [Ca^{++}] in the myocyte.

□ The cellular entry and exit of Ca^{++} occur by different pathways that are under physiologic control. The inward movement of Ca^{++} across the sarcolemma (cellular membrane) along its concentration gradient occurs through voltage-dependent channels (i.e., the movement of Ca^{++} through these pores is controlled by electrical potentials) and receptor-operated channels (i.e., the movement of Ca^{++} through these pores is controlled by cell membrane receptors sensitive to physiologic messengers and drugs). The outward movement of Ca^{++} across the sarcolemma depends on the Na^+/Ca^{++} exchange mechanism and on active pumping by a Ca^{++}-ATPase. The Na^+/Ca^{++} exchanger can operate in either direction (allowing either exit or entry of Ca^{++} and the opposite movement of Na^+) depending on the relative concentration of extracellular and intracellular Na^+ and Ca^{++}. Nevertheless, the downhill movement of Na^+ into the cell along its electrochemical gradient under physiologic conditions provides the energy (and mandates the direction of ion movement) for the translocation of Ca^{++} out of the cell against its concentration gradient. Calcium kinetics within the cell is modulated by several mechanisms that include: (1) uptake and release by intracellular structures such as the mitochondria, the internal surface of the sarcolemma, and the SR; (2) Ca^{++} buffering by intracellular proteins such as calmodulin, troponin C, and myosin-P light chains; and (3) a Ca^{++}-stimulated Mg^{++}-AT-Pase located within the membranes of the SR that extrudes Ca^{++} from the cytosol and sequesters it within these structures through an energy-requiring process.

---

618 What pharmacologic agents alter myocardial contractility due to effects on Ca^{++} kinetics?

☐ The improvement in myocardial contractility observed with cardiac glycosides, sympathomimetic amines (β_1 and α agonists), and phosphodiesterase inhibitors (e.g., aminophylline) is mediated by alterations in Ca^{++} kinetics in heart muscle that increase Ca^{++} availability to the myofilaments for contraction. In a comparable fashion, the diminished myocardial contractility observed with β-adrenoreceptor blockers, Ca^{++} antagonists, quinidine and other class I antiarrhythmic agents, and barbiturates are caused by drug-induced defects in Ca^{++} movement or concentration in heart muscle that decreases Ca^{++} availability to the myofilaments for contraction.

---

619 What are the effects of β-adrenergic agonists on cytosolic $[Ca^{++}]$ and on myocardial contraction and relaxation?

☐ β-adrenergic agonists increase Ca^{++} influx across the sarcolemma by recruiting Ca^{++} channels and such action increases myocardial contractility. The greater Ca^{++} influx occurs through activation of a membrane-bound enzyme, adenylate cyclase, that catalyzes the production of cyclic AMP from ATP. Cyclic AMP acts as a second messenger, activating protein kinases that phosphorylate a protein located near a Ca^{++} channel, which enhances its open state. Myocardial relaxation is also stimulated by cyclic AMP. Augmented Ca^{++} reuptake by the SR and decreased sensitivity of the myofilament to Ca^{++} explain the enhanced myocardial relaxation observed with β agonists.

620   How can inotropic agents be classified according to their effect on cytosolic [Ca^{++}] in the myocardium?

☐ Because the pharmacologic action of inotropic agents is largely mediated by changes in the myocardial handling of Ca^{++} and Ca^{++}-protein interactions, these drugs might be classified as: (1) agents that increase cytosolic Ca^{++}, by either a cyclic AMP-dependent process (e.g., cathecolamines, β agonists, phosphodiesterase inhibitors such as amrinone and milrinone, forskolin), or by a cyclic AMP-independent process (e.g., digitalis preparations); and (2) agents that do not significantly alter cytosolic Ca^{++} levels but augment the sensitivity of the contractile apparatus to this ion by effects on the low-affinity Ca^{++} binding site of troponin C (e.g., pimobendan, sulfamazole). It must be recognized that agents that increase cytosolic Ca^{++} (e.g., digitalis, β agonists, amrinone) only augment the so-called Ca^{++} transient (rapid release of Ca^{++} from the SR that transiently produces a 10,000-fold increase in cytosolic [Ca^{++}]) but not the resting [Ca^{++}] in myocardial cells; consequently, myocardial contractility is stimulated but relaxation is not adversely affected.

621   What are the mechanisms responsible for the increased cytosolic cyclic AMP levels with inotropic agents (e.g., catecholamines, amrinone, forskolin)?

☐ The mechanisms responsible for the increased cyclic AMP levels observed with positive inotropic drugs are: (1) effects on membrane receptors that activate adenylate cyclase through the stimulatory subunit (G$_s$) of guanine nucleotide-binding protein (GTP), leading to increased conversion of ATP to cyclic AMP (examples of this type include dobutamine, β agonists); (2) inhibition of phosphodiesterase III, the enzyme responsible for the degradation of cyclic AMP, thereby leading to an increase in cytosolic cyclic AMP levels (e.g., amrinone, milrinone); and (3) direct activation of the catalytic unit of adenylate cyclase (as opposed to the β agonist-induced activation of cell membrane receptors, which is mediated through the regulatory subunits G$_s$ and G$_i$ or by inhibiting degradation) producing an increase in cyclic AMP concentration (e.g., forskolin). The latter group of drugs appear to be promising agents for the future treatment of heart failure.

622 What are the effects of xanthines and those of acetylcholine on myocardial contractility?

☐ Theophylline and related xanthines (e.g., aminophylline) inhibit phosphodiesterase, an enzyme responsible for the breakdown of cyclic AMP, and thereby have positive inotropic effects on the myocardium that are comparable to those of β-adrenergic agonists. The sensitivity of the contractile elements to $[Ca^{++}]$ might be also increased with these agents. By contrast, acetylcholine reduces contractility and this effect is likely due to higher cyclic guanosine monophosphate (GMP).

623 What are the hemodynamic effects of IV administration of epinephrine, isoproterenol, norepinephrine, dopamine, and dobutamine?

☐ The sustained IV administration of isoproterenol and, to a lesser extent, epinephrine produces tachycardia and hypotension due to stimulation of β_1 adrenoceptors in the SA node and β_2 adrenoceptors in the systemic vascular bed, respectively. On the other hand, norepinephrine produces hypertension due to peripheral vasoconstriction mediated through stimulation of vascular α receptors (this catecholamine has only α-constrictor effects on arterioles without any β_2-dilator effects on these vessels) and cardiac stimulation (produces a powerful stimulation of β_1 receptors). Dopamine and dobutamine produce significant cardiac stimulation without intense tachycardia and have mild systemic vascular effects (described in the answer to a subsequent question).

624 What sympathomimetic amines are useful in the treatment of severe heart failure? Why are the natural catecholamines (epinephrine and norepinephrine) not useful in the management of this condition?

☐ Sympathomimetic amines that are useful in the treatment of severe heart failure include IV formulations of dopamine and dobutamine, as well as several oral compounds (e.g., levodopa, ibopamine, dopexamine, pirbuterol). The natural catecholamines epinephrine and norepinephrine are not useful for the treatment of heart failure because of: (1) rapid development of tolerance to these drugs; (2) down-regulation of β receptors with prolonged administration, which reduces the sensitivity of failing myocardium to β agonists; (3) norepinephrine depletion of cardiac sympathetic nerves (because sympathomimetic agents act, in part, by releasing endogenous norepinephrine); and (4) arteriolar constriction that increases cardiac afterload (e.g., norepinephrine). The previously mentioned mechanisms that account for the lack of efficacy of epinephrine also play some role in the limited response to the sympathomimetic amines currently used in the therapy of severe heart failure.

---

625 What are the cardiovascular effects of stimulation of β_1 (cardiac), β_2 (peripheral), and α (peripheral) adrenoceptors?

☐ Stimulation of β_1 adrenoceptors augments atrial and ventricular contractility (acting on the myocardium), increases heart rate (acting on the SA node), and enhances AV conduction (acting on the AV conduction system). Stimulation of β_2 adrenoceptors vasodilates systemic arterioles and causes bronchodilation. Stimulation of α adrenoceptors vasoconstricts peripheral arterioles.

---

626 Compare the effects on β_1- (cardiac), β_2- (peripheral), and α- (peripheral) adrenergic receptors of epinephrine, norepinephrine, dopamine, isoproterenol, dobutamine, and methoxamine.

☐ All of the above-mentioned sympathomimetic amines have intense (++++) β_1- (cardiac) stimulatory effects except for methoxamine that is devoid of such action. With respect to β_2- (peripheral) agonist action, norepinephrine and methoxamine have no such effects, dobutamine has only a mild action (+), epinephrine and dopamine have a moderate effect (++), and isoproterenol has an intense action (++++). The α- (peripheral) agonist effect is as follows: absent with isoproterenol, mild (+) with dobutamine, and intense (+ + ++) with the remaining drugs including epinephrine, norepinephrine, dopamine (high dosage), and methoxamine.

---

627   What properties of dopamine are most relevant for its use in severe heart failure?

□ Dopamine is an endogenous catecholamine that stimulates dopaminergic, α-adrenergic, and β-adrenergic receptors. This natural compound is either released from nerve terminals where it directly stimulates dopaminergic receptors or retained within nerve terminals to become the immediate biosynthetic precursor of norepinephrine. The vasodilation caused by dopamine is due to stimulation of specific dopaminergic receptors in blood vessels including those in the coronary, renal, mesenteric, and cerebral vascular beds. These effects are inhibited by phenothiazines (e.g., chlorpromazine) and butyrophenones (e.g., haloperidol) but not by β adrenoceptor blockers. Dopamine administration at relatively high dosage (5 μg/kg/min) produces the opposite effect on vascular tone, causing constriction of both arterioles and veins of all vascular beds. Dopamine increases cardiac contractility when used at both low and high dosages.

---

628   Provide details on the receptors responsible for the dopamine-induced vasodilation and vasoconstriction.

□ Dopamine interacts with receptors located on both the presynaptic (dopaminergic-2 or DA_2 receptor and α_2 adrenoceptor) and postsynaptic (dopaminergic-1 or DA_1 receptor, α_1 adrenoceptor, α_2 adrenoceptor) membranes of the sympathetic nerve terminals that reach the vascular walls of arterioles and veins. Administration of dopamine at a low dosage (less than 5 μg/kg/min) causes vasodilation due to activation of: (1) presynaptic dopaminergic-2 (DA_2) receptors, inhibiting norepinephrine release from storage granules of the nerve endings; and (2) postsynaptic dopaminergic-1 (DA_1) receptors, which directly dilate vascular smooth muscle (i.e., renal, splanchnic, and coronary vasodilation). Activation of dopaminergic receptors stimulates adenylate cyclase, which raises intracellular concentration of cyclic AMP. Administration of dopamine at high dosage (above 5 μg/kg/min) produces vasoconstriction due to more prominent effects on postsynaptic receptors (constriction) than on presynaptic (dilation) ones, as follows: (1) postsynaptic α_1 adrenoreceptor and α_2 adrenoceptor are activated, leading to direct vasoconstriction of vascular smooth muscle; and (2) presynaptic α_2 adrenoceptors are also stimulated, leading to reduced norepinephrine release. It must be recognized that norepinephrine exiting the presynaptic terminals also activates the two types of α adrenoceptors. The vasodilatory action of dopamine mediated by activation of dopaminergic-1 receptors is due to increased intracellular concentration of cyclic AMP in vascular smooth muscle cells.

---

629 Summarize the cardiac and renal effects of low and high dosages of dopamine.

□ The systemic infusion of dopamine at rates below 2 μg/kg/min dilates renal, mesenteric, and coronary vascular beds. Infusion rates of 2 to 5 μg/kg/min have effects on vascular beds that are similar to those of the lower dosage plus a positive inotropic effect (increased myocardial contractility and cardiac output with little change in heart rate) and either a reduction or no change in total peripheral resistance. At 2 to 5 μg/kg/min IV dopamine stimulates cardiac β_1 receptors, increasing myocardial contractility and cardiac output. The β_1-agonist effects of dopamine are more prominent at higher dosage but the concomitant activation of α_1 and α_2 receptors augments preload and afterload (due to constriction of venous and arterial beds, respectively). Dopamine-induced diuresis also occurs with dosages of up to 5 μg/kg/min and is due to a combination of positive inotropic effects, selective renal vasodilator action, and direct tubule effects (reducing salt and water reabsorption). Dosages of 5 to 10 μg/kg/min produce systemic vasoconstriction, decrease renal blood flow, and increase vascular peripheral resistance, arterial pressure, coronary vascular resistance, and heart rate.

630 What dopamine dosages should be used for the treatment of refractory heart failure?

☐ Patients with refractory heart failure (acute as well as chronic decompensated) and normal blood pressure should initially receive low dosage of IV dopamine (e.g., 0.5 to 2 μg/kg/min) that is gradually increased until the low cardiac output improves or diastolic pressure and heart rate rise. High dosages of dopamine are indicated in cardiogenic shock to achieve more intense positive inotropic effects. Infusion rates of 2 to 5 μg/kg/min in patients with heart failure increase left ventricular contractility, cardiac output, renal blood flow, GFR, and Na^+ excretion, without significant changes in heart rate and total body oxygen consumption, and decrease peripheral and pulmonary vascular resistance (if elevated). When even larger dosages of dopamine are required for its positive inotropic action, simultaneous infusion of nitroglycerin or nitroprusside might be necessary to counteract the vascular constrictor effects of dopamine.

631 What is the role of dopamine in the treatment of heart failure during and after cardiac surgery?

☐ Dopamine (or dobutamine or amrinone) is an effective drug for the treatment of acute heart failure following cardiopulmonary bypass. Any of these drugs, with or without intra-aortic balloon counterpulsation, might also allow discontinuation of cardiopulmonary bypass in patients with severe cardiac depression who cannot otherwise be weaned from the heart-lung machine. These drugs might help to overcome cardiogenic shock caused by myocardial stunning (postischemic depression of myocardial contractility) observed in the early postoperative period.

632 What are the main cardiovascular effects of dobutamine, and how do they differ from those of dopamine?

☐ Dobutamine is a synthetic sympathomimetic amine capable of stimulating β_1, β_2 and α adrenoreceptors. The inotropic effects of dobutamine are more intense than those of dopamine. Myocardial contractility increases with dobutamine due to stimulation of α_1 and β receptors (dopamine stimulates only the latter type); stimulation of each of these receptors in the peripheral vessels has counterbalancing effects so that the net action on vascular resistance is negligible. Nevertheless, dobutamine reduces systemic vascular resistance in patients with heart failure due to indirect effects of the increased cardiac output produced by this drug. This reduction in vascular resistance with dobutamine maintains arterial pressure relatively constant. In contrast to dopamine, dobutamine does not directly modify renal blood flow (lack of renal vasodilator effect) but causes a redistribution of cardiac output that preferentially increases coronary and skeletal muscle blood flow as compared to the mesenteric and renal blood flow. The usual dosage of dobutamine is identical to that of dopamine (e.g., moderate dosage of 2 to 5 μg/kg/min and high dosage of 5 to 10 μg/kg/min). A therapeutic regimen for the treatment of heart failure might combine a low dosage infusion of dopamine (to obtain a renal vasodilator effect) and dobutamine because the latter drug provides a stronger effect on cardiac contractility.

633 What are the indications for IV dopamine or dobutamine, and for how long should these drugs be used in the therapy of heart failure?

☐ Dopamine and dobutamine are effective drugs for the treatment of acute heart failure and decompensated advanced chronic cardiac failure. These agents might be combined with nitroprusside or nitroglycerin to optimize results by reducing cardiac afterload and preload, respectively, as well as to augment the diuretic response to loop diuretics. Dobutamine is recommended in low cardiac output states associated with ischemic heart disease. The duration of treatment with dopamine or dobutamine is generally up to 72 hours of continuous IV infusion, that may be repeated on a weekly basis (e.g., dilated cardiomyopathy, waiting period before cardiac transplantation). Such treatment might have favorable hemodynamic effects lasting weeks or even months after the drug(s) have been discontinued. Portable IV infusion devices might be used in ambulatory patients prescribed dopamine or dobutamine. These drugs are also effective in the treatment of acute heart failure after cardiac surgery.

---

634 What are the major adverse effects of dopamine and dobutamine infusion?

☐ Complications of therapy with dopamine or dobutamine include sinus tachycardia, supraventricular and ventricular arrhythmias, myocardial ischemia or infarction, gangrene of fingers or toes, and tissue necrosis (due to accidental extravasation of dopamine). The latter condition favorably responds to local infiltration with phentolamine.

---

635 What patients might respond better to dobutamine than to dopamine and vice versa in the therapy of heart failure?

☐ When the main goal of therapy is to improve ventricular function by direct inotropic stimulation, dobutamine is preferred to dopamine because this drug is a more cardioselective agent. The increase in cardiac output observed at any level of heart work (assessed as the product of heart rate and systolic pressure) is greater with dobutamine than with dopamine. Thus, in patients with acute or refractory heart failure, especially with sinus tachycardia but without hypotension, dobutamine is the preferred drug. On the contrary, dopamine is a better therapeutic choice in patients with heart failure and hypotension because this agent has significant direct vascular effects. The vasoconstrictor effects of a high-dosage regimen of dopamine might help to restore the undesirably low blood pressure of hypotensive patients. Once hypotension is corrected with high-dosage dopamine, decreasing its rate of administration can improve renal and mesenteric perfusion due to selective dopaminergic vasodilation (this property is absent with dobutamine administration).

636   What orally active sympathetic amines might be used to treat patients with heart failure, and what are the long-term results of
such therapy?

    □ Orally active sympathomimetic drugs used in heart failure
include levodopa (transformed by decarboxylation to
dopamine and thereby exerting effects similar to those
described previously for the IV the administration of
dopamine), ibopamine (a dopamine-like drug), dopexamine (a
dopamine analog), pirbuterol (a β_1 and β_2 agonist), terbutaline, and salbutamol (the last two agents are also β-
adrenergic agonists). Although hemodynamic status might
improve acutely in patients with heart failure, tolerance to
these drugs develops generally within a few weeks. In addition to drug tolerance, orally active β agonists predispose to
cardiac arrhythmias so that long-term salutary results are
unlikely. Furthermore, available evidence suggests that these
drugs have long-term deleterious effects in patients with heart
failure. The long-term salutary effect of β blockers (e.g.,
metoprolol) in hypertensive heart disease and idiopathic dilated cardiomyopathy is consistent with the possible
nonsalutary influences of prolonged treatment with β agonists
in heart failure.

637   What are the mechanism of action and the main hemodynamic effects of phosphodiesterase inhibitors (e.g., amrinone, milrinone,
enoximone, pimobendan) used in the therapy of heart failure?

    □ The phosphodiesterase inhibitors exert positive inotropic
and vasodilatory effects by increasing the intracellular cyclic
AMP concentration (due to inhibition of phosphodiesterase III,
an enzyme that breaks down cyclic AMP). Cytosolic $[Ca^{++}]$
increases during cardiac action potential with administration
of these drugs, augmenting myocardial contractility. Amrinone and milrinone, the prototype agents of this group, are
used IV for short periods in the management of severe congestive heart failure that is refractory to conventional measures. These drugs produce dose-dependent increases in
cardiac output and reduce right- and left-sided filling pressures as well as systemic vascular resistance. The effects of
phosphodiesterase inhibitors resemble those observed with a

combined infusion of dobutamine and nitroprusside (a positive inotropic agent and a mixed vasodilator, respectively). The pharmacologic action of phosphodiesterase inhibitors is synergistic to that of direct-acting sympathomimetic agents and is also additive to the effects of digitalis preparations.

---

638 Compare the mechanisms responsible for the inotropic effects of sympathomimetic amines with those of phosphodiesterase inhibitors.

☐ The inotropic effects of administered sympathomimetic amines (as well as circulating catecholamines and those released from adrenergic nerve terminals within the heart) might be secondary to stimulation of: (1) β adrenoceptors, which in turn activate adenylate cyclase, leading to increased cyclic AMP production that stimulates Ca^{++} influx through slow Ca^{++} channels (presumably because of activation of protein kinases that phosphorylate the slow Ca^{++} channel); and (2) α adrenoceptors, which increase cytosolic $[Ca^{++}]$ during myocardial contraction, presumably involving the slow Ca^{++} channel independently of changes in cyclic AMP. The inotropic effects of phosphodiesterase inhibitors (e.g., amrinone, milrinone, xanthines) are not mediated by the adrenergic receptors but are due to inhibition of cardiac phosphodiesterase, producing an increase in intracellular cyclic AMP that augments Ca^{++} influx (as described above for the augmented cyclic AMP caused by activation of adenylate cyclase).

---

639 What are the routes of administration, dosage, as well as short– and long-term effects of amrinone and milrinone in the therapy of heart failure?

☐ Amrinone and milrinone might be administered IV as well as PO. The IV infusion of amrinone consists of an initial bolus of 0.75 mg/kg followed by a dose of 5 to 10 μg/kg/min that can be maintained for several hours to several days in patients with severe heart failure (it is most useful in those with myocardial depression following cardiac surgery, acute exacerbations of chronic heart failure, left ventricular failure due to myocardial infarction, and severe heart failure awaiting cardiac transplantation). Milrinone has indications similar to amrinone and the recommended dosage is 10 to 30 mg/d. The hemodynamic actions of oral amrinone might resemble those following IV infusion and this   drug has multiple side effects (e.g., gastrointestinal symptoms, hepatotoxicity, hypotension, ventricular arrhythmias, fever, thrombocytopenia). The toxic profile for milrinone does not include thrombocytopenia. None of the phosphodiesterase inhibitors including amrinone and milrinone have salutary long-term effects with respect to either symptoms or survival (including patients who tolerate long-term oral administration of these drugs) of patients with heart failure.

---

640 At what stage of heart failure might IV inotropic agents be prescribed?

☐ IV inotropic agents (e.g., sympathomimetic amines, phosphodiesterase inhibitors) are generally prescribed to patients with heart failure who are symptomatic either at rest or with minimal activity despite optimal dosage adjustment of digitalis glycosides, diuretics, oral vasodilators, and maximal salt restriction (i.e., optimal therapy of abnormalities in preload, afterload, and myocardial function by means of conservative measures). These patients belong to NYHA functional class III or IV and might also require a more invasive therapeutic approach to their management including thoracentesis, paracentesis, ultrafiltration, ultrafiltration plus dialysis, and even the possible application of a circulatory assist device. Class IV heart failure patients might be also considered for cardiac transplantation if all relevant criteria are met (see pertinent questions).

---

641 What criteria must be satisfied before prescribing a course of IV therapy with vasodilators or inotropic drugs in patients with heart failure?

☐ A course of IV therapy for 2 to 3 days with a vasodilator, an inotropic agent (e.g., amrinone or dobutamine) or a combination of these drugs might be initiated only after: (1) the patient has been placed at bed rest and has received optimal dosages of cardiac glycosides, diuretics, and oral vasodilators;

(2) significant depletion of K^+ or Mg^{++} has been corrected; (3) large fluid accumulation in serous cavities that was not mobilized with diuretics has been mechanically removed; (4) precipitating causes of heart failure have been treated and the underlying cause of heart failure reassessed; and (5) every aspect of therapy has been thoroughly reconsidered. The combination of IV administration of nitroprusside or nitroglycerin with dobutamine or dopamine might be of benefit in patients with severe heart failure in whom the response to one of these drugs was insufficient.

642 Outline the various steps in the management of acute decompensation of congestive heart failure unresponsive to conventional therapy, as well as that of refractory or intractable heart failure.

□ Treatment of these functional states of congestive heart failure requires hospitalization as the initial step to allow for a regimen of IV medication. High-dosage furosemide (250 to 4000 mg/d) in combination with metolazone or other diuretics should be the first agent(s) prescribed immediately on admission. If the response to diuretics is insufficient, the level of systolic blood pressure (SBP) will determine whether dopamine at 3 to 20 μg/kg/min (if SBP less than 90 mmHg) or nitroprusside at 10 to 300 μg/min (if SBP greater than 90 mmHg) should be infused. IV infusion of vasodilators or inotropic agents generally mandates discontinuation of oral formulations of these or comparable agents. Patients who were given dopamine and had insufficient response but SBP increased over 90 mm Hg, might be additionally infused nitroprusside at 10 to 300 μg/min. On the other hand, patients who initially had SBP above 90 mm Hg and received nitroprusside but the response was insufficient might benefit from the addition of dobutamine 5 to 20 μg/kg/min or amrinone 5 to 10 μg/kg/min, if blood pressure support is necessary. After 24 to 48 hours of continuous IV therapy, oral drugs might be prescribed including captopril 6.25 to 50 mg t.i.d., or isosorbide dinitrate 40 to 60 mg every 4 to 6 hours plus hydralazine 10 to 40 mg every 6 hours.

643   What are the standard goals or desired levels for the various hemodynamic parameters when monitoring the response to therapy with IV vasodilators and diuretics in critically ill, hospitalized patients with heart failure?

☐ The hemodynamic goals during treatment of heart failure with vasodilators (e.g., nitroprusside) and diuretics are: (1) pulmonary capillary wedge pressure 15 mmHg or less; (2) systemic vascular resistance 1200 $dyn \cdot sec \cdot cm^{-5}$ or less; (3) right atrial pressure 8 mmHg or less; and (4) systolic blood pressure 80 mmHg or higher.

644   What arguments favor the use of inotropic therapy (e.g., digitalis) at both early and advanced stages of heart failure as compared to using these agents in only the late stages of this disorder?

☐ The best timing for initiation of inotropic therapy in congestive heart failure is controversial. Currently, inotropic therapy is generally used at late stages of congestive heart failure when its manifestations are no longer controlled by diuretics and vasodilators (e.g., loop diuretics, nitrates, and ACE inhibitors). At the late stage of heart failure, cardiac performance is significantly compromised, the left ventricle is considerably dilated, and inotropic agents might produce symptomatic relief in some patients. Because most inotropic agents increase cytosolic $[Ca^{++}]$, they might produce serious or lethal complications due to myocardial Ca^{++} overload. The use of inotropic agents in late stages of heart failure, when significant structural damage is already present, is not expected to have a meaningful impact on survival. Thus, at the late stage of congestive heart failure, the primary therapeutic goal of inotropic agents should be improvement of symptoms and quality of life without unduly shortening of life expectancy. An alternative approach is to use positive inotropic agents (e.g., digitalis preparations) early in the management of mild to moderate left ventricular dysfunction. Administration of these drugs at an early stage might improve left ventricular contractility enough to prevent the need for compensatory cardiac hypertrophy and dilation. Furthermore, such therapy might theoretically improve survival (especially with inotropic agents that sensitize the Ca^{++} pathway), although information that supports this view is currently not available. The digitalis-induced inhibition of counterregulatory mechanisms (e.g., sympathetic and renin-angiotensin activation) is compatible with long-term beneficial effects of these drugs in patients with congestive heart failure.

645 Might β blockers have a useful role in the management of heart failure?

☐ Yes. Because hyperactivity of the sympathetic nervous system might have deleterious long-term consequences in chronic heart failure, cardioselective β blockers might be beneficial in this population. β-Adrenergic blockers (e.g., metoprolol) can improve ventricular function, including myocardial contractility and relaxation. These drugs appear to be most effective in idiopathic dilated cardiomyopathy, whereas their beneficial effect is less evident in patients whose heart failure is due to ischemic heart disease. The improvement in congestive heart failure observed with β blockers might be due to: (1) the "protective" effect of β blockade against high levels of catecholamines that are deleterious in these patients; (2) β_1-adrenergic receptors are up-regulated in response to β-blockade therapy, and this "resensitizing" of receptors might be beneficial; (3) inhibition of sympathetically mediated vasoconstriction caused by the release of renin and certain prostaglandins; (4) a shift in substrate utilization from fatty acids to glucose, which increases the efficiency of the heart; and (5) the property of these drugs to reduce the risk of sudden death, especially after a myocardial infarction. It appears that the beneficial effects of β-adrenergic blockers are limited to those agents without any intrinsic agonist sympathetic activity (e.g., metoprolol). Administration of very low dosages of cardioselective β blockers to such patients (e.g., awaiting cardiac transplantation) with careful monitoring of the hemodynamic condition as well as slow titration of the medication as needed, might increase resting cardiac output, augment ventricular ejection fraction, and produce an overall clinical improvement. Nevertheless, β-blocker therapy should not be considered a component of the standard management of patients with heart failure.

646   When and how might β blockers be used in the treatment of heart failure?

□ Commercially available β-adrenergic blocking drugs generally carry a warning with respect to their possible detrimental effects in patients with left ventricular dysfunction. Furthermore, these drugs have not been approved for the standard treatment of heart failure. Yet, these agents might have salutary effects in some patients with this condition by antagonizing the detrimental effects of sympathetic agonists. Chronic activation of the sympathetic nervous system might have adverse effects on heart failure due to vasoconstriction, stimulation of the renin-angiotensin system, promoting myocardial ischemia, causing Ca^{++} overload, and increasing the risk of arrhythmias. Attenuation of the sympathetic effects by the use of β blockers with (e.g., bucindolol, celiprolol) or without (e.g., metoprolol) vasodilator properties might improve ventricular performance and clinical manifestations in some patients with congestive heart failure. If the clinician decides to add β blockers to the medical regimen of patients with congestive heart failure, these drugs should be prescribed with great caution. Initial dosage should be low because of the risks of hypotension, bradycardia, and ventricular decompensation. If tolerance to a low dosage is good, the dosage might be slowly titrated upward (e.g., using metoprolol). An initial regimen for patients with compensated heart failure is metoprolol 6.25 mg orally twice a day for one week followed, if tolerated, by a doubling of the dose every week up to 50 mg orally twice a day.

647   What is the specific treatment of acute heart failure?

□ The treatment of acute heart failure differs according to its clinical manifestations and cause. Management of common forms of acute heart failure uses different drugs as follows: (1) patients presenting with symptoms of backward failure (e.g.. pulmonary edema) without evidence of forward failure (e.g., absence of systemic underperfusion) might be treated with diuretics exclusively; (2) patients with evidence of left ventricular systolic dysfunction and normal or high blood pressure might be effectively treated with vasodilators;

(3) patients with normal blood pressure and forward plus backward heart failure might be prescribed diuretics and vasodilators concomitantly; (4) patients with low blood pressure, forward failure, and backward failure might be conveniently treated with three groups of drugs, namely diuretics, vasodilators, and inotropic agents; and (5) patients with myocardial ischemia as the cause of acute heart failure should not receive inotropic agents because these drugs generally increase myocardial oxygen demand, potentially aggravating ischemia; instead, these patients might respond better to vasodilators (e.g., afterload-reducing agents or nitrates).

---

648 What is the overall management of acute cardiogenic pulmonary edema?

☐ The treatment of acute cardiogenic pulmonary edema involves measures aimed at: (1) reversing the syndrome of cardiorespiratory failure; (2) controlling the precipitating factors of this condition; and (3) identifying the underlying heart disease for the long-term management of these patients. Most frequently it is possible to identify and treat precipitating causes of acute pulmonary edema (e.g., acute myocardial infarction, fluid overload, arrhythmias). Precipitating factors are managed concomitantly with the syndrome of cardiorespiratory failure. On the other hand, treatment of the underlying disease is generally initiated after institution of all emergency therapeutic measures.

---

649 What are the measures aimed at reversing the syndrome of cardiorespiratory failure in patients with acute cardiogenic pulmonary edema?

☐ Several measures should be immediately implemented in patients with acute cardiogenic pulmonary edema including: (1) oxygen-enriched inspired air by nasal cannula or facial mask in patients with adequate respiratory effort, or by mechanical ventilation after intubation in patients with poor/absent respiratory effort, hypercapnia, and those who have arterial oxygen tension of 60 mmHg or less despite inhalation of 100% O_2 at about 20 L/min; (2) an upright position of the patient's chest if respiratory effort is adequate; patient should sit up in the bed or in a chair with the legs hanging down to decrease venous return to the heart; (3) furosemide at a dosage of 40 to 60 mg IV over a 2-minute period; (4) morphine sulfate at a dosage of 3 to 5 mg IV over a 3-minute period while watching for possible respiratory depression; if respiratory depression develops, morphine should be discontinued and a morphine antagonist administered immediately; morphine should not be used in patients with poor respiratory effort or hypercapnia, abnormal mental status, intracranial bleeding, chronic pulmonary disease, or bronchial asthma; (5) rotating tourniquets, by applying blood pressure cuffs (inflated to 10 mmHg below diastolic pressure) or soft-rubber tubing to three of the four extremities and releasing one of the tourniquets every 15 to 20 minutes while applying it to the free extremity; the rotating tourniquets are effective measures that reduce cardiac preload, yet this technique is currently used less frequently because of the effectiveness of other measures, especially furosemide; (6) nitroglycerin (e.g., 0.3 to 0.6 mg sublingually or 5 μg/min IV titrated upward in 5 μg/min increments at 3-minute intervals as needed) or nitroprusside (same IV dosage as nitroglycerin) that reduces cardiac preload or afterload, relieving the symptoms of pulmonary edema; patients with hypertensive heart disease leading to pulmonary edema might be significantly improved with IV nitroprusside; arterial blood pressure should not fall below 100 mmHg during treatment with vasodilators; (7) digitalis might be useful in patients with atrial fibrillation/flutter or other supraventricular tachycardias and very high ventricular rate; in addition, this drug might improve patients with sinus rhythm who had not been taking this drug and who present with severe aortic valve disease, hypertension, or decreased ejection fraction; (8) aminophylline (theophylline ethylendiamine), at a loading dosage of 5 mg/kg injected IV over a 10-minute period followed by a constant infusion of 0.5 mg/kg/h (if renal and hepatic function are normal, otherwise, the maintenance dosage must be reduced) for up to 12 hours (thereafter dosage should be reduced to 0.1 mg/kg/h); determination of blood levels is useful because the rate of degradation of the drug is variable and toxicity is substantial (optimal blood level is 10 to 20 mg/L); (9) inotropic agents (e.g., dobutamine or amrinone) if there is no response to previous measures, presumably due to myocardial failure; and (10) ultrafiltration (intermittent or continuous), an effective modality for rapid fluid removal in patients who fail to respond to diuretics.

650 How does morphine provide symptomatic improvement in patients with acute pulmonary edema?

☐ The salutary actions of morphine in acute pulmonary edema are due to: (1) afterload-reducing effect on the left ventricle secondary to decreases in arteriolar resistance and blood pressure; and (2) diminished cardiac preload mediated by the combined effects of augmented capacitance of systemic veins ("pharmacologic phlebotomy") and depression of respiratory effort that reduces mean negative intrathoracic pressure; the reduced preload accounted for by the last two mechanisms causes a diminished venous return to the heart, ameliorating pulmonary edema.

651 What are the main indications for supplemental oxygen administration in patients with heart failure?

☐ Administration of supplemental oxygen in heart failure might be of significant therapeutic value in the following conditions: (1) pulmonary edema due to heart failure as well as that secondary to noncardiac conditions (e.g., fluid overload); (2) heart failure precipitated by pulmonary infection or infarction; (3) decompensated cor pulmonale with significant hypoxemia that worsens pulmonary hypertension; (4) heart failure due to any cause that is accompanied by arterial oxygen saturation below 90%; and (5) acute myocardial infarction in the initial 24 to 48 hours, but oxygen might be omitted if arterial oxygen tension is normal.

652 How should supplemental oxygen be administered?

☐ The method for supplemental oxygen delivery depends on whether the patient breathes spontaneously, is apneic, or is already undergoing mechanical ventilation. Supplemental oxygen might be satisfactorily administered to most patients breathing spontaneously by delivering 2 to 4 L/min of 100% O_2 by facial mask or nasal prongs/catheters. A higher administration rate might be used if the previous regimen fails to correct arterial hypoxemia. Oxygen-rich mixtures (FiO_2 of 60% or higher) might be provided with mechanically controlled ventilation after endotracheal intubation in patients with severe pulmonary edema refractory to more conservative measures or depression of spontaneous respiration (e.g., drug overdose, cerebrovascular accident). Application of positive pressure to the controlled ventilation might further improve the patient's oxygenation.

---

653   Might oxygen supplementation be harmful to patients with heart failure? What is the role of oxygen administration at night in patients with severe heart failure?

☐ Yes. Oxygen supplementation to patients without arterial hypoxemia or in the absence of significant tissue hypoxia due to heart failure might increase systemic vascular resistance and blood pressure (thereby augmenting left ventricular afterload), leading to a slight reduction in cardiac output. Tissue oxygen delivery does not significantly increase by augmenting the fraction of oxygen in the inspired air in the absence arterial hypoxemia. In addition, FiO_2 of 60% or higher has the potential for inducing oxygen toxicity in any patient independently of the presence of heart failure. Thus, oxygen supplementation should be prescribed when the potential advantages outweigh disadvantages. Hypoxemia, especially during sleep, is relatively common in severe heart failure. Such blood gas abnormality is generally secondary to the combined effects of pulmonary edema and Cheyne-Stokes respiration. Oxygen administration by nasal cannula or facial mask (e.g., 2 L/min) helps to correct hypoxemia, facilitates sleep, and reduces arousals caused by the carbon dioxide retention phase of the Cheyne-Stokes respiration.

---

654   How effective is IV vasodilator therapy in acute left ventricular failure and what are the guidelines for its use?

☐ Vasodilator therapy is very effective in patients with acute left ventricular pump failure with and without pulmonary edema. General guidelines for the use of IV vasodilators in this condition include: (1) start therapy with low initial dosages of the selected drug (e.g., nitroglycerin 5 to 10 μg/min, nitroprusside 5 to 10 μg/min, or phentolamine 0.1 mg/min) after measurement of initial hemodynamic parameters (blood pressure, heart rate, left ventricular filling pressure, cardiac output, and systemic vascular resistance) and repeat measurements during treatment; (2) maintain same dosage of drugs if cardiac output increases in response to the vasodilator-induced reduction in left ventricular filling pressure or systemic vascular resistance; (3) increase the dosage gradually every 5 to 15 min if blood pressure is maintained and the expected salutary hemodynamic effects of the vasodilators do not occur; (4) start inotropic agents (e.g., dopamine, dobutamine, or amrinone) in addition to either continuing or discontinuing the vasodilators if blood pressure decreases without salutary changes on cardiac output or left ventricular filling pressure (augmentation and reduction of parameter, respectively); and (5) substitute oral vasodilators for IV therapy when the clinical condition improves; attempts to wean the patient from the IV therapy should be made when cardiac output is more than 2.0 L/min/m^2 and left ventricular filling pressure is 15 mm Hg or lower, and oral medication is started. Thiocyanate levels must be monitored during prolonged infusions of nitroprusside.

---

655 What criteria might be used to decide whether digitalis should be administered to patients with acute pulmonary edema with sinus rhythm who have been receiving an unknown dosage of digitalis?

☐ Digitalis preparations should not be administered to patients with features consistent with digitalis intoxication, including paroxysmal atrial tachycardia with AV block, nonparoxysmal AV junctional tachycardia, frequent ventricular premature contractions, ventricular tachycardia, or a history of previous digitalis intoxication including nausea or vomiting. If these signs and symptoms are absent, digitalis preparations might be administered to patients with acute cardiogenic pulmonary edema. The decision to prescribe digitalis is usually based on clinical and ECG evaluation because measurement of plasma glycoside levels takes too long for results to be useful in the management of acute pulmonary edema.

---

656   What are the side effects of aminophylline therapy in acute pulmonary edema?

☐ Side effects of aminophylline include nausea and vomiting, headache, flushing, hypotension, palpitations, and precordial pain. Increased blood perfusion of poorly ventilated lung alveoli might produce hypoxemia. The most serious toxic effects of aminophylline include convulsions, hypotension (due to systemic vasodilation), and sudden death (complication of ventricular arrhythmias). Because aminophylline has the potential for inducing serious side effects, this drug should be used with caution in the management of patients with acute pulmonary edema.

---

657   What measures might be instituted for the management of precipitating factors of acute pulmonary edema?

☐ Specific therapeutic measures tailored to each recognized precipitating factor might be applied to reverse the syndrome of cardiorespiratory failure in patients with acute pulmonary edema. A bradyarrhythmia that fails to respond to pharmacotherapy might require a temporary cardiac pacemaker. A tachyarrhythmia that is not secondary to digitalis intoxication and that fails to respond to pharmacologic therapy might require cardioversion with DC countershock. A febrile syndrome might require measures to lower body temperature, whereas a hypertensive crisis must be treated with afterload-reducing drugs (e.g., nitroprusside). In a comparable fashion, recognition of acute myocardial ischemia, severe anemia, thyrotoxicosis, or any other precipitating factor of acute pulmonary edema should lead to implementation of measures aimed at correcting the specific process responsible for decompensated cardiac function.

658 What diagnostic and therapeutic procedures might be applied to determine the underlying condition responsible for acute pulmonary edema?

☐ Diagnostic procedures that might help to determine the underlying condition include a complete history and physical examination, ECG, chest x-ray, echocardiogram, catheterization of the right and left side of the heart, radioisotope angiography, blood cultures, creatine phosphokinase isoenzyme (CPK-MB) determinations, and other tests according to the presumptive diagnosis. The echocardiogram might reveal a previously unrecognized mitral stenosis, left atrial myxoma, hypertrophic obstructive cardiomyopathy, congestive cardiomyopathy, and other conditions. Cardiac catheterization might disclose a ventricular septal defect, mitral regurgitation, and other processes that require medical and surgical therapy. Although management of the underlying disease can be generally accomplished with nonsurgical procedures, this is not always the case. Patients with acute infective endocarditis, prosthetic valve dysfunction, prolapsing atrial myxoma, ventricular septal defect, critically severe aortic or mitral stenosis, or mitral regurgitation complicating acute myocardial infarction, might require surgical treatment of the underlying disease. Alternatively, balloon valvuloplasty might be performed in poor surgical candidates with aortic or mitral stenosis.

659 What are the potential salutary effects of mechanical ventilation in patients with cardiogenic and noncardiogenic pulmonary edema?

☐ Patients with pulmonary edema irrespective of its specific cause who also have poor respiratory effort are at risk of progressive respiratory failure with hypoxemia, hypercapnia, or respiratory arrest. For such patients, mechanical ventilation is a lifesaving procedure. In addition, mechanical ventilation might decrease the work of breathing by respiratory muscles, correct the blood gas abnormalities, decrease sympathetic activation, diminish whole body oxygen consumption, and thereby reduce circulatory stress. If hypoxemia is not corrected by standard mechanical ventilation, or if high/toxic levels of oxygen (e.g., 60% O_2 or more in inspired atmosphere) are necessary for prolonged periods, positive end-expiratory pressure (PEEP) might be added to help correct, at least in part, this blood gas abnormality. The increased intrathoracic pressure generated by mechanical ventilation, especially if PEEP has been applied, might be beneficial in patients with cardiogenic pulmonary edema because the associated higher alveolar pressure opposes fluid accumulation in the airways and decreases pulmonary vascular congestion due to the attendant increase in right ventricular afterload (that reduces right-sided cardiac output).

660   What are the potential nonsalutary or counterproductive effects of mechanical ventilation in patients with cardiogenic and noncardiogenic pulmonary edema?

☐ The relatively high pulmonary volume and airway pressure that accompany mechanical ventilation might be counterproductive because of hemodynamic and nonhemodynamic mechanisms. The hemodynamic complications might be caused by increased pulmonary vascular resistance due to lung volume expansion as well high alveolar pressure that augments right ventricular afterload, decreases systemic venous return, and reduces cardiac output. Such reduction in right-sided cardiac output will lead to a secondary decrease in left-sided cardiac output so that oxygen transport to peripheral tissues might be significantly reduced. The detrimental effect on oxygen transport to peripheral tissues is particularly relevant in patients with noncardiogenic pulmonary edema (we have previously explained the potential salutary effect of a decreased cardiac output by the right ventricle in patients with cardiogenic pulmonary edema). The decreased left ventricular output might also produce a fall in blood pressure accompanied by severe renal underperfusion (and possibly a reduction in cerebral and myocardial blood flow). Additional hemodynamic complications arising from the increased right ventricular pressure include displacement of the interventricular septum, which impedes left ventricular filling during diastole, as well as direct compression of the left ventricle by the inflated lung that also reduces diastolic filling. Nonhemodynamic complications of mechanical ventilation arise from barotrauma that might produce pneumomediastinum, pneumothorax, and subcutaneous emphysema.

---

661 What is the management of transient acute heart failure that follows cardiopulmonary bypass in the course of cardiac surgery?

☐ Effective treatment of acute heart failure following cardiopulmonary bypass consists of IV sympathomimetic agents or application of intra-aortic balloon counterpulsation. The former measure increases myocardial contractility, and the latter improves coronary and cerebral perfusion while reducing cardiac work load. Other therapeutic measures are generally not effective.

---

662 What are the goals and major indications for mechanical circulatory support?

☐ The major goals of mechanical circulatory support (e.g., left ventricular assist device, intra-aortic balloon counterpulsation) are to correct underperfusion of vital organs (most important goal) and to decrease cardiac work. The total combined blood flow of the patient's heart and the mechanical device (if applicable) must be sufficient to restore major organ function, overcome tissue hypoxia, and correct systemic acidosis. Because the most frequently used mechanical assist devices can provide flows higher than 2 $L/m^2/min$, they are capable of completely sustaining the circulation at rest. A reduction in myocardial oxygen consumption and higher coronary blood flow can be attained with mechanical circulatory support. The major indication for mechanical circulatory support is cardiogenic shock that occurs: (1) following heart surgery; (2) while awaiting cardiac transplantation; and (3) during acute myocardial failure with or without cardiac infarction.

---

663 What nonmedical factors are relevant to prescribing mechanical circulatory support, and what is the survival with this therapy?

☐ Important nonmedical factors to be considered before prescribing mechanical circulatory support include: (1) recognition of the complexity of even the simplest devices that require significant expertise of the health care team as well as the demanding nature of this therapy with respect to personnel time and resources; and (2) recognition that this management modality is very expensive. Thus, patients must be carefully selected and every effort should be made to improve the likelihood of their recovery. The survival rate for patients of all ages on the intra-aortic balloon ranges from 30% to 60% and the morbidity including limb ischemia is substantial. Survival is significantly lower in the elderly, being only 10% in patients older than 70 years who receive mechanical circulatory assistance (all types included).

---

664 What are the criteria (or inclusion criteria) for use of mechanical circulatory support?

☐ Criteria that must be satisfied for use of mechanical circulatory support in cardiogenic shock include: (1) persistence of circulatory crisis after correction of hypothermia, hypovolemia, blood gas abnormalities, cardiac arrhythmias, and provision of optimal pharmacologic support; (2) a potentially reversible cause of heart failure (e.g., postcardiotomy heart failure, transient acute myocardial failure with or without infarction) or use of support as a bridge to cardiac transplantation; (3) cardiac index lower than $1.8 \, L/m^2/min$ with a left or right atrial pressure higher than 20 mmHg; (4) systolic arterial pressure lower than 90 mmHg with systemic vascular resistance higher than $2100 \, dyn \cdot sec \cdot cm^{-5}$; and (5) systemic underperfusion manifested by oliguria (e.g., urine output less than 20 mL/h in an adult patient) and metabolic acidosis.

---

665 What are the exclusion criteria for mechanical circulatory support?

☐ Patients who have a concomitant disease that seriously limits their life expectancy (e.g., advanced malignancy, severe hepatic disease, serious infections resistant to therapy), or produces severe incapacitation (e.g., symptomatic cerobrovascular disease), or imposes a serious risk of death during application of the circulatory support (e.g., bleeding disorder, coagulopathy), or requires treatment to support patient's life that cannot be effectively provided (e.g., renal failure requiring maintenance hemodialysis or peritoneal dialysis) should be excluded as candidates for mechanical circulatory support. Consequently, only patients who satisfy all inclusion criteria and are free of any exclusion criteria should be considered as potential candidates for mechanical circulatory support.

---

666 How long is mechanical circulatory support generally needed for patients with acute myocardial failure or following cardiac surgery?

☐ Mechanical circulatory support is generally needed for a period of only hours or a few days (up to one week) in patients after cardiac surgery or with acute myocardial failure. Depression of left ventricular function after heart surgery (e.g., coronary artery bypass grafting) tends to spontaneously improve within 3 days and that observed after acute myocardial failure (e.g., stunned ventricle or cardiac ischemia) usually recovers within 3 to 7 days. Patients in whom myocardial recovery fails to occur within one week are unlikely to survive.

---

667 What effects on cardiac preload and afterload does each of the main models of nonsynchronized mechanical circulatory assist devices have?

☐ Heterotopic circulatory assist devices decrease preload but increase afterload of the assisted ventricle and might have opposite effects on the other ventricle. Thus, a left ventricular assist device (LVAD) decreases preload but increases afterload of the left ventricle, and increases preload and decreases afterload of the right ventricle. In a comparable fashion, a right ventricular assist device (RVAD) decreases preload but increases afterload of the right ventricle, and increases preload of the left ventricle without changing the afterload of the left chamber. Biventricular assist devices (BVAD) can modify the preload of both ventricles in both directions. The extracorporeal membrane oxygenators (ECMO) have effects on cardiac preload and afterload similar to those described above for the

LVAD except that they decrease right ventricular preload. Most assist devices can maintain blood flows of 2.5 L/m²/min.

---

668   What are the major characteristics and hemodynamic effects of intra-aortic balloon (IAB) counterpulsation?

□ IAB counterpulsation is the most commonly used mechanical device for circulatory support. It consists of a balloon (about 12 inches long) that is positioned within the thoracic aorta between the origin of the left subclavian artery and the renal arteries. The balloon is inflated during cardiac diastole to prevent peripheral blood "run off" through the abdominal aorta, thereby reducing perfusion of the abdominal viscera and lower body, and is deflated during systole. Consequently, diastolic blood pressure and diastolic coronary perfusion pressure (and possibly coronary blood flow) increase without augmenting left ventricular afterload because the higher blood pressure occurs when the ventricle is undergoing relaxation. The IAB is synchronized with the ECG to deflate during left ventricular contraction. The hemodynamic effects of IAB counterpulsation include increases in the following: diastolic aortic pressure (++), myocardial oxygen supply/demand ratio (+++), myocardial blood flow (++), cardiac output (+), and left ventricular stroke work index (+). In addition, IAB counterpulsation decreases left ventricular wall tension (+), diastolic left ventricular pressure (+), left ventricular volume (+), myocardial contractility as evaluated by dP/dt and V_{max} (+) (rate of force development and maximum velocity of shortening, respectively), and systolic aortic pressure (+). Although cardiac output might increase up to 40% with IAB counterpulsation, a more modest elevation of 10% to 20% is generally observed depending on extent of myocardial ischemia and severity of depression of cardiac contractility.

---

669   How useful is IAB counterpulsation among available devices of assisted circulation and mechanical hearts?

□ The IAB counterpulsation is a relatively simple and effective method that is used as initial choice in most patients with cardiogenic shock who require mechanical circulatory support.

Although many patients might be hemodynamically stabilized with this instrument, some of them (e.g., cardiac index lower than 1.5 L/m²/min) require more sophisticated and expensive mechanical support devices. The application of IAB counterpulsation is a well-established practice in the management of patients following cardiac surgery. A percutaneous technique for balloon insertion through the femoral or the axillary artery is currently used. This insertion technique allows immediate application of the IAB device in the emergency room, intensive care unit, or cardiac catheterization laboratory (as opposed to the surgical operation room), but has not diminished the complications caused by insertion (e.g., limb ischemia, bleeding, infection).

---

670 What are the main complications of assisted circulation and mechanical hearts?

☐ Serious complications might develop in patients receiving mechanical circulatory support including hemorrhage, ischemic necrosis of limbs, thromboembolism, hemolysis, infection, neurologic injury, and renal failure. The incidence and severity of these complications depend on the mechanical device being used, the duration of treatment, and the patient's condition.

---

671 What are the simplest and least expensive left ventricular and right ventricular assist devices available?

☐ The simplest and least expensive ventricular assist devices consist of an external roller pump or a centrifugal pump connected to cannulae inserted in the patient's circulatory system. In a right ventricular support system, blood is withdrawn from the right atrium and returned to the pulmonary artery. In a left ventricular support system, blood is removed from the left atrium or left ventricle and returned to the ascending aorta. These ventricular assist devices maintain the patient's pulmonary circulation so that oxygen uptake and carbon dioxide excretion occur in the lung alveoli; therefore an external oxygenator (cardiopulmonary bypass system) is not necessary in most circumstances. Surgical opening of the chest is usually required for any of these circulatory support systems. The external roller and centrifugal pumps are best suited for short-term (up to one week) support.

672   What resuscitative devices might be used to restore perfusion to vital organs in a patient who suffers a cardiac arrest refractory to conventional treatment?

□ Rapid restoration of perfusion to vital organs in a patient who sustained a cardiac arrest refractory to standard resuscitative maneuvers in the emergency room or cardiac catheterization laboratory might be accomplished with: (1) an ECMO system that involves a percutaneous cannulation of a femoral vein (for removal of venous blood) and femoral artery (for return of oxygenated blood that has circulated through a membrane oxygenator by means of a centrifugal pump); this device might be effective for a period of up to 48 hours; or (2) a left atrial-femoral artery system that might be most appropriate for patients whose cardiac arrest occurs in the catheterization laboratory. This system is inserted under fluoroscopic guidance and requires cannulation of the internal jugular or femoral vein for placement of a left atrial catheter by means of a transeptal puncture. Blood is withdrawn from the left atrium and returned with a pump (e.g., Hemopump that has a small spiral rotating pump) to the femoral artery. The gas exchange occurs in the patient's lungs because this device does not have an oxygenator. This circulatory assist device might be continuously used for a few days. It must be recognized that although ECMO systems might not significantly facilitate myocardial recovery, external pumps might offer better chances to overcome transient myocardial depression. In addition, the need for continuous anticoagulation with ECMO systems (as opposed to devices with external pumps that allow discontinuation of anticoagulation if necessary) imposes greater risks to the patient.

673   What factors predispose to arrhythmias and how are they managed in patients with heart failure?

□ Predisposing factors to cardiac arrhythmias in patients with heart failure, especially rhythm disturbances of ventricular origin, include fibrous scarring, ventricular aneurysms, left ventricular hypertrophy, myocardial ischemia, neurohormonal activation of the sympathetic and renin-angiotensin-systems, digitalis toxicity, and electrolyte disorders (K^+ and Mg^{++} depletion, hyponatremia). Patients with severe heart failure commonly exhibit multiform ventricular premature beats, couplets, and non-sustained ventricular tachycardia. The risk of sudden death is high in individuals having frequent multiform ventricular premature beats and ventricular tachycardia. The treatment of asymptomatic rhythm disturbances consists of optimizing therapy for heart failure, prevention of digitalis toxicity, and correction of electrolyte disturbances including severe hyponatremia and depletion of K^+ and Mg^{++}. Prophylactic antiarrhythmic therapy with verapamil, quinidine, or amiodarone is not recommended because the risks associated with these medications outweigh the potential benefits. The management of symptomatic arrhythmias is explained in the answer to a subsequent question.

---

674 What is the treatment of symptomatic ventricular tachyarrhythmias (causing syncope, hypotension, exacerbation of heart failure, or aborted sudden death) in patients with heart failure?

☐ Electrophysiologic testing in the cardiology laboratory helps to determine whether pharmacologic therapy might be of value, as well as to select the most adequate drug (e.g., amiodarone, quinidine, calcium antagonists, β blockers). Nonpharmacologic therapy might include implantation of an automatic cardioverter-defibrillator, catheter ablation of arrhythmogenic sites, and surgery (e.g., aneurysmectomy plus coronary artery bypass grafting, cardiac transplantation).

---

675 How might treatment efficacy of heart failure be assessed?

☐ Efficacy of therapeutic measures for heart failure include evaluation of: (1) symptoms; (2) fluid volume status; (3) functional capacity by exercise testing or comparable method; (4) ventricular function by noninvasive or invasive methods; and (5) survival. The most important short-term and long-term measures of treatment efficacy in heart failure are patient symptoms and survival, respectively. Nevertheless, response to treatment might be evaluated with other criteria in selected conditions as well as in the evaluation of drugs and other therapeutic regimens for heart failure.

676 When might hospital admission be required in the management of heart failure?

☐ The initial management of severe heart failure, acute and chronic, might require admission to the hospital. Patients with refractory or intractable heart failure should be also managed in the hospital. In addition, precipitating causes of heart failure (e.g., infective endocarditis), complications (e.g., acute pneumonia), or associated diseases (e.g., viral hepatitis) that require close follow-up of the patient's condition and parenteral administration of drugs generally require hospitalization.

677 Does therapy of congestive heart failure with diuretics, vasodilators, or digitalis impose a risk for worsening of renal function or inducing overt renal failure?

☐ Any diuretic or vasodilator (especially ACE inhibitors) might induce renal insufficiency of variable degree in patients with heart failure. Such renal insufficiency might be due to prerenal mechanisms (e.g., diuretic-induced volume depletion, renal underperfusion secondary to vasodilator-induced hypotension or dilation of renal efferent arterioles especially with ACE inhibitors) or to renal injury (e.g., acute tubular necrosis). The combination of ACE inhibitors, especially long-acting formulations (enalapril, lisinopril) with an intense regimen of diuretics, commonly leads to renal insufficiency in patients with heart failure. Consequently, renal function monitoring is of critical importance in the follow-up of patients receiving diuretics and vasodilators. Digitalis preparations are free of nephrotoxic effects, and these compounds do not produce renal insufficiency.

678 What are refractory and intractable forms of heart failure, and what conditions must be ruled out before establishing such diagnoses?

☐ Refractory heart failure is present if the patient's condition continues on a downhill course despite intensive therapy. Intractable heart failure refers to a state of the disease that is resistant to all regular therapeutic measures. Before establishing the diagnosis of both refractory and intractable heart failure, other reversible causes of clinical deterioration must be ruled out including: (1) low cardiac output state due to either diminished preload caused by overaggressive diuretic therapy or high afterload (e.g., hypertension); (2) digitalis toxicity, which might produce symptoms similar to those for refractory heart failure and be present in association with a serum glycoside level in the usual therapeutic range; (3) electrolyte imbalance such as hypokalemic metabolic alkalosis and hyponatremia, which might mimic the symptoms of heart failure; (4) inadequate therapy of heart failure that was aimed at systolic dysfunction when the main defect was diastolic dysfunction; and (5) an intercurrent or associated disease that mimics heart failure (e.g., viral illness, occult malignancy). It is therefore evident that a thorough assessment is required before concluding that refractory or intractable heart failure is present.

679 Name common causes of decompensated heart failure or apparent resistance to therapy (refractory heart failure).

☐ Common causes of decompensation as well as lack of response to therapy of heart failure include: (1) poor patient compliance to prescribed dietary salt restriction or medication; (2) suboptimal dosage of medication (e.g., need to titrate digitalis dosage upward); (3) drugs with negative inotropic effects (e.g., β blockers, Ca^{++} antagonists, disopyramide) that need to be titrated downward or discontinued; (4) concomitant drug therapy with agents that produce salt retention (e.g., aldosterone, fludrocortisone, estrogens, androgens, chlorpropamide, other corticosteroids, NSAIDs, minoxidil and other vasodialtors); (5) antiarrhythmic agents (e.g., amiodarone, disopyramide phosphate, quinidine) and psychotropic drugs (e.g., amitriptyline) can worsen cardiac function; (6) use of digitalis preparations in obstructive cardiomyopathy (this drug might worsen outflow obstruction of the ventricle and cause heart failure); (7) intake of ethanol or other drugs with potential cardiodepressant effects (e.g., adriamycin); and (8) unrecognized associated disease (e.g., anemia, pulmonary infection, pulmonary emboli, infective endocarditis, thyrotoxicosis, viral hepatitis, hepatic cirrhosis, occult neoplasms). Consequently, a thorough evaluation of the patient is required to rule out these potential causes of cardiac decompensation or apparent resistance to therapy.

---

680 What drugs are considered as first-line agents in the management of congestive heart failure?

☐ Diuretics, vasodilators (e.g., ACE inhibitors, nitrates such as isosorbide dinitrate, hydralazine), and digitalis are all first-line agents in the management of congestive heart failure. Whether a diuretic, vasodilator or digitalis preparation is selected for the initial treatment of this condition depends on factors described in detail elsewhere in this chapter. However, two of these drugs (e.g., diuretic plus vasodilator) are commonly selected to be simultaneously used at the start of therapy of heart failure. If the response to the initial treatment falls short of goals, an additional drug is added. Failure to respond to the first-line agents might lead to the use of more potent inotropic agents such as dopamine, dobutamine, or phosphodiesterase inhibitors (for which hospitalization is necessary). Calcium antagonists or β blockers might be of value in patients with predominant diastolic dysfunction (e.g., hypertrophic cardiomyopathy) because of their salutary effects on left ventricular relaxation.

---

681 Compare the expected hemodynamic responses to diuretics, vasodilators, and inotropic agents evaluated with the Frank-Starling curve in patients with congestive heart failure.

☐ The expected hemodynamic responses to various therapies in congestive heart failure are as follows: (1) diuretics reduce end-diastolic pressure without altering pump performance; (2) vasodilators (e.g., nitroprusside) markedly reduce filling pressure and increase stroke volume; and (3) inotropic agents increase stroke volume as do vasodilators, but the reduction in filling pressure is less intense and predictable than with vasodilators.

---

682 What is the treatment of left-sided heart failure with predominant diastolic dysfunction?

☐ The treatment of left-sided heart failure due to predominant diastolic dysfunction involves measures aimed at correction of: (1) pulmonary congestion or edema by means of diuretics and venodilator drugs (e.g., furosemide and sublingual/transdermal nitroglycerin); (2) abnormal diastolic ventricular relaxation by means of Ca^{++} antagonists and β blockers; (3) hypertension, if present, to secure adequate systolic ventricular emptying that will facilitate diastolic filling, and to prevent further ventricular hypertrophy, which worsens diastolic dysfunction; and (4) very rapid heart rate or abnormal rhythm, which might compromise ventricular filling if diastole is too short because of tachycardia or the atrial contribution is diminished or lost (e.g., normal atrial and ventricular synchrony is of critical importance for adequate filling of the ventricle in diastole). Inotropic agents including digitalis preparations have no value in patients with diastolic dysfunction and well-preserved ventricular ejection fraction. In addition, excessive reduction of cardiac preload with diuretics or venodilators might have deleterious effects in patients with diastolic dysfunction because maintenance of adequate stroke volume requires high filling pressures.

---

683 What is the importance of selecting a specific group of drugs (e.g., diuretics, vasodilators, inotropic agents) in the management of acute heart failure as opposed to prescribing all of them to all patients?

☐ The need for selecting a specific group of drugs in the management of acute heart failure as opposed to prescribing all three groups to all patients is largely based on the distinct possibility of inducing harm to some patients with the latter therapeutic option. A representative example is a patient with heart failure and severe hypotension who would most likely be harmed if vasodilators are prescribed as the exclusive therapy due to further blood pressure reduction caused by these agents. Another example is a patient with a ventricular arrythmia who would most likely be harmed if inotropic agents are prescribed because of the possibility of inducing ventricular fibrillation.

---

684   Which one of the three types of drugs, vasodilators, digitalis, or diuretics, is best for the treatment of patients with symptomatic heart failure and diminished ventricular ejection fraction (normal about 0.67, and a value less than 0.50 indicates moderately severe myocardial depression)?

□   A therapeutic regimen that combines vasodilators, digitalis, and diuretics appears to be the best plan for the management of symptomatic heart failure and diminished ventricular ejection fraction (ratio of stroke volume and end-diastolic volume or SV/EDV). Each of the three groups of drugs might be required at different times in the course of treatment in a given patient. In addition, some patients with heart failure might be initially treated with a diuretic (e.g., acute pulmonary edema with generalized fluid retention), while the initial treatment for others might be a digitalis preparation (e.g., acute heart failure due to atrial fibrillation with a very fast ventricular rate), or a vasodilator (e.g., symptomatic heart failure associated with severe hypertension). Consequently, none of these types of drugs is superior to the other because their different pharmacologic effects preclude the use of one of them in replacement of the other.

---

685   Outline an effective sequence for the use of each type/class of drugs in the management of chronic heart failure.

□   Because the management of patients with heart failure must be always individualized, tailoring the various measures to the patient's characteristics (e.g., age, occupation, life-style, ability and motivation to cooperate, associated diseases, response to prior therapy), it is not possible to outline a strict order for the use of drugs in the therapy of this illness. Yet, therapeutic regimens for the following conditions might be: (1) ACE inhibitors as initial therapy in most patients with hypertensive or ischemic heart disease with or without diuretics or digitalis preparations; (2) digitalis glycosides as initial therapy if chronic atrial fibrillation is present (and attempts to revert to sinus rhythm are not contemplated) with or without ACE inhibitors or diuretics; (3) digitalis should not be used in patients at risk of serious side effects (e.g., patients with ventricular arrhythmias, previous evidence of propensity to digitalis toxicity); (4) vasodilators other than ACE inhibitors (e.g., hydralazine, nitrates) might be used in early stages of heart failure if ACE toxicity is documented, precluding use of the latter group of drugs; and (5) nitroglycerin patches or ointment might be used as an effective venodilator in the prevention of paroxysmal nocturnal dyspnea.

---

686 What therapeutic measures are of importance in the follow-up of outpatients with advanced heart failure?

□ Therapeutic measures that might be enforced in patients with advanced heart failure include: (1) maintenance of digoxin levels of 1.0 to 2.0 ng/mL unless contraindications are present; (2) titration of oral vasodilators to maximal dosages (e.g., captopril 400 mg/d, isosorbide dinitrate 320 mg/d, hydralazine 300 mg/d); (3) adjustment of diuretic regimen as dictated according to body weight measured daily and signs/symptoms of heart failure; (4) progressive walking program modified as needed; and (5) detailed patient education and close follow-up by the health care team.

---

687 A 57-year-old woman with increasing peripheral edema and complete inability to perform her daily duties (mostly typing) is admitted to the hospital for evaluation of her whole body composition (clinical research study) before heart surgery (mitral value replacement). She had acute rheumatic fever at age 17, and was essentially asymptomatic until age 50 at which time she began experiencing exertional dyspnea. Since the age of 53 she had noticed peripheral edema and had been treated with a low-salt diet, diuretics, and a digitalis preparation. During the last 5 years her weight decreased from 71 to 46 kg. On admission to the hospital the patient appears severely ill, with an acute and chronic disease state. Physical examination reveals a cachectic woman, with severe orthopnea and the following vital signs:

rectal temperature 37.2°C, pulse 118/min, respiratory rate 24/min, blood pressure 116/82 mmHg. Other physical findings included neck vein distention, marked hepatomegaly, and generalized edema involving the trunk and all extremities. Dullness and rales are detected over the lung bases, bilaterally. Significant cardiomegaly is evident clinically and roentgenologically. Auscultation of the heart discloses mitral valve disease (stenosis and insufficiency). The ECG shows atrial fibrillation, right axis deviation, and biventricular hypertrophy.

<u>What alterations in body composition are expected?</u>

☐ We can predict significant alterations in this patient's body composition, but the severity of these abnormalities must be quantified to establish with certainty the percent deviation from normal levels. The major weight loss in association with a state of anasarca indicates that this patient has lost fat tissue as well as cellular tissue (lean body mass) but the ECF volume is greatly enlarged. It can be predicted that the plasma volume is increased, and the ratio of total body Na^+ (and exchangeable Na^+ or Na_e) to total body K^+ (and exchangeable K^+ or K_e) would be also augmented because this ratio is indicative of the relationship between ECF and ICF volumes, respectively.

688 Compare the whole body composition of this typical patient having advanced congestive heart failure with that of a normal individual of identical gender and age.

☐ The cachectic state is evident by the total body fat of 4.1 kg or 8.9% body weight as compared to a normal level of about 25% body weight. The measured values and the percent comparison with the normal levels of several parameters are as follows: (1) plasma volume 3080 mL or 150% normal; (2) ECF volume 19.1 liters or 168% normal; (3) total exchangeable Na^+ (Na_e) 2920 mEq or 153% normal (the abnormally high Na_e reflects the expansion of ECF but not an abnormally high serum [Na^+], which was 137 mEq/L); (4) total exchangeable Cl^- (Cl_e) 2240 mEq or 161% normal; (5) total body water 30.5 liters or 126% normal; (6) ICF volume 11.4 liters or 92% normal; (7) total exchangeable K^+

(K_e) 1608 mEq or 84% normal; (8) Na_e / K_e (mEq/mEq) 1.82 or 178% normal; and (9) $Na_e + K_e$ 4528 mEq or 120% normal. Examination of the patient's data and comparison with normal values demonstrate expansion of ECF and plasma volume, reduction of fat content and lean body mass, and changes in the total content of Na^+, Cl^-, and K^+ that are closely related to the abnormal fluid volume characteristic of advanced congestive heart failure.

689   A 70-year-old man with a previous history of hypertension and arteriosclerotic heart disease is brought to a hospital emergency room with severe shortness of breath, central cyanosis, and diaphoresis. He had three "small" myocardial infarctions in the previous 6 years, and he had been in stable congestive heart failure for 18 months preceding the current episode. Over the 48 hours before being brought to the hospital he had remained indoors, sitting up on a sofa, because of dyspnea of increased intensity. Current medication included verapamil 180 mg and hydrochlorothiazide 25 mg daily. On arrival to the emergency room, he is gasping for air, with extreme cyanosis, and severe agitation. His blood pressure is 164/114 mmHg, pulse 110/min and regular. Neck veins are distended, and examination of the heart reveals a diffuse apical impulse in the anterior axillary line, and a protodiastolic as well as a presystolic gallop (combined S_3 and S_4 gallop). Prominent moist rales are present throughout both lung fields. Presacral and pretibial (+++) edema is present. The room air arterial blood gases and other laboratory data are as follows:

pH	7.36
PCO_2	44 mmHg
$[HCO_3^-]_p$	24 mEq/L
PO_2	32 mmHg

Plasma chemistries

[Na$^+$]	130 mEq/L
[K$^+$]	3.2 mEq/L
[Cl$^-$]	84 mEq/L
total CO_2	26 mmol/L
glucose	152 mg/dL
BUN	59 mg/dL
creatinine	2.6 mg/dL
anion gap	20 mEq/L

The ECG reveals an "old" inferior wall myocardial infarction and diffuse anterolateral ischemia. Cardiac enzymes (CPK-MB) are within normal limits.

What is the most likely cause of this patient's symptoms?

☐ The severe shortness of breath, central cyanosis, and diaphoresis present on arrival to the emergency room are most likely due to severe left ventricular failure with acute cardiogenic pulmonary edema. The profound impairment in alveolar gas exchange is responsible for the hypoxemia (PO_2 32 mmHg) and central cyanosis (evident on examination of the tongue). The persistent and intense respiratory effort is secondary to postcapillary pulmonary hypertension with alveolar transudate accumulation as well as to the accompanying hypoxemia and accounts for the shortness of breath. The sympathetic activation that accompanies the patient's hemodynamic crisis explains the diaphoresis.

---

690   What is the cause of this patient's left ventricular failure and cardiogenic pulmonary edema?

☐ The left ventricular failure and cardiogenic pulmonary edema present on arrival at the hospital emergency room are best explained by a combination of hypertensive and ischemic heart disease. The high blood pressure (i.e., 164/114 mmHg) observed in association with symptomatic left ventricular failure and diminished cardiac output indicate a severe increase in systemic vascular resistance. Thus, the augmented left ventricular afterload has played a role in the precipitation of symptomatic heart failure. The previous history of myocardial infarction with a current ECG documenting this earlier injury, in association with acute ischemic changes (likely due to the sum of effects of coronary artery disease, increased oxygen consumption secondary to augmented left ventricular afterload, and decreased arterial PO_2), support a role of cardiac ischemia in the pathogenesis of acute pulmonary edema. An additional factor that might partly account for the presence of pulmonary edema as well as the state of overall ECF volume expansion is the associated renal insufficiency (as demonstrated by BUN of 59 mg/dL and creatinine of 2.6 mg/dL), which further predisposes to salt and water retention in this patient with congestive heart failure.

691   What is the most likely explanation for the room air arterial blood gases obtained at the emergency room?

☐   The severe hypoxemia (i.e., PO_2 32 mmHg) indicates a major impairment of alveolar gas exchange due to extensive alveolar edema. The expected response to this degree of hypoxemia is primary hyperventilation causing hypocapnia (decreased PCO_2), yet this patient exhibits hypercapnia (a PCO_2 of 44 mmHg is clearly abnormally high in association with a PO_2 of 32 mmHg). Carbon dioxide retention might be explained by the combined effects of respiratory fatigue following prolonged hyperventilation and a severe abnormality in alveolar gas exchange due to pulmonary edema. Because this patient is known to have had congestive heart failure for 18 months, he should have developed a chronic respiratory alkalosis due to sustained hyperventilation; thus $[HCO_3^-]_p$ should have been substantially lower than 24 mEq/L (level measured on arrival to the emergency room). Although the acute carbon dioxide retention due to pulmonary edema superimposed on chronic respiratory alkalosis increases the $[HCO_3^-]_p$ somewhat, its level should still be below normal. Consequently, it appears that chronic diuretic treatment with hydrochlorothiazide has produced a mild metabolic alkalosis that properly explains the measured $[HCO_3^-]_p$ of 24 mEq/L.

692   What is the cause of this patient's renal insufficiency?

☐ The cause of renal insufficiency in this 70-year-old man is likely multifactorial. The severe left ventricular failure decreases renal perfusion, producing prerenal azotemia (the high BUN to creatinine ratio of about 23, since BUN and creatinine are 59 mg/dL and 2.6 mg/dL, respectively, is consistent with this pathogenesis). This patient's long-standing hypertension is likely to have produced arteriolar nephrosclerosis that might also be playing a role in the observed renal insufficiency. In addition, the possibility of other superimposed mechanisms such as obstructive uropathy (e.g., prostatic hypertrophy in this elderly man), or allergic interstitial nephritis (e.g., drugs) must be considered.

693   How should this patient's pulmonary edema be managed?

☐ The patient's pulmonary edema requires immediate application of multiple measures including: (1) oxygen-rich mixtures such as 2 to 4 L/min oxygen by nasal cannula, with close observation for the possibility of respiratory depression requiring laryngeal intubation and mechanical ventilation; (2) IV administration of 40 mg furosemide to reduce left ventricular preload and induce natriuresis and diuresis; (3) IV infusion of nitroprusside at initial rate of 5 to 10 μg/kg/min and further adjustments as needed to decrease afterload and reduce systolic blood pressure to under 120 mm Hg; (4) nitroglycerin administration by either sublingual or IV routes; and (5) IV aminophylline at a dose of loading dose of 5 mg/kg followed by a maintenance dose of 0.3 to 0.5 mg/kg/min, which might help to maintain the patient's respiratory effort, preventing ventilatory depression and need for laryngeal intubation and mechanical ventilation. The relatively high PCO_2 (i.e., 44 mmHg) observed in this patient contraindicates the use of morphine because this drug will most likely produce further ventilatory depression.

694   A 56-year-old-woman with a long-standing history of chronic obstructive pulmonary disease (COPD) is admitted to the hospital because of worsening congestive heart failure. She has a 30-year history of one to two packs of cigarettes daily, sputum production

for at least 6 months per year in the past 5 years, home-oxygen use for 3 years, and congestive heart failure over the last 2 years. Two days before admission she has noticed chills and subjective fever (body temperature not measured), yellowish bronchial secretions, a major decrease in urine production, persistent epigastric discomfort, marked swelling of the lower extremities, and progressive somnolence. Physical examination on admission to the hospital reveals an obtunded patient with mild cyanosis. Rectal temperature and respiratory rate are 38.2°C and 22/min, respectively. Her blood pressure is 142/82 mmHg, pulse 162/min and regular. Neck examination reveals jugular vein distention, and cardiac evaluation discloses a prominent retrosternal and epigastric impulse indicative of right ventricular hypertrophy. Diminished air flow and diffuse wheezing are present in both lung fields. Examination of the abdomen reveals the liver edge at 15 cm below the costal margin, accompanied by hepatojugular reflux and moderate diffuse epigastric pain elicited with palpation of the right upper abdominal quadrant. The liver span in the midclavicular line is 18 cm. Neurologic examination reveals flapping tremor and funduscopic evaluation discloses bilateral papilledema. Room air arterial blood gases and other laboratory data are as follows:

pH	7.28
PCO_2	66 mmHg
$[HCO_3^-]_p$	30 mEq/L
PO_2	38 mmHg
Plasma chemistries	
$[Na^+]$	137 mEq/L
$[K^+]$	4.1 mEq/L
$[Cl^-]$	93 mEq/L
total CO_2	32 mmol/L
glucose	118 mg/dL
creatinine	1.1 mg/dL
BUN	18 mg/dL
hematocrit	57%
white cell count	12,800 cells/mm^3
neutrophils	78%
lymphocytes	16%
monocytes	2%
eosinophils	0%

The ECG reveals multifocal atrial tachycardia and low voltage in peripheral and precordial leads. Microscopic examination of the sputum reveals an abundant mixed flora that contains a mixture of positive and negative organisms on Gram strain.

What is the most likely cause of this patient's decompensated heart failure?

☐ A respiratory tract infection is the most likely explanation for worsening of heart failure in this patient with long-standing chronic lung disease. This diagnosis is supported by the recent history of chills and fever (although body temperature elevation was not confirmed), fever on admission, yellow bronchial secretions (indicative of an inflammatory reaction with accumulation of white cells), abundance of both Gram-positive and Gram-negative bacteria on microscopic examination of bronchial secretions, leukocytosis, and neutrophylia. This infectious process increases airway resistance and augments the work of respiratory muscles per liter of minute ventilation, producing a more intense dyspnea. The increased tissue oxygen demands as well as increased carbon dioxide production that accompanies a febrile state further augments the shortness of breath. Consequently, hypoxemia and hypercapnia either develop or, if previously present, are aggravated, producing further elevation in pulmonary artery pressure, which promotes the right-sided heart failure observed in this patient.

695   **What might be the cause of this patient's persistent epigastric discomfort on admission?**

☐ Congestive hepatomegaly due to right-sided heart failure is the most likely cause for the persistent epigastric pain. This diagnosis is supported by physical examination that demonstrates an enlarged liver that is painful on gentle palpation, accompanied by hepatojugular reflux. This presumptive diagnosis, if correct, would be confirmed by amelioration and disappearance of epigastric pain in response to correction of overall visceral congestion that accompanies right-sided heart failure.

696 Is this patient's cardiac arrhythmia, a multifocal atrial tachycardia, most likely responsible for the state of decompensated heart failure?

☐ No. Supraventricular tachyarrhythmias are exceedingly common in patients with chronic pulmonary diseases (e.g., COPD), do not generally produce significant hemodynamic compromise, do not require specific treatment, and are most likely due to the blood gas abnormalities and other factors (e.g., drugs) present in these patients. Successful management of the cardiorespiratory failure without any maneuvers aimed at correcting the arrhythmia (e.g., digitalis, antiarrhythmic drugs), reverses the disturbance of heart rhythm in most instances. Furthermore, the application of measures primarily aimed at correcting the cardiac arrhythmia are generally counterproductive because they fail to correct the rhythm disturbance and might increase the patient's morbidity or mortality.

697 How important is this patient's abnormal blood gases in the decompensated heart failure?

☐ The blood gas abnormalities documented on admission (i.e., PO_2 38 mmHg, PCO_2 66 mmHg, pH 7.28) most likely play a prominent role in this patient's decompensated heart failure. Hypoxemia, hypercapnia, and acidemia increase pulmonary vascular resistance, thereby augmenting right ventricular afterload that might precipitate decompensation of cardiac function. The abnormally high airway resistance in a patient with COPD also augments right ventricular afterload. In addition, the increased cardiac output secondary to hypoxemia worsens pulmonary hypertension, and therefore might precipitate right ventricular failure. The critical importance of abnormal blood gases and respiratory dysfunction on the decompensated heart failure becomes apparent by the immediate salutary effects of correction of hypoxemia and hypercapnia on cardiac function.

698   What might account for the somnolence, flapping tremor of upper extremities, and bilateral papilledema?

☐ Hypercapnic encephalopathy might properly explain the somnolence, flapping tremor (also known as asterixis, a neurologic sign that might be observed in patients with hepatic encephalopathy or uremia), and bilateral papilledema. These manifestations are not present in patients with congestive heart failure without hypercapnia. Effective treatment of cardiorespiratory failure is accompanied by the disappearance of these signs and symptoms.

699   What is the most appropriate management of the above patient?

☐ The most important therapeutic measures aimed at ameliorating the state of cardiorespiratory failure include: (1) controlled administration of 24% or 28% O_2 with a venturi mask (or by nasal cannula at 2 L/min) to improve PO_2 with periodic evaluation of arterial blood gases. Because this patient has hypercapnic encephalopathy, the possibility of further respiratory depression in response to oxygen administration is high; thus, the likelihood of the need for laryngeal intubation and mechanical ventilation is substantial; (2) bronchodilator agents including β-adrenergic agonists, aminophylline, and corticosteroids might play a critical role to improve the patient's signs and symptoms; (3) loop diuretics to promote a negative salt and water balance, ameliorating the congestive hepatomegaly, peripheral edema, as well as the abnormal alveolar-capillary gas exchange; and (4) antibiotics to eradicate the pulmonary infection (and the febrile syndrome), which appears as the main cause of deterioration of the patient's condition, leading to the syndrome of cardiorespiratory failure.

700   What major elements must be considered in the selection of a patient as a potential recipient of heart or heart-lung transplantation?

☐ Major elements for selecting a patient as an adequate potential candidate for heart or heart-lung transplantation include: (1) end-stage heart disease (the most frequent indication is cardiomyopathy) that failed to respond to all conventional medical and surgical therapies, and all pertinent diagnostic procedures including endomyocardial biopsy have been performed to rule out any other unsuspected etiologies that might respond to conventional management of the disease; (2) the patient is free of any other serious disease (e.g., active infection, systemic disease that will significantly limit survival or rehabilitation, severe vascular disease, malignancy with uncertain prognosis, insulin-requiring diabetes mellitus, advanced irreversible hepatic or renal dysfunction, psychiatric disease) and has good chances of a prolonged and productive life (advanced age is a contraindication, arbitrarily taken as older than 60 years); and (3) candidate has been thoroughly informed about all the risks involved in this therapy, the need of continuous follow up by the health care team, and compliance with a strict therapeutic regimen that includes daily intake of medication for life, and the patient was considered as an acceptable candidate after a comprehensive psychosocial evaluation by a psychologist and/or a clinical social worker. Whether the candidate might be considered to receive heart or heart-lung transplantation is dependent on other factors including the level of pulmonary-vascular resistance (this parameter must be low in patients who might receive orthotopic cardiac transplantation).

SELECTED REFERENCES

1. Adrogué HJ and Wesson DE: Potassium. Libra & Gemini Publications, Houston, 1992.

2. Adrogué HJ and Wesson DE: Salt and Water. Libra & Gemini Publications, Houston, 1993.

3. Braunwald E (ed): Heart Disease. W.B. Saunders Co., Philadelphia, 1992.

4. Katz AM: Physiology of the Heart. Raven Press, New York, 1992.

5. Singh BN, Dzau VT, Vanhoutte PM, Woosley RL (eds): Cardiovascular Pharmacology and Therapeutics. Churchill Livingstone, New York, 1994.

INDEX

Numbers after index entries indicate question numbers.

cardiac, 320, 321, 325, 328
 major clinical features of, 322
cause of, 323
noncardiac, 321
paroxysmal nocturnal, 331
pulmonary, 322, 325, 328
use of diuretics in diagnosis of, 326

Eccentric hypertrophy, use of digitalis,
 605
Echocardiography
 in evaluation of heart failure, 401,
  403, 658
 of high output heart failure: from
  anemia, 385
  from thyrotoxicosis, 387
Eclampsia, mechanisms responsible for
 acute pulmonary edema in, 235
 two-dimensional, measurement of
  ejection fraction, 63
Edema
 alveolar, radiologic findings, 349
 brawny, 304
 classification of, 203
  renal mechanisms and, 204
 combined use of loop diuretics and
  thiazides in management of,
  470
 distribution of, cause and, 306
 examples of formation of, with and
  without preceeding fluid
  retention, 205, 206
 factors that protect lung against, 225
 generalized: examination of fluid in
  evaluation of, 308
  main causes of, 209, 305
  net filtration pressure of and, 210,
   211
 interstitial pulmonary, radiologic
  findings, 349
 localized: causes of, 305
  examination of fluid in evaluation
   of, 308
  physical findings helpful in
   diagnosis of, 306, 307
 main characteristics of, in heart
  failure, 300
 measures important in treatment of,
  421, 422

mechanisms of formation of,
 Starling's law of fluid exchange
 and, 212-214
mild, low-NaCl foods and, 426
nonpitting, 304
peripheral, 301, 687
 assessment of presence or severity
  of, 309
 detection of, on physical
  examination, 310
pitting, 302-304
 demonstration of, 303
primary, 204
pulmonary (*see* Pulmonary edema)
secondary, 204
Effective circulating blood volume,
 179, 180, 186, 187
Effective refractory period (ERP), 87
Efferent mechanisms
 of neural control of cardiovascular
  function, 126
 in regulation of ECF volume, 175
Efferent renal nerve activity, urinary
 salt and water excretion and, 191
Efficacy of digitalis, drug interactions
 and, 604
Ejection fraction, 38
 reliability in measurement of, 63
 supernormal, 155
Ejection phase, evaluation of
 myocardial contractility during, 62
Elasticity, passive and active of
 myocardium, 37
Electric circuit theory, 17
Electrical stimulation, paired, 58
Electrocardiogram (ECG)
 of high output heart failure: from
  anemia, 385
  from thyrotoxicosis, 387
 impact of hyperkalemia on, 92-96
 poor prognosis in heart failure from
  findings of, 411
Electrogenic transport, 76, 105
Electrolyte(s)
 abnormalities in, 397, 398
  sudden death in patients with
   heart failure and, 259
  ventricular arrhythmias and, 259
 acetazolamide and, 461